HANDBOOK OF CRITICAL CARE OBSTETRICS

HANDBOOK OF CRITICAL CARE OBSTETRICS

Edited by

Steven L. Clark, MD

Professor of Obstetrics and Gynecology
University of Utah
Salt Lake City, Utah

David B. Cotton, MD

Professor and Chairman
Department of Obstetrics and Gynecology
Wayne State University
Detroit, Michigan

Gary D. V. Hankins, MD

Department of Obstetrics and Gynecology
Wilford Hall Medical Center
Lackland Air Force Base
San Antonio, Texas

Jeffrey P. Phelan, MD

Pasadena, California

b

**Blackwell
Science**

Blackwell Science
Editorial offices:
238 Main Street, Cambridge, Massachusetts 02142, USA
Osney Mead, Oxford OX2 0EL, England
25 John Street, London WC1N 2BL, England
23 Ainslie Place, Edinburgh EH3 6AJ, Scotland
54 University Street, Carlton, Victoria 3053, Australia
Arnette SA, 1 rue de Lille, 75007 Paris, France
Blackwell-Wissenschaft-Verlag GmbH Kurfürstendamm 57, 10707 Berlin,
Germany
Feldgasse 13, A-1238 Vienna, Austria

Distributors:

North America
Blackwell Science, Inc.
238 Main Street
Cambridge, Massachusetts 02142
(Telephone orders: 800-215-1000 or
  617-876-7000)
Australia
Blackwell Science Pty., Ltd.
54 University Street
Carlton, Victoria 3053
(Telephone orders: 03-347-5552)

Outside North America and Australia
Blackwell Science, Ltd.
c/o Marston Book Services, Ltd.
P.O. Box 87
Oxford OX2 0DT
England
(Telephone orders: 44-865-791155)

Typeset by Huron Valley Graphics, Ann Arbor, Michigan
Printed and bound by Braun-Brumfield, Ann Arbor, Michigan

© 1994 by Blackwell Scientific Publications
Printed in the United States of America
95 96 97 5 4 3 2

Library of Congress Cataloging-in-Publication Data
Handbook of critical care obstetrics / edited by Steven L. Clarke . . .
    [et al.].
        p.   cm.
    Includes bibliographical references and index.
    ISBN 0-86542-351-2
    1. Obstetrical emergencies—Handbooks, manuals, etc.
    2. Pregnancy—Complications—Handbooks, manuals, etc.   I. Clark,
    Steven L.
        [DNLM: 1. Critical Care—in pregnancy—handbooks. 2.
Pregnancy
    Complications—therapy—handbooks.   WQ 39 H23553 1994]
    RG571.H299   1994
    618.2'025—dc20
    DNLM/DLC
    for Library of Congress   94-8611
                                                                    CIP

CONTENTS

PREFACE

Since the publication of the second edition of *Critical Care Obstetrics,* interest in this field has continued to grow. The editors have received numerous favorable comments regarding the usefulness of this text, not only as a reference source, but on labor and delivery suites as well. The management protocols outlined in the clinical chapters appear to be especially useful.

The *Handbook* was developed with the above comments in mind. Each chapter has been condensed, with a de-emphasis of theory and pathophysiology and a focus upon practical clinical management. Key figures and tables have been retained; management protocols have been updated, as needed. In addition, the *Handbook* contains a newly developed appendix, containing over 40 new figures and tables, including normal lab values, formulas, charts, treatment recommendations and many other pieces of information we, as practicing clinicians felt would be useful to have together in one place. Protocols for advanced cardiac life support (ACLS) are also included, and the management protocols have been collated together in the appendix for quick reference.

The *Handbook* will fit in most lab coat pockets; we feel it will be an invaluable tool for the house officer as well as the experienced clinician who cares for complicated obstetric patients.

ACKNOWLEDGMENTS

The editors of this *Handbook* gratefully acknowledge the efforts of all the contributors listed in the second edition of *Critical Care Obstetrics*. Their original contributions formed the framework by which the Handbook was shaped. They are: Drs. Steven J. Allen, William Barthe, Jr., Thomas J. Benedetti, Gerald G. Briggs, Michael Burnhill, Robert C. Cefalo, William H. Daily, Gary A. Dildy, Patrick Duff, Thomas R. Easterling, Joe C. Files, Thomas J. Garite, Anita Giezentanner, Steven H. Golde, Bernard Gonik, Jeffrey S. Greenspoon, Robert H. Hayashi, Susan Hou, Monica Jones, Thomas H. Joyce III, Wesley Lee, William C. Mabie, James N. Martin, Jorge H. Mestman, Kenneth J. Moise, Jr., John C. Morrison, C. Paul Morrow, Susan E. Rutherford, David A. Sacks, Andrew J. Satin, Carl V. Smith, John M. Thorp, Jr., Steven A. Vasilev, and Carl P. Weiner.

HANDBOOK OF CRITICAL CARE OBSTETRICS

PART
I

Basic Principles

CHAPTER ONE

Cardiorespiratory Changes During Pregnancy

BLOOD VOLUME

Maternal plasma volume increases by 11% as early as the seventh week of pregnancy. This increase reaches a plateau at 32 weeks, remaining stable thereafter until delivery. Although wide variations are recognized, the increase in plasma volume at term averages approximately 45%–50%. Placental production of chorionic somatomammotropin, of progesterone, and possibly of prolactin stimulates maternal erythropoiesis, but it results in a smaller (20% less) red cell mass increase. These changes account for the physiologic anemia that is often observed in pregnant patients despite adequate iron stores. The maximal hemodilution occurs by approximately 30–32 weeks.

The absolute increase in blood volume is positively correlated with the number of fetuses. Pritchard observed that the overall increase in blood volume for singleton pregnancies was estimated to be 1570 mL, which represented a 48% increase over nonpregnant values. The same study noted that twin pregnancies resulted in an average of 1960 mL.

Several studies emphasize the significance of maternal blood volume expansion for good pregnancy outcome. Plasma volume has been found to be more closely related to fetal weight than to maternal body stature or height, and a relationship between large babies and large plasma volumes has been confirmed. Conversely, an association was reported between low-birth-weight babies and low postpartum maternal plasma volume. Perinatal morbidity related to prematurity also occurs in women whose maternal heart volume (estimated by chest radiographs) fails to expand in the usual manner. Collectively, these findings suggest that gestational hypervolemia is an important determinant of fetal well-being. Women who do not exhibit the typical hormonal, metabolic, and hemodynamic changes during early pregnancy appear to be at increased risk of embryonic demise.

BLOOD PRESSURE

Systolic and diastolic blood pressure decreases during pregnancy until midpregnancy, with gradual recovery to nonpregnant values by term gestation. Intra-arterial and manual blood pressure measurements differ during pregnancy. Recently, Kirshon and colleagues found automated cuff systolic blood pressures to be significantly lower than direct intra-arterial measurements in postpartum patients. However, no differences were observed between radial artery and automated cuff diastolic blood pressure measurements.

The etiology of maternal blood pressure changes is likely to be related to hormonal and cardiovascular changes during pregnancy. Phippard et al. studied these alterations in pregnant baboons. Early peripheral vasodilatation and cardiac output augmentation were found to precede gestational hypervolemia. The increased cardiac output did not completely compensate for decreased afterload, thereby providing a reasonable explanation for mean arterial blood pressure decreases seen as early as the first trimester. In fact, mean arterial blood pressure decreases by nearly 10% as early as the seventh week of pregnancy.

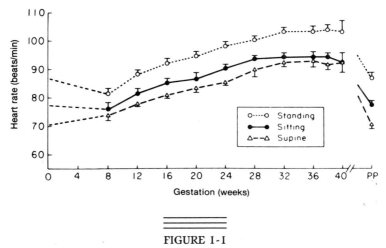

FIGURE 1-1

Sequential changes in mean heart rate in three positions throughout pregnancy (*n* = 69 patients with standard errors of the mean). (Reproduced by permission from Wilson M et al. Blood pressure, the renin–aldosterone system, and sex steroids throughout normal pregnancy. Am J Med 1980;68:97.)

HEART RATE

Maternal heart rate increases occur as early as the seventh week of pregnancy, and, by late pregnancy, maternal heart rate averages approximately 20% over postpartum values (Figure 1-1).

STROKE VOLUME AND CARDIAC OUTPUT

Cardiac output is the product of heart rate and stroke volume. This parameter reflects the overall functional capacity of the left ventricle to maintain satisfactory blood pressure and organ perfusion. There is convincing evidence that maternal cardiac output increases as early as 10 weeks' gestation and peaks at 30%–50% over control values by the latter part of the second trimester. This rise, from approximately 4.5 to 6.0 L/min, is sustained for the remainder of the pregnancy if cardiac output is measured in the lateral decubitus position.

Recently, investigators have validated Doppler ultrasound with direct Fick or thermodilution methods for studying maternal cardiac output. In one study, heart rate increased significantly by 5 weeks' gestation and continued to do so until stabilizing at 32 weeks (+17% above prepartum values). Stroke volumes increased by 8 weeks of pregnancy, with maximal values (+32% over prepartum values) obtained by 16–20 weeks. Overall, cardiac output increased as early as 5 weeks' gestation from 4.88 L/min to 7.21 L/min (+48%) by 32 weeks. The second trimester was associated with significant increases of left atrial and left ventricular end-diastolic dimensions, suggesting an increase in venous return. Recent invasive studies performed in the late third trimester confirm approximately equal contributions of heart rate and stroke volume to the increased cardiac output seen in late pregnancy.

There have been several theories attempting to explain the mechanism responsible for the stroke volume increases that contribute to higher cardiac output during early pregnancy. Burwell has proposed that the increased plasma volume, cardiac output, and heart rate during pregnancy are similar to the hemodynamic changes following the development of an arteriovenous fistula in the uteroplacental circulation. Metcalfe and associates have suggested that the left ventricular dilatation is related to hormonal factors and is analogous to decreased venous tone observed with normal pregnancy or after the administration of oral contraceptives. Based on animal studies, they have suggested that the early increase in stroke volume results from a "shift to the right" of the left ventricular pressure-volume curve, as a result of the Frank-Starling mechanism.

REGIONAL BLOOD FLOW

Significant increases in regional blood flow have been observed to the uterus, kidneys, and skin during pregnancy. Renal blood flow increases to approximately 30% over nonpregnant values by midpregnancy. This increase in renal blood flow remains stable until term gestation when measurements are taken in the lateral decubitus position. However, a remarkable decrease in renal blood flow can be measured in the supine position later in pregnancy due to the mechanical effects of the gravid uterus on the vena cava. The glomerular filtration rate increases 30%–50% over control values as a result of elevated renal plasma flow; however, the actual cause of these changes is unknown.

Uterine blood flow increases from approximately 50 mL/min at 10 weeks' gestation to 500 mL/min at term—a figure that represents more than 10% of systemic cardiac output. Skin perfusion begins to increase slowly in early pregnancy up to 18–20 weeks' gestation and is followed by a sharp rise between 20 and 30 weeks. Earlier studies have documented the increased skin temperature that results from dilatation of dermal capillaries. This may serve as a mechanism by which the excessive heat of fetal metabolism is allowed to dissipate via the maternal circulation. Significant changes in blood flow to the brain or liver have not been confirmed during pregnancy.

EFFECT OF POSTURE ON MATERNAL HEMODYNAMICS

Prior to the 1960s, investigators had not been aware of the clinical significance of maternal posture on changes in cardiac output, and their patients were studied in the supine position. The unique angiographic studies of Bieniarz et al. indicate that the gravid uterus is associated with significant obstruction of caval blood flow in approximately 90% of women studied in the supine position. Central venous return is reduced in supine gravidas and may result in decreased cardiac output, a sudden drop in blood pressure, bradycardia, and syncope. In 1953, these clinical changes were first described by Howard and are now commonly referred to as the "supine hypotensive syndrome." Holmes was able to document significant supine hypotension in 8.2% of 500 women during late pregnancy.

Vorys et al. first described the reduction of venous return to the heart due to the mechanical effects of the gravid uterus on the vena cava during late pregnancy. A 16% cardiac output reduction from the lateral position was observed in the dorsal lithotomy position. The relationship of gestational age on the maternal cardiovascular response to posture was subsequently studied by Ueland et al., as seen in Figure 1-2. Maternal heart rate was maximal (range +13%–20%) by 28–32 weeks' pregnancy, especially in the sitting position. Stroke volume increased early, with maximal values by 20–24 weeks (range +21%–33%), followed by a progressive decline toward term gestation that was quite striking in the supine position. In fact, assumption of the supine position at term led to stroke volume

---

FIGURE 1-2

Effect of posture on maternal hemodynamics. (Reproduced by permission from Ueland K, Metcalfe J. Circulatory changes in pregnancy. Clin Obstet Gynecol 1975;18:41. Modified from Ueland K, Novy MJ, Peterson EN, Metcalfe J. Maternal cardiovascular dynamics. IV. The influence of gestational age on the maternal cardiovascular response to posture and exercise. Am J Obstet Gynecol 1969;104:856.)

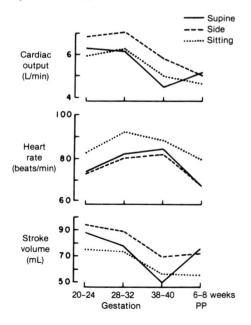

and cardiac output values that were even below their corresponding postpartum measurements. Clark et al. have shown that assumption of the motionless standing position results in decreases in cardiac output that exceed those seen while supine.

ANTEPARTUM HEMODYNAMIC VALUES FOR LATE PREGNANCY

Clark and colleagues recently conducted normative studies of maternal cardiovascular hemodynamics. Ten primiparous women underwent right heart catheterization during late pregnancy (35–38 weeks) and again postpartum (11–13 weeks) to establish normal values for central maternal hemodynamics (Table 1-1). When compared to the postpartum state, late pregnancy was associated with significant increases in the following parameters (measured in the left lateral recumbent position): heart rate (+17%), stroke volume (+23%), and cardiac output (+43%). Significant decreases occurred in late pregnancy in systemic vascular resistance (SVR) (−21%), pulmonary vascular resistance (PVR) (−34%), serum colloid osmotic pressure (COP) (−14%), and COP-PCWP (pulmonary capillary wedge pressure) gradient (−28%). No significant changes were found in PCWP, central venous pressure (CVP), or mean arterial pressure (MAP). Normal late third-trimester pregnancy was not associated with hyperdynamic left ventricular function as determined by Starling function curves (left ventricular stroke work index/PCWP).

HEMODYNAMIC CHANGES DURING LABOR

Repetitive and forceful uterine contractions can have a significant effect on the cardiovascular system during labor. The quantity of blood expressed by each uterine contraction has been estimated to be approximately 300–500 mL. During labor contractions, angiographic studies suggest that the ball-shaped uterus improves blood flow from pelvic organs and lower extremities back to the heart.

TABLE 1-1
Central hemodynamic changes associated with late pregnancy
($n = 10$)

	Nongravid	Gravid	Change (%)
Mean arterial pressure (mm Hg)	86 ± 8	90 ± 6	NS
Pulmonary capillary wedge pressure (PCWP) (mm Hg)	6 ± 2	8 ± 2	NS
Central venous pressure (CVP) (mm Hg)	4 ± 3	4 ± 3	NS
Heart rate (beats/min)	71 ± 10	83 ± 10	+17%
Cardiac output (L/min)	4.3 ± 0.9	6.2 ± 1.0	+43%
Systemic vascular resistance (SVR) (dyne/s/cm^{-5})	1530 ± 520	1210 ± 266	−21%
Pulmonary vascular resistance (dyne/s/cm^{-5})	119 ± 47	78 ± 22	−34%
Serum colloid osmotic pressure (COP) (mm Hg)	20.8 ± 1.0	18.0 ± 1.5	−14%
COP-PCWP gradient (mm Hg)	14.5 ± 2.5	10.5 ± 2.7	−28%
Left ventricular stroke work index (LVSWI) (g/m/m^2)	41 ± 8	48 ± 6	NS

Measurements from the lateral decubitus position are expressed as mean ± standard deviation.

Significant changes are noted at the $p < 0.05$ level, paired two-tailed t test; NS = nonsignificant.

(Adapted with permission from Clark SL, Cotton DB, Lee W, et al. Central hemodynamic assessment of normal term pregnancy. Am J Obstet Gynecol 1989;161:1439–1442.)

The first stage of labor is associated with progressive increases in cardiac output. Kjeldsen found cardiac output to increase by 1.10 L/min in the latent phase of labor, 2.46 L/min in the accelerating, and 2.17 L/min in the decelerating phase. Ueland and Hansen also described an increase in cardiac output between early and late first stage of labor in the supine position. The increases in cardiac output during the first and second stages of labor were not as pronounced when the patient was given caudal anesthesia compared with local anesthesia (paracervical or pudendal). These investigators concluded that the relative lack of pain and anxiety in patients receiving caudal analgesia may limit the absolute increase in cardiac output encountered at delivery.

Robson and colleagues reported the first use of Doppler ultrasound for serial maternal cardiac output measurements during labor. Serial cardiac output values were taken from 15 women in the left semilateral position under meperidine labor analgesia. Prelabor cardiac output (between contractions) increased from 6.99 to 7.88 L/min (+13%) by 8 cm cervical dilatation, primarily as a result of stroke volume augmentation. During contractions, there were even further cardiac output increases due to augmentation of both heart rate and stroke volume. The magnitude of these contraction–induced cardiac output changes increased with progression of labor: ≤3 cm (+17%); 4–7 cm (+23%); and ≥8 cm (+34%). Lee and coworkers have also used Doppler and M-mode echocardiography to study parturients with epidural analgesia in the left lateral decubitus position. The cardiac output increases during firm contractions under epidural labor analgesia were similar to Robson's observations: A 16% increase in left ventricular stroke volume was associated with an overall 11% cardiac output increase during firm contractions in the first stage of labor. Under epidural anesthesia, however, heart rate was minimally influenced by uterine contractions.

POSTPARTUM HEMODYNAMICS

Significant hemodynamic fluctuations may occur during the postpartum period. These cardiovascular changes reflect the net effect of blood loss at delivery and the body's physiologic compensation to peripartum hemorrhage. Similar to the findings of other investigators employing different methodology, Pritchard and colleagues used chromium-labeled red blood cells to quantitate blood loss associated with vaginal delivery (505 mL) and cesarean section (1028 mL). They found that normal pregnant women can lose up to 30% of the predelivery blood volume as a result of parturition, with little change in postpartum hematocrit.

In 1976, Ueland compared intrapartum blood volume and hematocrit changes between vaginal delivery ($n = 26$) and elective cesarean section ($n = 34$) (Figure 1-3). The percentage changes in venous hematocrit and blood volume were serially measured in both groups. The average blood loss from vaginal delivery was 610 mL, compared to 1030 mL with cesarean section. Blood volume decreased steadily from one hour postpartum until the third day following vaginal delivery, whereas

FIGURE 1-3

Percentage changes in blood volume and venous hematocrit following vaginal delivery or cesarean section. (Reproduced by permission from Metcalfe J, Ueland K. Heart disease and pregnancy. In Fowler NO (ed). Cardiac Diagnosis and Treatment ed 3. Hagerstown, MD: Harper & Row, 1980:1153–1170.)

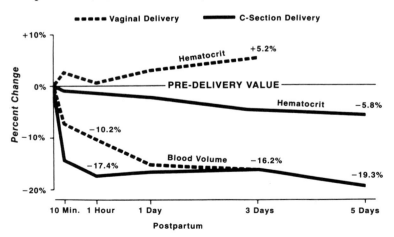

it remained fairly stable in the surgical group. Similar blood volume decreases (-16.2%) were observed in both groups by the third postpartum day. However, differences in hematocrit changes in vaginal ($+5.2\%$) versus cesarean (-5.8%) patients indicated that most of the volume loss by the former was due to postpartum diuresis.

During the first week after delivery, Chesley et al. reported a 2-liter decrease in the sodium space compartment associated with 3 kilograms of weight loss. This well-known postpartum diuresis usually occurs between the second and fifth day and provides a physiologic mechanism by which increased extracellular fluid accumulated during pregnancy may be dissipated. The potential clinical significance of this phenomenon is illustrated by Hankins and coworkers, who performed serial invasive hemodynamic measurements in eight eclamptic women. Typically, these patients were found to have initial low biventricular filling pressures, elevated SVR, and hyperdynamic left ventricular function. Three women who did not demonstrate a significant diuresis by 48–72 hours postpartum were noted to develop an elevated PCWP (mean 16.7 mm Hg). Their wedge pressures eventually normalized following postpartum diuresis. These investigators suggested that this phenomenon was due to mobilization of extracellular extravascular fluid prior to diuresis. In this regard, postpartum pulmonary edema may develop in high-risk patients who fail to diurese before mobilization of extravascular fluid.

The puerperium has also been characterized by changes in cardiac output, stroke volume, and heart rate. Ueland and Hansen measured these parameters in 13 patients who received caudal anesthesia and found a 59% and a 71% increase respectively in cardiac output and stroke volume by 10 minutes postpartum. By one hour postpartum, cardiac output was elevated 49% above baseline values, which paralleled the 67% increase in stroke volume. At that time, a 15% decrease in pulse rate was observed, although no statistically significant changes in blood pressure were noted. The postpartum high cardiac output state probably results from increased venous return to the heart secondary to the following: 1) a shift of blood from the uterus to the intravascular space, 2) the release of caval compression from the gravid uterus, and 3) the mobilization of extravascular fluid into the intravascular compartment.

Postpartum cardiac output has also been studied at a time remote from delivery. As late as four to five days postpartum, cardiac output has been elevated approximately 18%–29% from prelabor values. The return of cardiac output to nonpregnant values has been variably reported to range from two to four weeks postpartum.

CARDIORESPIRATORY INTERACTIONS DURING PREGNANCY

The maternal respiratory system is extremely important for the maintenance of fetal oxygenation during pregnancy. A relative hyperventilation of pregnancy begins in the first trimester and increases 42% by term gestation (Figure 1-4). Because hyperventilation has been observed during the luteal phase of the menstrual cycle and progesterone can induce similar changes in nonpregnant women, it is likely that this phenomenon results from hormonal factors. Although the mechanism of progesterone-induced hyperventilation has not been clearly defined, it has been suggested that this hormone acts as a primary respiratory center stimulant. Because respiratory rate remains essentially unchanged during pregnancy, the relatively greater increase in minute volume over oxygen consumption or basal metabolic rate can be attributed to an increase in tidal volume.

The hyperventilation of pregnancy is associated with a resting arterial carbon dioxide tension below 30 mm Hg. This chronic respiratory alkalosis is partially compensated by increased renal bicarbonate excretion into the urine. According to Awe and associates, there appears to be a postural effect on arterial oxygen tension during term pregnancy. In their study of 23 pregnant women, arterial oxygen tensions were found to be greater than 90 mm Hg in the sitting position. A moderate hypoxemia (arterial oxygen tension less than 90 mm Hg) occurred in 25% of their supine patients. The supine position was also associated with a much greater likelihood for the alveolar-arterial oxygen tension gradient to be abnormal (greater than 10 mm Hg) when compared with the upright position. There was,

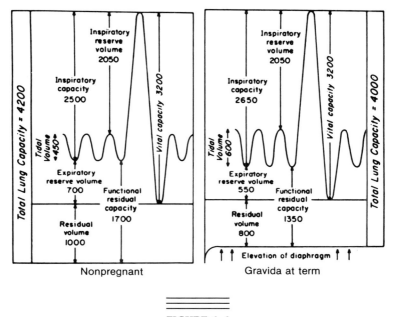

FIGURE 1-4

Respiratory changes during pregnancy. (Reproduced with permission from Bonica JJ. Principles and Practice of Obstetrical Analgesia and Anesthesia. Philadelphia: FA Davis Company, 1962.)

however, significant improvement in this gradient when women shifted from the supine to the sitting position.

CARDIORESPIRATORY SIGNS AND SYMPTOMS DURING PREGNANCY

Functional changes in the cardiorespiratory system are responsible for signs and symptoms that may simulate heart disease during normal pregnancy. Milne and associates found the incidence of dyspnea to increase from 15% in the first trimester to approximately 50% by 19 weeks and 75% by 31 weeks' gestation. Easy fatigability and decreased exercise tolerance are common during pregnancy. Occasionally, the mechanical effects of the uterus may reduce venous return to the heart, leading to dizziness or even syncope. The increased venous pressure distal to this partial obstruction contributes to the dependent lower-extremity edema commonly seen during pregnancy. A mild amount of pulmonary atelectasis from the enlarging uterus adjacent to the diaphragm occasionally leads to the presence of basilar rales by auscultation. All of these changes may make the confirmation of functional heart disease during pregnancy very difficult by history and physical exam alone.

Cutforth and associates carefully compared cardiac auscultatory findings with phonocardiograms in 50 normal primigravid women during pregnancy. They documented a loud and widely split first heart sound in 88% of their patients from early closure of the mitral valve. The only significant change noted in the second heart sound was a tendency for persistent expiratory splitting. A third heart sound was heard in 84%. Systolic ejection murmurs were found in 92% of their subjects. By contrast, only nine patients demonstrated an early soft diastolic murmur (often transient), which was thought to result from increased flow through the atrioventricular valve. The changes in heart sounds and murmurs during pregnancy began between 12 and 20 weeks gestation and usually disappeared by one week postpartum.

The radiographic changes in the chest roentgenogram during pregnancy have been the subject of much debate and controversy. Turner reviewed 200 chest films from pregnant women in an attempt to characterize changes specific to this condition. Aside from cardiac enlargement, there was no documentation of any specific changes in cardiac contour or pulmonary vascularity when compared with nonpregnant women. It was recommended that the same criteria for interpretation of chest films should be applied to both pregnant and nonpregnant women.

In the 1940s, Hollander and Crawford followed 18 pregnant women with serial chest films (posteroanterior with oblique views) and esophagrams. Aside from the enlargement of the heart in response to the hypervolemia of pregnancy, they were able to document another consistent radiographic change—an indentation of the anterior esophageal wall by the enlarged left atrium.

   Hollander and Crawford also followed 18 pregnant women for electrocardiographic changes. They found the development of a deep Q wave and a negative T wave in lead III. Additionally, the QRS axis changed an average of 15 degrees to the left. According to a more recent statistical analysis of electrocardiograms taken from 102 pregnant patients at Grady Memorial Hospital, the pattern of QRS axis change was not predictable for a given individual. Mean electrocardiographic values during pregnancy are summarized in Table 1-2.

TABLE 1-2
Mean ECG (electrocardiogram) measurements during normal pregnancy, delivery, and postpartum in 102 patients

	ITM	2TM	3TM	D	PP
Heart rate (bpm)	77	79	87	80	66
QT interval (s)	0.378	0.375	0.361	0.362	0.406
QT_c interval (s)	0.424	0.427	0.431	0.414	0.423
PR interval (s)	0.160	0.160	0.155	0.155	0.160
P wave					
Duration (s)	0.092	0.092	0.091	0.091	0.096
Amplitude (mm)	1.9	1.9	2.0	2.0	1.9
Axis (degrees)	40	38	38	41	35
QRS complex					
Duration (s)	0.074	0.074	0.074	0.076	0.077
Amplitude (mm)	11.5	11.5	12.4	12.2	11.2
Axis (degrees)	49	46	40	44	44
T wave					
Duration (s)	0.168	0.171	0.165	0.166	0.176
Amplitude (mm)	3.4	3.5	3.4	3.6	3.5
Axis (degrees)	27	25	22	33	34

ITM, 2TM, and 3TM = first, second, and third trimesters.
D = 1–3 days after delivery.
PP = 6–8 weeks postpartum.
(Reproduced by permission from Carruth JE, Mirvis SB, Brogan DR, et al. The electrocardiogram in normal pregnancy. Am Heart J 1981;6:1075.)

━━━━━━━

SUGGESTED READING

Carruth JE, Mirvis SB, Brogan DR, et al. The electrocardiogram in normal pregnancy. Am Heart J 1981;6:1075.

Clark SL, Cotton DB, Lee W, et al. Central hemodynamic assessment of normal term pregnancy. Am J Obstet Gynecol 1989;161:1439.

Clark SL, Cotton DB, Lee W, et al. Position change and central hemodynamic profile during normal third trimester pregnancy and postpartum. Am J Obstet Gynecol 1991;164:883.

James CF, Banner T, Caton D. Cardiac output in women undergoing cesarean section with epidural or general anesthesia. Am J Obstet Gynecol 1989;160:1178.

Kirshon B, Lee W, Cotton DB, et al. Indirect blood pressure monitoring in the obstetric patient. Obstet Gynecol 1987;70:799.

Lim VS, Katz AI, Lindheimer MD. Acid–base regulation in pregnancy. Am J Physiol 1976;231:1764.

Lucius H, Gahlenbeck H, Kleine HO, et al. Respiratory functions, buffer system, and electrolyte concentrations of blood during human pregnancy. Respir Physiol 1970;9:311.

Pritchard JA. Changes in the blood volume during pregnancy and delivery. Anesthesiology 1965;26:393.

Prowse CM, Gaensler EA. Respiratory and acid–base changes during pregnancy. Anesthesiology 1965;26:381.

Robson SC, Hunter R, Boys W, Dunlop W, Bryson M. Changes in cardiac output during epidural anaesthesia for caesarean section. Anaesthesia 1989;44:475.

Schrier RW. Medical progress: pathogenesis of sodium and water retention in high-output and low-output cardiac failure, nephrotic syndrome, cirrhosis, and pregnancy. N Engl J Med 1988; 319:1127.

Templeton A, Kelman GR. Maternal blood-gases, $(P_AO_2-P_aO_2)$, physiologic shunt, and VD/VT in normal pregnancy. Br J Anaesth 1976;48:1001.

Turner AF. The chest radiograph during pregnancy. Clin Obstet Gynecol 1975;18:65.

Ueland K. Maternal cardiovascular dynamics. VII. Intrapartum blood volume changes. Am J Obstet Gynecol 1976;126:671.

Wilson M, Morganti AA, Zervodakis I, et al. Blood pressure, the renin-aldosterone system, and sex steroids throughout normal pregnancy. Am J Med 1980;68:97.

CHAPTER TWO

Colloid Osmotic Pressure and Pregnancy

The osmotic pressure of a fluid is a relative property and can be demonstrated only when two solutions of differing colloid concentrations are separated by a semipermeable membrane. Those molecules that are unable to pass through the membrane are referred to as "colloids" and are responsible for the oncotic pressure of a solution.

Plasma is composed of three major proteins: albumin, globulin, and fibrinogen. The plasma concentration of albumin is twice that of the globulin concentration and 15 times that of fibrinogen. Osmotic pressure is related to the number of molecules rather than the size of the molecules; therefore, it becomes apparent that albumin is responsible for up to 75% of the oncotic pressure of plasma. The majority of the remaining oncotic effect is exerted by the globulin fraction. Fibrinogen plays a minor role. Because the net protein charge of plasma proteins is negative at physiological pH, positively charged ions (mainly sodium cations) become trapped with the protein molecules in order to maintain electroneutrality across the capillary membrane. This phenomenon is referred to as the Gibbs-Donnan effect. The resulting colloid osmotic pressure (COP_p) is approximately 50% greater than would result from the proteins alone.

STARLING'S LAW AND THE LUNG

The Starling law of the capillary can be expressed by the equation

$$Q_f = K_f[(P_c - P_i) - R(COP_p - COP_i)]$$

where

Q_f = the total flow of fluid across a capillary membrane,
K_f = the fluid filtration coefficient,
P_c = the capillary hydrostatic pressure,
P_i = the interstitial hydrostatic pressure,
R = the reflection coefficient,
COP_p = the capillary osmotic pressure of the plasma, and
COP_i = the osmotic pressure of the interstitial fluid.

1. Forces affecting fluid movement out of the pulmonary capillary:

Capillary hydrostatic pressure	7 mm Hg
Interstitial fluid colloid osmotic pressure	+ 16 mm Hg
Total outward force	23 mm Hg

2. Forces affecting fluid movement into the pulmonary capillaries:

Plasma colloid osmotic pressure	25.4 mm Hg
Interstitial hydrostatic pressure	− 6.0 mm Hg
Total inward force	19.4 mm Hg

3. Net mean filtration force:

Total inward force	23.0 mm Hg
Total outward force	− 19.4 mm Hg
Net force	3.6 mm Hg

The total net filtration pressure at the pulmonary capillary is felt therefore to be slightly positive and thus results in a net movement of fluid into the interstitial spaces.

NORMAL STARLING FORCES IN PREGNANCY

Oian and coworkers measured Starling forces in 10 normal patients in the first trimester of pregnancy and in 10 additional normal women in the third trimester. Values for COP_p, in early pregnancy (23.2 ± 0.8 mm Hg) were noted to be statistically higher than values obtained in the third trimester (21.1 ± 1.2 mm Hg). These workers also quantitated interstitial fluid COP and hydrostatic pressure.

The authors proposed that, as pregnancy progressed, an increase in capillary filtration secondary to elevated capillary hydrostatic pressure initially would lead to a fall in COP_i by simple dilution. To account for the greater decline in COP_i as compared with COP_p, with advancing gestation, proteins would have to be removed from the interstitium at an increased rate. The authors proposed that an increase in lymphatic flow would effect such a reduction in the protein concentration of the interstitium.

Having measured three of the four Starling forces in the pregnant patient, the Norwegian group then calculated capillary hydrostatic pressure (P_c) from the Starling equation. It would appear that pregnancy is associated with a moderate fall in COP_p and a rise in P_c. Such alterations of these Starling forces would tend to increase fluid filtration from the intravascular compartment to the interstitium. A progressive fall in the COP of the interstitium exerts a protective effect. Increasing P_c in late gestation probably overwhelms this mechanism, however, allowing for increased fluid egress from capillaries. When lymphatic drainage is no longer capable of removing this fluid, edema formation results. Higher P_c in the lower extremity may well explain why edema commonly occurs in the legs of the pregnant patient.

MEASUREMENT AND CALCULATION OF COP_p

Although the various Starling forces have been measured with experimental techniques, only COP_p can be measured with any degree of practicality.

Several commercial devices are now available for the determination of COP_p. In situations where an osmometer is not available, COP_p can be calculated after determination of serum albumin or total protein concentrations where the COP_p is expressed in mm Hg and TP is the total protein concentration in g/dL. Weil et al. reported poor correlation with COP_p and serum albumin and total protein concentrations. However, since then, computerized analysis of serum albumin, total protein, and COP_p in groups of normotensive gravid patients and patients with pregnancy-induced hypertension has resulted in two new equations for the calculation of COP_p during pregnancy:

$$COP_p \text{ (mm Hg)} = 5.21 \times \text{Total serum protein} - 11.4$$

and

$$COP_p \text{ (mm Hg)} = 8.1 \times \text{Serum albumin} - 8.2$$

These two equations are thought to be accurate, with a 10% range of error in 75% and 80% of cases, respectively.

NORMAL VALUES

The COP_p in the fetus appears to increase during intrauterine life and achieves a value of 10 ± 2.3 mm Hg at 40 weeks of gestation. Weil and associates reported that the mean COP_p in healthy ambulatory adult volunteers was 25.4 ± 2.3 mm Hg. A slightly lower COP_p has been noted in female patients when compared with their male counterparts. A downward trend in values is noted with advancing age.

Maternal COP_p values in normal pregnancy decrease and reach a nadir at approximately 34–36 weeks of gestation. This trend closely parallels the decrease in maternal serum albumin concentrations. A mean value at term is reported to be 22.4 ± 0.54 mm Hg. Oian et al. found hematocrit, serum albumin concentration, and total serum protein concentration to be significantly lower in the third trimester as compared with the first trimester. The authors concluded that reduction of the COP_p in the third trimester was the result of a dilution of plasma proteins secondary to a rise in plasma volume. Because albumin is thought to be the major protein responsible for plasma oncotic pressure, Robertson et al. have proposed that the fall in albumin concentration that occurs in pregnancy is the probable explanation for declining COP_p in the gravid state.

VARIATIONS IN COP_p

Factors that can affect COP_p are detailed in Tables 2-1 and 2-2.

TABLE 2-1
Factors associated with increased COP_p

Prolonged use of tourniquet prior to drawing sample
Hemolysis of sample
Plasma > serum
Increases in blood pressure
Increases in pH

TABLE 2-2
Factors associated with decreased COP_p

Decreases in blood pressure
Decreases in pH
Supine position
Age
Male > female
Pregnancy
Normotensive pregnancy > pregnancy-induced hypertension
Antepartum > postpartum
Tocolytic therapy
Excessive use of crystalloid fluids
Disease states associated with protein loss: sepsis, peritonitis

━━━━━━━

FLUIDS AND COP$_p$

Intravenous fluids can be divided into crystalloids and colloids. Information on the effect of crystalloids on COP$_p$ is limited to normal saline and lactated Ringer's solution. They contain only cations and anions mixed in various combinations with water. Because the capillary membrane is permeable to such low-molecular-weight molecules as sodium and chloride, the addition of crystalloids to the intravascular compartment would be expected to lower COP$_p$. Haupt and Rackow found that one liter of normal saline administered to patients in hypovolemic shock effected a 12% decrease in COP$_p$ from baseline levels. Continued use of saline was associated with further declines in the COP$_p$. Colloids include products derived from human plasma (albumin and plasma protein fraction) as well as such synthetic products as Hespan (Du Pont Ltd.).

Human serum albumin is available in concentrations of 5% and 25%. The 5% solution is composed of 50 g albumin in one liter of normal saline and has a COP of approximately 20 mm Hg, and the 25% solution has a COP of 100 mm Hg. The clearance of exogenous albumin is understood poorly but probably involves multiple sites, including kidneys, liver, and intestines. The effect of albumin has been found to last for approximately 24 hours.

Plasma protein fraction (PPF) is a 5% solution of human albumin and globulins in a buffered electrolyte solution. Albumin comprises the majority of the protein in this solution. For this reason, PPF is expected to have a COP slightly greater than albumin.

Hetastarch (Hespan) is a synthetic colloid consisting of hydroxyethyl-substituted, branched-chain polysaccharides with an average molecular weight of 69,000. The COP of hetastarch is 20 mm Hg. Larger particles are degraded by the liver and excreted in the stool and urine. Low-molecular-weight particles are eliminated from the vascular space by diffusion through systemic capillaries or filtration through the kidneys. The volume-expanding effect of hetastarch has been found to last from 24 to 36 hours.

In vitro analysis comparing the synthetic colloid solutions with 4.5% albumin have revealed that hetastarch showed the least capability for diffusion across capillary membranes. This property is probably related to this substance's high-molecular-weight particles. In vivo comparisons of various colloid solutions and their effect on COP_p has revealed that use of one liter of hetastarch results in a 36% increase and use of one liter of 5% albumin results in an 11% increase. In this study, patients initially given either one of these colloids, followed by maintenance crystalloid therapy, had continued elevation of their COP_p for 48 hours. Patients treated only with saline showed depressed COP_p values when compared with baseline levels. The lowered levels continued for up to five days.

COP_p VALUES IN PREGNANCY-INDUCED HYPERTENSION

Measurements of COP_p at term in patients with pregnancy-induced hypertension (PIH) have revealed values that are lower than those from a similar group of normotensive patients (17.9 ± 0.68 mm Hg versus 22 ± 0.48 mm Hg). The degree of hypertension, however, does not seem to correlate with the magnitude of reduction in the COP_p.

Chesley first proposed that proteinuria was the etiology for decreased COP_p in preeclampsia, but recent studies have shed new light on the mechanism for reduced COP_p. Bhatia et al. measured fibronectin levels in 12 patients with mild PIH and 20 patients with severe PIH and compared these values with a control gravid population. Fibronectin levels in both the mild and severe PIH groups were significantly higher than those in controls (444 ± 122, 401 ± 102, and 217 ± 61 μg/mL, respectively). Using fibronectin as a sensitive indicator of capillary damage, these authors proposed that altered capillary permeability to plasma proteins was the etiology of decreased COP_p in PIH patients. Statistical analysis revealed that vascular damage was fourfold more important than proteinuria in explaining decreased COP_p.

Therefore, experimental evidence indicates that lowered COP_p in the patient with PIH is the result of loss of serum proteins across capillary membranes. Urinary protein loss also contributes to lowering the COP_p.

COP_p IN THE POSTPARTUM PERIOD

When compared with intrapartum values, values of COP_p measured in the first 24 hours postpartum have revealed a significant reduction. Cotton et al. reported a COP_p value of 15.4 ± 2.1 mm Hg postpartum as compared with a value of 21.0 ± 2.1 mm Hg in the intrapartum period in a group of 72 normal patients at term. The nadir of the COP_p appears to occur from 6 to 16 hours after delivery. After 24 hours postpartum, a trend toward recovery of the COP_p to intrapartum levels has been noted.

Patients with PIH show a similar decrease in COP_p values in the postpartum period. Benedetti et al. found COP_p values of 17.9 ± 0.68 mm Hg in the postpartum period. This decline in COP_p in the first 24 hours after delivery was noted to be of similar magnitude to the postpartum decline seen in normotensive pregnant patients.

Explanations for the postpartum decrease in COP_p included 1) supine positioning during the labor and delivery process, 2) blood loss at delivery, 3) administration of large amounts of crystalloid intravenous fluids during labor, and 4) mobilization of extravascular fluid to the intravascular space.

Jones et al. have studied the effect of crystalloid versus colloid therapy on postpartum COP_p. Patients given 5% albumin were noted to have less fall in the postpartum COP_p when compared with patients who were administered PlasmaLyte A. In addition, the colloid group returned to baseline COP_p levels within 36 hours of delivery; continued reduction in the COP_p was noted in the crystalloid group for 48 hours postpartum (see Table 2-3).

Although the administration of albumin has been demonstrated to result in less reduction in COP_p after delivery, its routine use is not warranted in the normal parturient. The use of colloid therapy in patients at high risk to subsequently develop pulmonary edema after delivery remains controversial. The administration of large volumes of crystalloid should, however, be avoided in these patients.

TABLE 2-3
Normal values for COP_p

Variable	COP (mm Hg, Mean ± SD)
Condition	
Ambulatory	25.4 ± 2.3
Supine	21.6 ± 3.6
Age (years)	
<50	21.6 ± 4.7
50–70	20.7 ± 4.2
70–89	19.7 ± 3.7
Sex	
Male	21.6 ± 4.8
Female	19.6 ± 4.2
Normotensive pregnancy	
Antepartum (at term)	22.4 ± 0.5
Postpartum (first 24 hours)	15.4 ± 2.1
Pregnancy-induced hypertension	
Antepartum (at term)	17.9 ± 0.7
Postpartum (first 24 hours)	13.7 ± 0.5

SD = standard deviation.

COP_p AND BETAMIMETIC THERAPY

COP_p is noted to fall slightly when betamimetic therapy is used for tocolysis in the pregnant patient. Long-term betamimetic therapy has been associated with dramatic reduction in COP_p values (25.1–19.3 mm Hg). Goyert and coworkers studied 15 patients in premature labor who were treated with intravenous ritodrine. COP_p was noted to fall from preinfusion levels of 15.4 ± 2.1 mm Hg to 14.3 ± 1.7 mm Hg after 12 hours of ritodrine infusion. Using serum fibronectin as a sensitive indicator of capillary endothelial damage, no increase in fibronectin levels could be detected before, as compared to during, ritodrine therapy (292 ± 86 vs. 284 ± 101 μg/mL). These investigators concluded that the decreased COP_p associated with ritodrine therapy was not secondary to leakage of serum proteins across damaged capillary membranes. The more likely explanation for the decline in COP_p noted with betamimetic therapy is an increase in plasma volume.

CLINICAL APPLICATION OF COP_p

COP_p TO PULMONARY CAPILLARY WEDGE PRESSURE GRADIENT

With the advent of the pulmonary artery catheter in 1970, the measurement of pulmonary capillary hydrostatic pressures became a reality. Early clinical and radiographic signs of pulmonary congestion are noted to occur at a pulmonary capillary wedge pressure (PCWP) of 18–22 mm Hg. Frank pulmonary congestion is noted at a value of 22–25 mm Hg. Subsequently, cases of pulmonary edema have been reported with normal or only slightly elevated levels of PCWP. Weil's group discovered that low COP_p values were commonly found in this subset of patients. They postulated that a decrease in the normal forces keeping fluid in the pulmonary microvasculature (COP_p) or an increase in the forces moving fluid out of the pulmonary capillaries (i.e., PCWP) could result in the formation of pulmonary edema. Therefore, the concept of a critical COP_p-PCWP gradient was proposed. This explanation for the etiology of pulmonary edema is probably an oversimplification of the complex Starling forces in the lung. The other components of the Starling equation are ignored (capillary permeability, interstitial hydrostatic pressure, and the COP_i). In addition, other protective mechanisms—such as alveolar endothelial permeability, pulmonary lymphatic flow, and surfactant—play vital roles in preventing the accumulation of excess lung water. Because COP_p and capillary hydrostatic pressure are the only two Starling forces that can be measured by current clinical methodology, the COP_p-PCWP gradient is probably the closest approximation of the net Starling interactions in the lung currently available.

Recent studies in pregnant patients with PIH have noted that pulmonary edema also may be related to reductions in the COP_p-PCWP gradient. Cotton et al. noted a negative COP_p-PCWP in five patients with severe PIH and pulmonary edema. Benedetti and coworkers measured COP_p and hemodynamic parameters in 10 patients with severe PIH who developed pulmonary edema in the postpartum period. The authors proposed that, in half the patients, mild to moderate reduction in COP_p coupled with an elevation in PCWP was the etiology for the pulmonary edema. Increased pulmonary capillary permeability was thought to be the etiology of pulmonary edema in three patients, while left ventricular dysfunction was proposed as the etiology in the remaining two patients in the series.

COP_p AND ACUTE RESPIRATORY DISTRESS SYNDROME

Colloid osmotic pressure has been used to distinguish the leaky-membrane pulmonary edema found in patients with acute respiratory distress syndrome (ARDS) from other forms of pulmonary edema. Acute respiratory distress syndrome can occur in a variety of conditions associated with pregnancy, including sepsis, pre-eclampsia, amniotic fluid embolism, and betamimetic-associated pulmonary edema. In pulmonary edema related to elevated capillary hydrostatic pressure, the endobronchial fluid (edema fluid from endotracheal tube suctioning) has a COP of less than 60% of that of simultaneously measured plasma. In pulmonary edema secondary to increased permeability of pulmonary capillary membranes, the COP of endobronchial fluid exceeds 75% of that of plasma. In more advanced stages, the oncotic pressure of the two determinations may be identical.

The role of colloid versus crystalloid therapy is controversial in patients with ARDS. Proponents of colloid therapy argue that increasing COP_p will prevent extravasation of fluid into the interstitium. Those opposed to the use of colloids in ARDS patients maintain that pulmonary interstitial edema is worsened as colloid extravasates into the interstitium, leading to further fluid movement out of the capillary. Despite these theoretical concerns, a recent study using radiolabeled tracers has failed to demonstrate a significant increase in the microvascular flux of albumin into pulmonary edema fluid in patients with ARDS. Appel and Shoemaker studied the use of various colloids in patients with ARDS and found that optimization of the COP_p-PCWP gradient with these solutions improved the cardiorespiratory status. Metildi and coworkers randomized 46 patients with ARDS to receive either crystalloid or albumin therapy for resuscitation. Although the intrapulmonary shunt did not improve to the same degree in the crystalloid group as compared with the albumin group, no difference in survival between the two groups was detected. The authors concluded that, because colloid therapy did not provide a clear advantage over crystalloids and is much more costly, the latter should be the preferred fluid therapy for the patient with ARDS.

SUGGESTED READING

Benedetti TJ, Kates R, Williams V. Hemodynamic observations of severe preeclampsia complicated by pulmonary edema. Am J Obstet Gynecol 1985;152:330.

Clark SL, Cotton DB, Lee W, et al. Central hemodynamic assessment of normal term pregnancy. Obstet Gynecol 1989;161:1439.

Cotton DB, Gonik B, Dorman K, Harrist R. Cardiovascular alterations in severe pregnancy-induced hypertension: relationship of central venous pressure to pulmonary capillary wedge pressure. Am J Obstet Gynecol 1985;151:762.

Cotton DB, Gonik B, Spillman T, Dorman KF. Intrapartum to postpartum changes in colloid osmotic pressure. Am J Obstet Gynecol 1984;149:174.

Gonik B, Cotton D, Spillman T, Abouleish E, Zavisca F. Peripartum colloid osmotic changes: Effects of controlled fluid management. Am J Obstet Gynecol 1985;151:812.

Guyton AC. Textbook of medical physiology, 6th ed. Philadelphia: WB Saunders Co, 1981:363–382.

Laks H, O'Connor NE, Anderson W, Pilon RN. Crystalloid versus colloid hemodilution in man. Surg Gynecol Obstet 1976;142:506.

McHugh TJ, Forrester JS, Adler L, Zion D, Swan HJ. Pulmonary vascular congestion in acute myocardial infarction: hemodynamic and radiologic correlations. Ann Intern Med 1972;76:29.

Morissette MP. Colloid osmotic pressure: its measurement and clinical value. CMA J 1983;116:897.

Nguyen HN, Clark SL, Greenspoon J, Diesfield P, Wu PY. Peripartum colloid osmotic pressures: correlation with serum proteins. Obstet Gynecol. 1986;68:807.

Oian P, Maltau JM, Noddeland H, Fadnes HO. Oedema-preventing mechanisms in subcutaneous tissue of normal pregnant women. Br J Obstet Gynecol 1985;92:1113.

Prather JW, Gaar KA, Guyton AC. Direct continuous recording of plasma colloid osmotic pressure of whole blood. J Appl Physiol 1968;24:602.

Taylor AE. Capillary fluid filtration: starling forces and lymph flow. Circ Res 1981;49:557.

Webb AR, Barclay SA, Bennett ED. In vitro colloid osmotic pressure of commonly used plasma expanders and substitutes: a study of the diffusibility of colloid molecules. Intensive Care Med 1989;15:116.

Weil MH, Carlson RW. Colloid osmotic pressure and pulmonary edema. Chest 1977;72:692.

CHAPTER THREE

The Pulmonary Artery Catheter: Insertion Technique and Complications

CATHETER PLACEMENT

The procedure for catheter placement involves two phases. The initial phase in pulmonary artery catheterization is establishing venous access with a large-bore sheath. Access is most commonly obtained via the internal jugular or subclavian veins; however, under certain circumstances (e.g., where access to the neck or thoracic region is difficult or in a patient with a coagulopathy where bleeding from a major artery could be hazardous), peripheral veins—including cephalic or femoral—can be used. Insertion of the introducer sheath via the right internal jugular vein is described here.

INSERTION OF THE SHEATH

To catheterize the internal jugular vein, place the patient supine with the head turned to the left in mild Trendelenburg position.

The landmark for insertion is the junction of the clavicular and sternal heads of the sternocleidomastoid muscle. When this junction is indistinct, its identification can be facilitated by having the patient raise her head slightly. When the landmark has been identified, 1% lidocaine is infiltrated into the skin and superficial subcutaneous tissue.

The internal jugular vein is entered first with a finder needle, consisting of a 21-gauge needle on a 10-mL syringe. The skin is punctured at the junction of the two clavicular heads, and the needle is directed with constant aspiration toward the ipsilateral nipple at an angle approximately 30 degrees superior to the plane of the skin. Free flow of venous blood confirms the position of the internal jugular vein. Next, the needle is withdrawn and the vein once again entered with a 16-gauge needle and syringe. Then a guide wire is placed through the needle and into the jugular vein. This placement is perhaps the most crucial part of the entire procedure; it is vital that the guide wire pass freely without any resistance whatsoever. Free passage confirms entrance into the vein.

Next, the needle is removed and the guide wire left in place. The incision is widened with a scalpel, and the introducer-sheath-vein-dilator apparatus is introduced over the guide wire. During introduction of introducer-sheath-vein dilator, it is crucial that the proximal tip of the guide wire be visible at all times to avoid inadvertent loss of the guide wire into the central venous system. The introducer-sheath-vein-dilator apparatus is advanced with a slight turning motion along the guide wire. In general, the point of entry into the vein is felt clearly by a sudden decrease in resistance. The sheath apparatus then is advanced to the hilt. The conscious patient is instructed to hold her breath to prevent negative intrathoracic pressure and inadvertent air embolism, and the guide wire and trocar are quickly removed and the sheath left in place.

Most current introducer systems contain an accessory port, which attaches to the proximal end of the introducer sheath and includes a one-way valve that prevents air introduction into the central venous system during removal of the guide wire and trocar. To keep the line open, the sheath then is infused with a crystalloid solution containing one unit of heparin per milliliter and secured in place with suture.

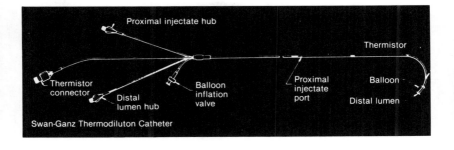

FIGURE 3-1

The pulmonary artery catheter. (Reproduced with permission from American Edwards Laboratories.)

INSERTION OF THE CATHETER

Phase two involves the actual placement of the pulmonary artery catheter (Figure 3-1). Pay careful attention to maintaining sterile technique as the catheter is removed from the package. The distal and proximal ports are flushed to assure patency. The balloon then is tested with 1 mL of air. When the catheter has been attached to the physiologic monitor and the air completely flushed from the system, minute movements in the catheter tip should produce corresponding oscillations on the monitor. The catheter tip is introduced through the sheath and advanced approximately 20 cm. At this point, the balloon is inflated and the catheter advanced through the introducer sheath into the central venous system. Occasionally, portable real-time sonography may be helpful in guiding central venous cannulation.

WAVEFORMS AND CATHETER PLACEMENT

Once within the superior vena cava, the balloon on the tip of the catheter will advance with the flow of blood into the heart. Characteristic waveforms and pressure observed are detailed in Figure 3-2.

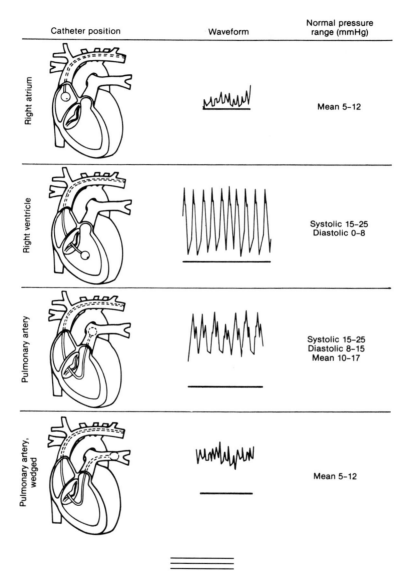

Catheter position	Waveform	Normal pressure range (mmHg)
Right atrium		Mean 5–12
Right ventricle		Systolic 15–25 Diastolic 0–8
Pulmonary artery		Systolic 15–25 Diastolic 8–15 Mean 10–17
Pulmonary artery, wedged		Mean 5–12

FIGURE 3-2

Pulmonary artery catheter placement—catheter tip position, corresponding waveforms, and normal pressure ranges are demonstrated. (Reproduced with permission from American Edwards Laboratories.)

Entrance into the right ventricle is signaled by a high spiking waveform with diastolic pressures near zero. This is the time of maximum potential complications during the catheter placement because most arrhythmias occur as the catheter tip impinges on the interventricular septum. For this reason, the catheter must be rapidly advanced through the right ventricle and into the pulmonary artery. If premature ventricular contractions occur during this process and the catheter does not advance promptly out of the right ventricle, the balloon should be deflated and the catheter withdrawn to the right atrium. As soon as the catheter enters the pulmonary artery, the waveform has two notable characteristics. First, and most important, is the rise in diastolic pressure from that seen in the right ventricle. Second, a notching of the peak systolic waveform often is seen and represents closure of the pulmonic valve. After entrance into the pulmonary artery has been confirmed (in most pregnant women, this occurs between 40 and 45 cm of catheter length), the catheter is advanced farther until the tip reaches a point within the pulmonary vasculature where the balloon diameter exceeds that of the corresponding pulmonary arterial branch. At this point, a wedge tracing is observed. If the balloon is deflated, the tracing should return to a pulmonary artery pattern.

COMPLICATIONS

Most complications actually seen in patients undergoing pulmonary artery catheterization are a result of obtaining central venous access. Such events include pneumothorax and insertion site infection and occur in 1%–5% of patients undergoing this procedure. Potential complications of pulmonary artery catheterization per se include air embolism, thromboembolism, pulmonary infarction, catheter-related sepsis, and direct trauma to the heart or pulmonary artery. Such complications occur in 1% or less of patients. Arrhythmias, consisting of transient premature ventricular contractions, occur during catheter insertion in 30%–50% of patients and are generally of no clinical consequence. The remaining complications can be minimized or eliminated by careful attention to proper insertion and maintenance techniques.

Recently, a Food and Drug Administration (FDA) task force has summarized recommendations regarding methods to minimize complications of central venous catheterization procedures. Numerous recent studies have documented the frequent discrepancy between measurements of pulmonary capillary wedge pressure and central venous pressure. In such circumstances, clinical use of the central venous pressure would be misleading. For these reasons, in a modern perinatal intensive care unit, central venous monitoring is seldom, if ever, indicated. Where proper equipment and personnel exist, the vast amount of additional information obtainable by pulmonary artery catheterization far outweighs the slight potential increase in risk attributable to catheter placement and is nearly always preferable.

SUGGESTED READING

Clark SL, Cotton DB. Clinical opinion: clinical indications for pulmonary artery catheterization in severe pregnancy induced hypertension. Am J Obstet Gynecol 1988;158:453.

Clark SL, Horenstein JM, Phelan JP, et al. Experience with the pulmonary artery catheter in obstetrics and gynecology. Am J Obstet Gynecol 1985;152:374.

Lee W, Leduc L, Cotton DB. Ultrasonographic guidance for central venous catheterization. Am J Obstet Gynecol 1989;161:1012.

Patel C, Labby V, Venus B, et al. Acute complications of pulmonary artery catheter insertion in critically ill patients. Crit Care Med 1986;14:195.

Scott WL. Complications associated with central venous catheters. Chest 1988;91:1221.

Swan JHC, Ganz W, Forrester J, et al. Catheterization of the heart in man with use of a flow-directed balloon-tipped catheter. N Engl J Med 1970;283:447.

U.S. Food and Drug Administration. Precautions necessary with central venous catheters, FDA Drug Bulletin. July 1989;15.

CHAPTER FOUR

Principles of Invasive
Hemodynamic Monitoring

There are four basic parameters necessary to describe comprehensively the hemodynamic status of any pregnant patient: preload, afterload, contractility, and heart rate.

PRELOAD

Preload refers to the volume of blood contained within a ventricle at cardiac end-diastole. Preload is determined by blood return to the ventricle and thus is directly related to intravascular volume. If increased amounts of blood enter the heart during diastole, the normal heart will respond with increased velocity of contraction and thus increased stroke volume. This is termed Starling's law of the heart. After the physiologic limit of adaptation is reached, however, the heart's pumping ability levels off and subsequently decreases in response to further increasing preload. The central venous pressure is a measurement of right ventricular preload. Left ventricular preload is approximated clinically as pulmonary capillary wedge pressure.

AFTERLOAD

Afterload represents the downstream resistance offered to each ventricle during cardiac systole. Cardiac output is inversely related to afterload (Figure 4-1). Clinically, afterload is assessed as systemic vascular resistance, a derived parameter based upon blood pressure, central venous pressure, and cardiac output. Right ventricular afterload is represented by pulmonary vascular resistance, and left ventricular afterload by systemic vascular resistance.

FIGURE 4-1

Cardiac output (CO) versus mean arterial pressure (MAP). Increasing systemic vascular resistance (SVR) is demonstrated by isometric lines.

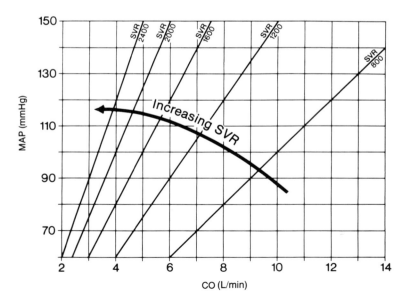

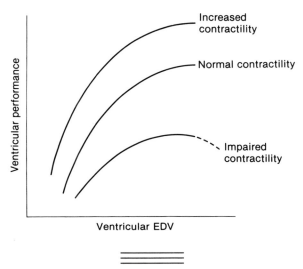

FIGURE 4-2

Ventricular end-diastolic volume versus ventricular performance. Increased, normal, and impaired contractility are demonstrated.

CONTRACTILITY

Contractility refers to the intrinsic contractile property of the myocardium. While alterations in preload affect the movement of stroke volume along a given Starling curve, alterations in contractility affect the Starling curve upon which the cardiac output operates (Figure 4-2). Contractility may be altered by various disease states or by pharmacologic agents that have positive or negative inotropic effects. One of the most useful measures of contractility is stroke work index, a derived parameter (Figure 4-3).

HEART RATE

Cardiac output is also directly affected by heart rate, independent of either Starling's forces or alterations in contractility. In the

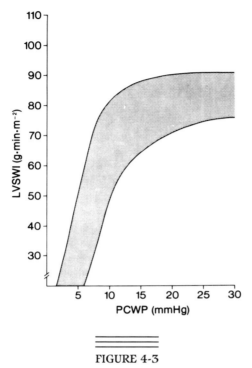

FIGURE 4-3

Pulmonary capillary wedge pressure (PCWP) versus left ventricular stroke work index (LVSWI): Normal relationship represented by shaded area.

normal heart, cardiac output generally increases with normal heart rate to the limits of physiologic tachycardia. However, at extremely rapid rates, ventricular filling and end-diastolic volume will be diminished because of inadequate diastolic filling time; under these circumstances, cardiac output will decrease. In addition, in the patient with a diseased heart, for example, mitral stenosis, even mild degrees of tachycardia may decrease diastolic filling time sufficiently to adversely affect stroke volume and cardiac output. Thus, while tachycardia is most often a response to physiologic stress, tachycardia itself may have adverse hemodynamic effects in certain types of structural or ischemic heart disease.

CLINICAL ASSESSMENT

In practice, blood pressure, pulse, and body surface area are measured in standard clinical fashion. Central venous and pulmonary capillary wedge pressures are measured from the proximal and distal ports of pulmonary artery catheter. Cardiac output is measured using thermodilution technique associated with the pulmonary artery catheter and a cardiac output computer. Once these parameters have been obtained clinically, derived parameters such as systemic and pulmonary vascular resistance and left ventricular stroke work index may be calculated in putting together the complete hemodynamic picture of the patient.

Once the above parameters have been determined, it is possible to identify and address the origin of the hemodynamic instability in a critically ill patient. The first step in management should always be to optimize cardiac preload. While a normal capillary wedge pressure is in the range of 6–10 mm Hg, Starling's law of the heart dictates continued improvement in ventricular contractility in most patients up to a wedge pressure of 14–16 mm Hg. Thus, for many patients in shock, achievement of this degree of preload may allow sufficiently improved cardiac output to avoid the need for inotropic agents.

If further cardiac output augmentation is necessary after preload has been optimized, increases in contractility (with inotropic agents) or decreases in systemic vascular resistance (afterload reduction) may be accomplished as clinically appropriate in order to approach optimal hemodynamic performance in any given patient.

BLOOD PRESSURE

True interarterial pressures obtained by direct arterial line measurements are more accurate than cuff pressures. As a rule, interarterial catheters result in pressures from 4–8 mm higher than corresponding cuff pressures. This principle, however, is generally valid only in normal patients; in certain subsets of critically ill patients, interarterial pressures may be up to 30 mm Hg higher than those obtained from a peripheral cuff. In circumstances characterized by severe vasoconstriction and resultant low cardiac output, cuff pressures may be even less accurate; under such circumstances, differences of up to 50 mm Hg have been reported. Thus, for patients in shock, interarterial catheters are preferred. In many clinical circumstances, however, either manual or automatic cuff assessment of blood pressure will prove satisfactory.

MIXED VENOUS OXYGEN SATURATION (SVo_2) MONITORING

SVo_2 may be assessed either periodically by direct sampling from the distal port of pulmonary artery catheter or continuous use of a pulmonary artery catheter equipped with fiberoptic oximetry sensor. SVo_2 is determined by four parameters: cardiac output, hemoglobin concentration, arterial oxygen saturation, and oxygen consumption. Normal SVo_2 ranges from approximately 66%-77%. Because changes in any single parameter contributing to SVo_2 may be compensated for by alterations in other parameters, there is poor direct correlation between SVo_2 and any single parameter. Decreases in SVo_2 of greater than 10% are clinically significant and indicate an imbalance between oxygen supply and demand; however, the cause of such imbalance cannot be explained by SVo_2 changes alone. Simultaneous knowledge of arterial oxygen saturation, hemoglobin, and cardiac output nevertheless provides the clinician with the tools necessary to evaluate significance of changes in SVo_2.

Alterations in hemoglobin produce only very small changes in SVo_2 until the hemoglobin reaches critically low levels. Similarly, alterations in arterial oxygen saturation (Sao_2) produce minimal effects on SVo_2 over the broad range of normal Sao_2 measurements. However, in the presence of sufficient arterial hypoxemia to produce frank arterial desaturation, SVo_2 will fall significantly. Under conditions of steady-state oxygen consumption, arterial oxygen saturation, and hemoglobin concentration, alterations in SVo_2 are proportionate to cardiac output; continuous assessment of SVO_2 may thus serve as an early warning indicator for significant decreases in cardiac output.

PULSE OXIMETRY

Pulse oximetry is based upon the principle of differential light transmittance by oxygenated and nonoxygenated hemoglobin and depends upon the use of two light-emitting diode (LED) sources: one red (660 nanometers) and one infrared (940 nanometers). Using a spectrophotometric device and an associated microprocessor, pulse oximeters will evaluate O_2 saturation with each pulse. In critically ill pregnant patients with tenuous physiologic oxygenation, pulse oximetry is an invaluable technique. The use of this technique often allows the clinician to avoid multiple arterial blood gases and, at the same time, provides a continuous rather than an intermittent method of patient evaluation. This technique should be a routine part of the management of any critically ill patient whose oxygen status is or may be compromised. Recent investigations into the use of fetal pulse oximetry may also prove clinically fruitful.

SUGGESTED READING

American College of Obstetricians and Gynecologists Technical Bulletin #175, Invasive Hemodynamic Monitoring in Obstetrics and Gynecology, Dec. 1992.

Clark SL, Cotton DB, Lee W, et al. Central hemodynamic assessment of normal third trimester pregnancy. Am J Obstet Gynecol 1989;161:1439.

Diurtie MB, McMichan JC. Continuous monitoring of mixed venous saturation. Chest 1984;85:423.

Gaasch WH, Levine HJ, Quinones MA, et al. Left ventricular compliance: mechanism and clinical implications. Am J Cardiol 1976;38:645.

Veille JC, Morton MJ, Burry KJ. Maternal cardiovascular adaptations to twin pregnancy. Am J Obstet Gynecol 1985;153:261.

CHAPTER FIVE

Maternal-Fetal Physiological Interactions in the Critically Ill Pregnant Patient

OXYGEN TRANSPORT

Each step in the process of oxygen transport from maternal lung to fetal tissue results in a progressive decrease in the partial pressure of oxygen (PO_2) (see Table 5-1). However, the oxygen uptake per unit body weight by the fetus exceeds that of the adult.

The human placenta functions as a venous equilibrator. Maternal blood and fetal blood run through two channels in the same direction (Figure 5-1). Exchange of oxygen occurs across the semipermeable membrane of the placenta. As the two bloodstreams move toward the end of their channels, the PO_2 in the uterine venous circulation is lower than the arterial systems. The PO_2 in the umbilical vein rises until the PO_2 is equal in each system. The umbilical venous stream cannot exit with a higher PO_2 than the uterine venous stream. The system attempts to equilibrate the PO_2 of fetal blood with the PO_2 of blood in the maternal circulation.

From the concept of venous equilibration, it is obvious that the uterine venous PO_2 is the major determinant of umbilical venous PO_2. If uterine venous PO_2 is elevated, there is an increase

TABLE 5-1

Stepwise decrement of P_{O_2} from inspired air to
fetal tissue*

Site	P_{O_2} (mm Hg)
Inspired air	120
Alveolar air	90
Maternal artery	80
Uterine vein	48
Umbilical vein	30
Umbilical artery	20

*This table demonstrates the stepwise decrement of P_{O_2} as
oxygen is transported from the atmosphere to the fetus.

in umbilical venous P_{O_2}. Likewise, a reduction in uterine venous
P_{O_2} will result in a similar fall in umbilical venous P_{O_2}.

The oxygen saturation of uterine venous blood is affected by
three major variables: 1) the oxygen saturation of maternal arterial blood, 2) the oxygen-carrying capacity of maternal blood,
and 3) the uterine blood flow. A decrease in the P_{O_2} of maternal
blood (which would occur in a hypoxemic mother, in an anemic
mother with reduced oxygen-carrying capacity, or in a mother
with reduced uterine blood flow, as it would if she were
hypotensive) will reduce uterine venous P_{O_2} and ultimately reduce umbilical venous P_{O_2}.

FETAL ADAPTATION TO LOW P_{O_2}

Despite a low P_{O_2}, fetal blood delivers large amounts of oxygen
to the fetal tissues to enable normal growth and development.
This is accomplished by two mechanisms: 1) the high affinity of
fetal hemoglobin for oxygen and 2) the high rate of perfusion of
vital fetal organs.

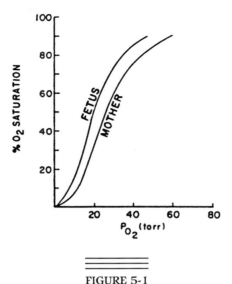

FIGURE 5-1

Maternal and fetal oxyhemoglobin dissociation curves: this figure demonstrates the high affinity of fetal hemoglobin toward oxygen, relative to adult hemoglobin. (Modified from Battaglia FC, Meschia G. An Introduction to Fetal Physiology. New York: Academic Press, 1986.)

The increased affinity of fetal hemoglobin for oxygen is demonstrated by comparing the oxyhemoglobin saturation curves of maternal and fetal hemoglobin (Figure 5-1, Table 5-2). It can be seen that, at the same Po_2, fetal hemoglobin has a higher affinity for oxygen than does maternal hemoglobin. For example, at a Po_2 of 34 mm Hg, fetal hemoglobin is 80% saturated with oxygen.

The fetus also has a relatively high heart rate and stroke volume, resulting in an increased relative cardiac output. A comparison of the perfusion rates of adults and fetal brain has shown that the fetal brain receives 2.5 times more blood per milliliter of oxygen consumed than does the adult organ. The fetus accomplishes this by having blood bypass the fetal lungs via the ductus arteriosus and having a biventricular cardiac output supply the systemic circulation. Despite the low fetal Po_2, the fetus has adequate oxygen to supply its energy needs and cannot be considered hypoxemic.

TABLE 5-2
Effect of transfusion of adult red blood cells on fetal sheep*

	% of Adult red blood cells	Po$_2$ (mm Hg)	% of O$_2$ saturation
Pretransfusion	0	29	83
Posttransfusion	80	32	54

*This table demonstrates that replacement of fetal red blood cells with adult red blood cells results in a diminished oxygen saturation. (Modified from Battaglia FC, Bowes W, McGaughey HR, et al. The effect of fetal exchange transfusions with adult blood upon fetal oxygenation. Pediat Res 1969;3:60.)

UTERINE PERFUSION PHYSIOLOGY

Blood flow to the uterus depends on systemic blood pressure. Autoregulation, the ability of an organ to change its vascular resistance in response to changes in perfusion pressure, has not been clearly demonstrated in the uteroplacental circulation, and the uterine vasculature acts as if it were continually maximally dilated. Uterine contractions result in a decrease in uterine blood flow that is proportional to the magnitude and duration of the contraction. As intrauterine pressure rises, intervillous blood slows and ultimately ceases.

EFFECTS OF HYPOXIA ON THE FETUS

Oxygen delivery to the fetus is determined by uterine blood flow and the level of the uterine venous Po$_2$. As umbilical venous oxygen is reduced, the fetus goes through three major stages of acute hypoxemia.

In the first stage, the oxygen content of fetal blood may be reduced up to 50% without the development of acidosis. The fetus initially compensates for this hypoxemia by redirecting even more of cardiac output to the heart and brain. Although this degree of hypoxemia is not life-threatening, the fetus is in a precarious state and will not tolerate further diminution of oxygen supply.

In the second stage, the fetus uses anaerobic metabolism, ultimately resulting in a base deficit and metabolic acidosis. There is an outpouring of catecholamines within the fetus that diminishes blood flow to every organ but the brain, heart, and placenta. If the uterus containing a fetus in the second stage of hypoxia begins to contract, uterine blood flow will slow as the intrauterine pressure rises and intermittently further impair fetal oxygenation. The fetal brain stem and heart will respond to this insult with brief episodes of bradycardia (late decelerations).

The third stage of hypoxia occurs when oxygen content is reduced by over 75%. Perfusion of the brain cannot be adequately maintained, and central nervous system damage may ensue if this stage persists. This degree of hypoxia will ultimately result in fetal death.

INTERVENTIONS TO IMPROVE FETAL OXYGENATION

A wide array of conditions in the mother can impair oxygen delivery to the fetus. Any state that lowers the Po_2 of the uterine vein will result in diminished oxygen transport. The Po_2 of the blood in the uterine vein will be lowered by any disease that 1) lowers maternal oxygen-carrying capacity, 2) decreases the Po_2 of the maternal blood, or 3) diminishes uterine blood flow.

In the anemic gravida, the oxygen-carrying capacity of her blood is diminished. Also, maternal acidosis and fever shift the hemoglobin saturation curve to the right and lower the oxygen-carrying capacity. Treatment must be aimed at increasing the oxygen-carrying capacity of maternal blood by replacement of red blood cells, maintenance of intravascular volume, and correction of metabolic derangements.

If a mother has diminished Po_2 due to pulmonary dysfunction or injury, fetal oxygenation will also be impaired. Even in mothers with normal arterial Po_2, increasing this value by increasing the Po_2 of inspired air may have favorable effects for the fetus. This effect is demonstrated in Figure 5-2, which shows blood oxygen content plotted against Po_2 for maternal arterial Po_2 (step a) with an increase in maternal O_2 content (step b). Using the Fick principle, uterine venous O_2 content should rise by the same amount (step c). Concurrently, uterine venous Po_2 will rise (step d), albeit by an amount much less than that of the uterine artery, because the change takes place at a different point on the hemoglobin dissociation curve. Increasing uterine venous Po_2 is followed by an identical increase in umbilical venous Po_2 (step e). This shifts the umbilical venous O_2 content upward (step f). The umbilical artery O_2 content moves upward in the same fashion (step g), ultimately resulting in increased umbilical

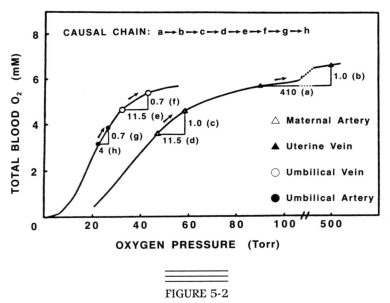

FIGURE 5-2

The effect on fetal oxygenation of increasing the Po_2 of maternal inspired air: Note that a large increase in the Po_2 of inspired air in the mother ultimately results in an increase of O_2 content in the fetus. See text for details. (Reprinted by permission from Battaglia FC, Meschia G. An Introduction to Fetal Physiology. New York: Academic Press, 1986.)

artery Po_2 (step h). Thus, small changes in fetal Po_2 theoretically result in proportionately larger changes in O_2 content because the fetus is operating on the steep portion of the O_2 dissociation curve. In a similar manner, decreases in maternal arterial Po_2 below 60 mm Hg result in an even more dramatic decline in fetal O_2 content. The oxygenation of critically ill patients is often monitored with pulse oximetry. Although O_2 saturation values of 85%–90% may be adequate to provide for maternal physiologic needs, in the gravid patient, an O_2 saturation of 95% or greater is essential to guarantee a $Po_2 > 60$ mm Hg and adequate fetal oxygenation.

Because oxygenation depends on flow, uterine blood flow should be maximized in the critically ill gravida to ensure adequate fetal oxygenation. Avoidance of the supine position, with its potential to occlude the maternal vena cava, diminish preload, and lower cardiac output, is essential in maintaining uterine blood flow.

SUGGESTED READING

Assali NS. Dynamics of the uteroplacental circulation in health and disease. Am J Perinatology 1989;6:105–109.

Meschia G. Evolution of thinking in fetal respiratory physiology. Am J Obstet Gynecol 1978;37:806–812.

Meschia G. Safety margin of fetal oxygenation. J Repro Med 1985;30:308–311.

Rankin J, Meschia G, Makowski EL, Battaglia FC. Relationship between uterine and umbilical Po_2 in sheep. Am J Physiology 1971;220:1688–1692.

Sheldon RE, Peters LH, Jones M, et al. Redistribution of cardiac output and oxygen delivery in the hypoxemic fetal lamb. Am J Obstet Gynecol 1979;135:1071–1075.

PART II

Clinical Management

CHAPTER SIX

Structural Cardiac Disease
in Pregnancy

COUNSELING THE PREGNANT
CARDIAC PATIENT

Table 6-1 represents a synthesis of current maternal mortality estimates for various types of cardiac disease. Group I includes conditions that, with proper management, should have negligible maternal mortality (<1%). Cardiac lesions in group II carry with them a 5%–15% risk of maternal mortality, either secondary to the cardiac disease itself or to the need for anticoagulation during pregnancy and associated thromboembolic phenomena. In individual cases and after appropriate counseling, this risk may prove acceptable to some women. Patients with cardiac lesions in group III are subject to a mortality risk exceeding 25%. In all but exceptional cases, this risk proves unacceptable to the patient, and prevention or interruption of pregnancy should be recommended strongly.

TABLE 6-1
Mortality risk associated with pregnancy

Group I: Mortality <1%

Atrial septal defect, uncomplicated
Ventricular septal defect, uncomplicated
Patent ductus arteriosus, uncomplicated
Pulmonic/tricuspid disease
Corrected tetralogy of Fallot
Porcine valve
Mitral stenosis, NYHA classes I and II

Group II: Mortality 5%–15%

Mitral stenosis with atrial fibrillation
Artificial valve
Mitral stenosis, NYHA classes III and IV
Aortic stenosis
Coarctation of aorta, uncomplicated
Uncorrected tetralogy of Fallot
Previous myocardial infarction
Marfan's syndrome with normal aorta

Group III: Mortality 25%–50%

Pulmonary hypertension
Coarctation of aorta, complicated
Marfan syndrome with aortic involvement

ATRIAL SEPTAL DEFECT

Atrial septal defect (ASD) is the most common congenital lesion seen during pregnancy and, in general, is asymptomatic. The hypervolemia associated with pregnancy results in an increased left-to-right shunt through the ASD, and thus a significant burden is imposed on the right ventricle. Although this additional burden is tolerated well by most patients, congestive failure and death with ASD have been reported. The majority of patients with ASD tolerate pregnancy, labor, and delivery without complication.

VENTRICULAR SEPTAL DEFECT

The size of the septal defect is the most important determinant of clinical prognosis during pregnancy. Small defects are tolerated well; larger defects are associated more frequently with congestive failure, arrhythmias, or the development of pulmonary hypertension. In addition, a large ventricular septal defect (VSD) often is associated with some degree of aortic regurgitation, which can add to the risk of congestive failure. Pregnancy, labor, and delivery generally are tolerated well by patients with uncomplicated VSD.

PATENT DUCTUS ARTERIOSUS

Although patent ductus arteriosus is one of the most common congenital cardiac anomalies, its almost universal detection and closure in the newborn period makes it uncommon during pregnancy. As with uncomplicated ASD and VSD, most patients are asymptomatic, and PDA generally is tolerated well during pregnancy, labor, and delivery.

EISENMENGER'S SYNDROME

Eisenmenger's syndrome develops when, in the presence of a congenital left-to-right shunt, progressive pulmonary hypertension leads to shunt reversal or bidirectional shunting. Although the syndrome can occur with ASD, VSD, or PDA, the low-pressure/high-flow shunt seen with ASD is far less likely to result in pulmonary hypertension and shunt reversal than is the condition of high pressure and high flow seen with VSD and PDA. Whatever the etiology, pulmonary hypertension carries a grave prognosis during pregnancy. During the antepartum period, the decreased systemic vascular resistance associated with pregnancy increases the likelihood or degree of right-to-left shunting. In such a patient, systemic hypotension leads to decreased right ventricular filling pressures; in the presence of fixed pulmonary hypertension, such decreased right heart pressures may be insufficient to perfuse the pulmonary arterial bed. Such hypotension can result from hemorrhage or complications of conduction anesthesia and can lead to sudden death.

Maternal mortality in the presence of Eisenmenger's syndrome is reported as 30% to 50%. In addition to the previously discussed problems associated with hemorrhage and hypovolemia, thromboembolic phenomena have been associated with up to 43% of all maternal deaths in Eisenmenger's syndrome. Sudden delayed postpartum death, occurring 2 to 6 weeks after delivery, is also seen.

Because of the high mortality associated with continuing pregnancy, abortion is the preferred management for the woman with pulmonary hypertension of any etiology. Dilatation and curettage in the first trimester or dilatation and evacuation in the second trimester are the methods of choice. Hypertonic saline and F-prostaglandins are contraindicated. The hemodynamic effect of E-prostaglandins in patients with pulmonary hypertension are not documented. This paucity of data and the lack of immediate reversibility of this agent should be considered when contemplating the use of E-prostaglandins in a pregnant patient with cardiac disease.

The use of epidural or intrathecal morphine sulfate, a technique devoid of effect on systemic blood pressure, represents the best approach to anesthetic management of these patients.

COARCTATION OF THE AORTA

Patients having coarctation of the aorta uncomplicated by aneurysmal dilation or associated cardiac lesions who enter pregnancy as class I or II have a good prognosis and a minimal risk of complications or death. On the other hand, in the presence of aortic or intervertebral aneurysm, known aneurysm of the circle of Willis, or associated cardiac lesions, the risk of death may approach 15%; therefore, therapeutic abortion must be considered strongly.

TETRALOGY OF FALLOT

Several published reports attest to the relatively good outcome of pregnancy in patients with corrected tetralogy of Fallot or transposition of the great vessels; however, there is a 15% mortality with an uncorrected lesion.

PULMONIC STENOSIS

Obstruction with pulmonic stenosis can be valvular, supravalvular, or subvalvular. The degree of obstruction, rather than its site, is the principal determinant of clinical performance. A transvalvular pressure gradient exceeding 80 mm Hg is considered severe and mandates surgical correction. A compilation (totaling 106 pregnancies) of three series of patients with pulmonic stenosis revealed no maternal deaths.

FETAL CONSIDERATIONS

Perinatal outcome in patients with cyanotic congenital cardiac disease correlates best with hematocrit; successful outcome in patients with a hematocrit exceeding 65% is unlikely. Such patients have an increased risk of spontaneous abortion, intrauterine growth retardation, and stillbirth. Maternal partial pressure of oxygen (Po_2) below 60% results in markedly decreased fetal O_2 saturation; thus Pao_2 should be kept above this level during pregnancy, labor, and delivery. Serial antepartum sonography for the detection of growth retardation and antepartum fetal heart rate testing are important in many patients with significant cardiac disease. Of equal concern in patients with congenital heart disease is a 5%–10% risk of fetal congenital cardiac anomalies. In such women, fetal echocardiography is indicated for prenatal diagnosis of congenital cardiac defects.

PULMONIC AND TRICUSPID LESIONS

Isolated right-sided valvular lesions of rheumatic origin are uncommon; however, such lesions are seen with increased frequency in intravenous drug abusers, where they are secondary to valvular endocarditis. Pregnancy-associated hypervolemia is far less likely to be symptomatic with right-sided lesion than with those involving the mitral or aortic valves. Even following complete tricuspid valvectomy for endocarditis, pregnancy, labor, and delivery generally are well tolerated.

MITRAL STENOSIS

Mitral stenosis is the most common rheumatic valvular lesion encountered during pregnancy. The principal hemodynamic aberration involves ventricular diastolic filling obstruction, resulting in a relatively fixed cardiac output.

Cardiac output in patients with mitral stenosis is largely dependent on two factors. First, these patients depend on adequate diastolic filling time. In order to avoid hazardous tachycardia, the physician should consider oral beta-blocker therapy for any patient with severe mitral stenosis who enters labor with a pulse exceeding 90–100 beats per minute.

A second important consideration is left ventricular preload. Such patients often require high-normal or elevated pulmonary capillary wedge pressure in order to maintain adequate filling pressure and cardiac output.

Potentially dangerous intrapartum fluctuations in output can be minimized by using epidural anesthesia; however, the most hazardous time for these women appears to be the immediate postpartum period. Such patients often enter the postpartum period already operating at maximum cardiac output and cannot accommodate the volume shifts that accompany delivery. A study of patients with severe mitral stenosis found that a postpartum rise in wedge pressure of up to 16 mm Hg could be expected in the immediate postpartum period (Figure 6-1). Because frank pulmonary edema generally does not occur with wedge pressures below 28–30 mm Hg, it follows that the optimal predelivery wedge pressure for such patients is 14 mm Hg or lower. Such a preload may be appropriated cautiously by intrapartum diuresis and with attentive maintenance of adequate cardiac output.

With careful monitoring, it is generally unnecessary to resort to midforceps deliveries for other than standard obstetric indications.

FIGURE 6-1

Intrapartum alterations in pulmonary capillary wedge pressure (PCWP) in eight patients with mitral stenosis. **A:** first-stage labor. **B:** second-stage labor, 15–30 minutes before delivery. **C:** 5–15 minutes postpartum. **D:** 4–6 hours postpartum. **E:** 18–24 hours postpartum. Reproduced by permission from Clark SL, Phelan JP, Greenspoon J, et al. Labor and delivery in the presence of mitral stenosis: central hemodynamic observations. Am J Obstet Gynecol 1985;152:986.

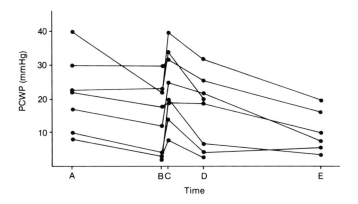

MITRAL INSUFFICIENCY

Hemodynamically significant mitral insufficiency is usually rheumatic in origin and most commonly occurs in conjunction with other valvular lesions. This lesion generally is tolerated well during pregnancy, and congestive failure is an unusual occurrence. More significant is an increased risk of atrial enlargement and fibrillation during pregnancy.

MITRAL VALVE PROLAPSE

Congenital mitral valve prolapse (MVP) is much more common during pregnancy than is rheumatic mitral insufficiency. When strict diagnosis criteria are applied, the prevalence of this condition is approximately 2%. Mitral valve prolapse generally is asymptomatic. The midsystolic click and murmur associated with congenital mitral valve prolapse syndrome are characteristic; however, the intensity of this murmur, as well as that associated with rheumatic mitral insufficiency, may decrease during pregnancy because of decreased systemic vascular resistance. It appears appropriate to reserve subacute bacterial endocarditis (SBE) prophylaxis for women with clinical or echocardiographic evidence of regurgitation associated with MVP.

AORTIC STENOSIS

In contrast to mitral valve stenosis, aortic stenosis generally does not become hemodynamically significant until the orifice has diminished to one-third or less of normal. The major problem experienced by patients with valvular aortic stenosis is maintenance of cardiac output. Because of the relative hypervolemia associated with gestation, such patients generally tolerate pregnancy well. However, with severe disease, cardiac output will be relatively fixed and, during exertion, may be inadequate to maintain coronary artery or cerebral perfusion. This inadequacy can result in angina, myocardial infarction, syncope, or sudden death. Thus, limitation of physical activity is vital to patients with severe disease. If activity is limited and the mitral valve is normal, pulmonary edema will be rare during pregnancy.

Delivery and pregnancy termination appear to be the times of greatest risk for patients with aortic stenosis. The maintenance of cardiac output is crucial; any factor leading to diminished venous return will cause an increase in the valvular gradient and diminished cardiac output. Blood loss, ganglionic blockade from epidural anesthesia, or supine vena caval occlusion by the pregnant uterus can all result in severe hypotension.

The cardiovascular status of patients with aortic stenosis may be complicated further by the coexistence of ischemic heart disease. Because hypovolemia is a far greater threat to the patient than is pulmonary edema, the wedge pressure should be maintained at or near 16 mm Hg to maintain a margin of safety against unexpected peripartum blood loss.

AORTIC INSUFFICIENCY

Aortic insufficiency generally is tolerated well during pregnancy because the increased heart rate seen with advancing gestation decreases time for regurgitant flow during diastole.

PERIPARTUM CARDIOMYOPATHY

Peripartum cardiomyopathy is defined as cardiomyopathy developing in the last month of pregnancy or the first 6 months postpartum in women without previous cardiac disease and after exclusion of other causes of cardiac failure. It is a diagnosis of exclusion that should not be made without a concerted effort to identify valvular, metabolic, infectious, or toxic causes of cardiomyopathy.

The incidence of peripartum cardiomyopathy is estimated at between 1 in 1500 to 1 in 4000 deliveries in the United States. The peak incidence of peripartum cardiomyopathy occurs in the second postpartum month, and there appears to be a higher incidence among older, multiparous black females. Other suggested risk factors include twinning and pregnancy-induced hypertension. Up to 50% of patients with peripartum cardiomyopathy may manifest evidence of pulmonary or systemic embolic phenomena. Overall mortality ranges from 25% to 50%.

Therapy includes digitalization, diuretics, sodium restriction, and prolonged bed rest. In refractory cases, concomitant afterload reduction with hydralazine or nitrates may be useful. Early endomyocardial biopsy has been suggested to identify a subgroup of patients who have a histologic picture of inflammatory myocarditis and who may be responsive to immunosuppressive therapy. Such patients may represent up to 29% of women with peripartum cardiomyopathy.

A notable feature of peripartum cardiomyopathy is its tendency to recur with subsequent pregnancies. Several reports have suggested that prognosis for future pregnancies is related to heart size. Patients whose cardiac size returned to normal within 6 to 12 months had an 11%–14% mortality rate in subsequent pregnancies; those patients with persistent cardiomegaly had a 40%–80% mortality rate.

HYPERTROPHIC CARDIOMYOPATHY

Hypertrophic cardiomyopathy involves primarily left ventricular hypertrophy, typically involving the septum to a greater extent than the free wall. The hypertrophy results in obstruction to left ventricular outflow and secondary mitral regurgitation. Although the increased blood volume associated with normal pregnancy should enhance left ventricular filling and improve hemodynamic performance, this positive effect of pregnancy is counterbalanced by the fall in arterial pressure and vena caval obstruction that are found in late pregnancy. In addition, tachycardia resulting from pain or fear in labor diminishes left ventricular filling and aggravates the relative outflow obstruction, an effect also resulting from second-stage Valsalva's maneuver.

The keys to successful management of the peripartum period in patients with hypertrophic cardiomyopathy involve avoidance of hypotension (resulting from conduction anesthesia or blood loss) and tachycardia, as well as labor in the left lateral recumbent position. The use of low or outlet forceps to shorten the second stage may also be considered. Cesarean section should be reserved for obstetric indications.

Despite the potential hazards, maternal and fetal outcome in patients with hypertrophic cardiomyopathy is generally excellent. Although beta-blocking agents were used routinely in these patients, currently they are reserved for patients with angina, recurrent supraventricular tachycardia, or occasional beta-blocker-responsive arrhythmias.

MARFAN'S SYNDROME

Marfan's syndrome is an autosomal dominant disorder characterized by generalized weakness of connective tissue; the weakness results in skeletal, ocular, and cardiovascular abnormalities. The increased risk of maternal mortality during pregnancy stems from aortic root and wall involvement, which may result in aneurysm formation, rupture, or aortic dissection. Prognosis is best individualized and should be based on echocardiographic assessment of aortic root diameter and postvalvular dilation. It is important to note that enlargement of the aortic root is not demonstrable by chest x-ray until dilation has become pronounced. Women with an abnormal aortic valve or aortic dilation may have up to 50% pregnancy-associated mortality rate; women without these changes and having an aortic root diameter less than 40 mm have a mortality less than 5%. Even in patients meeting these echocardiographic criteria, however, special attention must be given to signs or symptoms of aortic dissection because even serial echocardiographic assessment is not invariably predictive of complications. The routine use of oral beta-blockers to decrease pulsatile pressure on the aortic wall may be considered. If cesarean section is performed, retention sutures should be used because of general connective tissue weakness.

MYOCARDIAL INFARCTION

The prognosis for pregnant patients with myocardial infarction worsens with infarction in late pregnancy. Antepartum care of women with prior myocardial infarction centers upon bed rest to minimize myocardial oxygen demands. In women with angina, nitrates have been used without adverse fetal effects. Delivery within 2 weeks of infarction is associated with increased maternal mortality; therefore, if possible, attempts should be made to allow adequate convalescence prior to delivery. Labor in the lateral recumbent position, the administration of O_2, and pain relief with epidural anesthesia are essential.

CARDIOVASCULAR SURGERY

There are numerous reports of cardiovascular surgery during pregnancy; this surgery includes successful correction of most types of congenital and acquired cardiac disease and coronary artery bypass surgery.

Initiation of cardiopulmonary bypass is followed generally by fetal bradycardia, correctable by high flow rates. With the use of continuous electronic fetal heart rate monitoring, flow rate can be adjusted to avoid or correct fetal hypoperfusion and bradycardia, and fetal mortality can be reduced to less than 10%. Maternal mortality is, of course, highly dependent on the specific nature of the procedure being performed and does not appear influenced significantly by pregnancy. High-flow/high-pressure normothermic perfusion and continuous electronic fetal heart rate monitoring appear to be optimal for the fetus.

Severe valvular cardiac disease*

Goals of Therapy

Avoid hypotension, hypoxia, fluid overload.

Management Protocol

1. Admit patient at term with favorable cervix.
2. Place pulmonary artery catheter and optimize hemodynamics $\times$ 24 hours.
3. Oxytocin induction of labor.
4. Labor on left or right side.
5. Administer O_2 at 4–6 L/min.
6. I.V. 5% dextrose solution.
7. Use epidural anesthesia.
8. Intrapartum hemodynamic manipulation.
    A. Mitral stenosis—no pulmonary hypertension.
       1. Keep heart rate below 100 bpm with oral/I.V. beta-blocker.
       2. Diuresis to wedge pressure 12 to 14 mm Hg.†
    B. Aortic stenosis or pulmonary hypertension: Adjust wedge pressure to approximately 16 mm Hg.‡
9. Bacterial endocarditis prophylaxis.

Critical Laboratory Tests

Arterial blood gas, complete blood count, electrolytes, electrocardiogram, chest x-ray.

Consultation

Cardiology.

---

*For patients who are NYHA classes I or II throughout pregnancy, without prior myocardial infarction or pulmonary hypertension, steps 1 to 3 and 8 may be omitted.

†This must be done with careful attention to maintenance of blood pressure and cardiac output. In some patients, this optimal level cannot be achieved.

‡To maintain a margin of safety against unexpected hypotension or blood loss.

SUGGESTED READING

Abboud JK, Raya J, Noueihed R, et al. Intrathecal morphine for relief of labor pain in a parturient with severe pulmonary hypertension. Anesthesiology 1983;59:477.

Clark SL, Phelan JP, Greenspoon J, et al. Labor and delivery in the presence of mitral stenosis: central hemodynamic observations. Am J Obstet Gynecol 1985;152:986.

Easterling TR, Chadwick HS, Otto CM, et al. Aortic stenosis in pregnancy. Obstet Gynecol 1988;72:113.

Gleicher N, Midwall J, Hochberger D, et al. Eisenmenger's syndrome and pregnancy. Obstet Gynecol Surv 1979;34:721.

Hankins GDV, Berryman GK, Scott RT, et al. Maternal arterial desaturation with 15-Methyl prostlandier F_2 alpha for uterine atony. Obstet Gynecol 1988;72:367.

Hankins GDV, Wendel GD, Leveno KJ, et al. Myocardial infarction during pregnancy: a review. Obstet Gynecol 1985;65:139.

Hibbard LT. Maternal mortality due to cardiac disease. Clin Obstet Gynecol 1975;18:27.

Pyeritz RE, McKusick VA. The Marfan syndrome: diagnosis and management. N Engl J Med 1979;300:772.

Szekely P, Turner R, Snaith L. Pregnancy and the changing pattern of rheumatic heart disease. Br Heart J 1973;35:1993.

Ueland K. Cardiovascular surgery and the OB patient. Contemp OB/GYN Oct 1984;117.

Ueland K, Akamatsu TJ, Eng M, et al. Maternal cardiovascular dynamics. VI. Cesarean section under epidural anesthesia without epinephrine. Am J Obstet Gynecol 1972;114:755.

Veille JC. Peripartum cardiomyopathies: a review. Am J Obstet Gynecol 1984;148:805.

CHAPTER SEVEN

Arrhythmias, Artificial Valves, and Anticoagulation in Pregnancy

ANTICOAGULATION

Anticoagulation in the patient with an artificial heart valve and/ or atrial fibrillation during pregnancy is controversial, and focuses on the known teratogenic effects of oral anticoagulants weighed against a potential increased risk of thrombosis and thromboembolism incurred by using heparin rather than warfarin. Nevertheless, the use of heparin rather than coumarin during pregnancy is currently recommended by most experts in the United States.

A patient requiring anticoagulation when not pregnant should be treated during pregnancy, although the medication used may be different. Pregnant women having prosthetic heart valves should be treated with adjusted dose subcutaneous heparin from conception until delivery. During the postpartum period, coumarin may be reinstituted.

The adjusted-dose regimen employs heparin given subcutaneously every 12 hours in a dose sufficient to prolong the activated partial thromboplastin time (aPTT) obtained 6 hours after the dose (midinterval) to 1.5–2.0 times the normal control. This heparin regimen should provide plasma heparin levels of 0.2–0.4 units per milliliter if measured by heparin assay.

COMPLICATIONS OF ANTICOAGULATION

Patients are advised of the risks and options for oral anti-coagulant therapy. Patients seen before conception are given the option of changing to subcutaneous adjusted-dose heparin prior to conception. If the patient is already pregnant, she is informed of the option to terminate the pregnancy. In order to avoid an anomalous fetus, patients generally prefer to accept a possible small increased risk of thromboembolism and utilize heparin.

The patient is instructed in self-injection of heparin by the coagulation nurse who will monitor therapy and adjust the dose of heparin. Sodium heparin is used in the 20,000 U/mL concentration. The high concentration minimizes the volume injected and decreases the likelihood of local hematoma. Patients are advised to avoid using aspirin or any other medication without a physician's express permission.

The patient is instructed to withhold her injection and come to the hospital immediately if she thinks she is in labor. During labor, heparin is withheld. Epidural anesthesia may be administered, if appropriate, 12 hours or more after the last dose or when the patient is no longer anticoagulated. Following vaginal delivery, heparin is resumed 6 hours postpartum. The optimal time for resumption of heparin anticoagulation following cesarean delivery is unknown; however, serious bleeding complications are unusual if therapy is resumed in 18–24 hours. When therapy is resumed, the drug should be given intravenously. Postpartum anticoagulation can be continued then with warfarin.

PREVENTION OF BACTERIAL ENDOCARDITIS IN PATIENTS WITH ARTIFICIAL VALVES

American Heart Association recommendations for endocarditis prophylaxis are outlined in Table 7-1. Controversy persists regarding the need for prophylaxis with vaginal delivery. One

TABLE 7-1
American Heart Association SBE recommendation

Regimens for Genitourinary/Gastrointestinal Procedures

Drug	Dosage Regimen
Standard Regimen	
Ampicillin, gentamicin, and amoxicillin	Intravenous or intramuscular administration of ampicillin, 2 g, plus gentamicin, 1.5 mg/kg (not to exceed 80 mg), 30 min before procedure; followed by amoxicillin, 1.5 g, orally 6 h after initial dose; alternatively, the parenteral regimen may be repeated once 8 h after initial dose
Ampicillin/Amoxicillin/Penicillin-Allergic Patient Regimen	
Vancomycin and gentamicin	Intravenous administration of vancomycin, 1 g over 1 h plus intravenous or intramuscular administration of gentamicin, 1.5 mg/kg (not to exceed 80 mg), 1 h before procedure; may be repeated once 8 h after initial dose
Alternate Low-Risk Patient Regimen	
Amoxicillin	3 g orally 1 h before procedure; then 1.5 g 6 h after initial dose

(Reproduced by permission from Dajani AS, Bisno AL, Chung KJ, Durack DT, Freed M, Gerber MA, et al. Prevention of bacterial endocarditis: recommendations of the American Heart Association. JAMA 1990;264:2919–2922.)

TABLE 7-2
Characteristics of patients at risk for bacterial
endocarditis

Prosthetic heart valves (including bioprostheses)
Most congenital cardiac malformations
Surgical systemic-pulmonary shunts
Rheumatic and other acquired valvular dysfunction
Idiopathic hypertrophic subaortic stenosis (IHSS)
Previous history of bacterial endocarditis
Mitral valve prolapse with insufficiency

---

approach is to administer the high-risk regimen to patients with
systemic-pulmonary shunts, artificial valves, or a history of
endocarditis, reserving the low-risk regimen for pregnant patients with other structural abnormalities (Table 7-2).

DYSRHYTHMIAS

The use of antiarrhythmic therapy has been reviewed extensively
by Rotmensch and associates. Many of these medications have
been used to treat fetal dysrhythmias as well. Digoxin, procainamide, and quinidine may be used for the usual indications and in
therapeutic doses have not been shown to be harmful to the
fetus. A digoxinlike immunoreactive substance appears in some
normal and preeclamptic patients during the second trimester
and can be identified in many patients during the third trimester.
If serum monitoring of digoxin levels is anticipated, a pretreat-
ment level should be obtained in order to improve interpretation
of results.

The use of beta-blockers is appropriate in some tachyarrhythmias, in idiopathic hypertrophic subaortic stenosis (IHSS), and for the control of hyperthyroid symptoms. In a critical review, Ruben concluded that beta-blocker therapy is not associated with adverse neonatal outcome. Neonatal hypoglycemia and brady-cardia may occur, although they are usually not serious. Intrauter-ine growth retardation may be a consequence of the disease for which the beta-blockers are prescribed rather than a complication of therapy itself. Beta-blockers such as atenolol and acebutolol have lower degrees of plasma binding and are excreted in breast milk at higher concentrations, sufficient to cause bradycardia, hypotension, and poor perfusion in the infant. Verapamil is a calcium-entry-blocking drug that is effective in the conversion of a superventricular tachycardia to sinus rhythm. Although there are no reports of its adverse effect on the fetus, there is little experience with it in pregnancy. Amiodarone has been used with-out apparent ill effects on the fetus in the few cases in which it was indicated.

Women with life-threatening arrhythmias should have them evaluated prior to conception to determine the appropri-ateness of: 1) surgical or catheter ablation, 2) an antitachycardia pacemaker, or 3) an automatic implantable cardiovert-defibrillator. The issue of anticoagulation for atrial fibrillation in pregnancy has not been addressed specifically. However, it seems reasonable to anticoagulate a pregnant patient with the subcutaneous adjusted-dose heparin regimen if she meets the criteria described for nonpregnant patients. These include atrial fibrillation with a history of thromboembolic complications, atrial fibrillation in the presence of valvular disease such as mitral stenosis or regurgitation, atrial fibrillation in cardiomyo-pathy, or atrial fibrillation with thyrotoxic heart disease. An-ticoagulation is recommended for 3 weeks prior to cardioversion of atrial fibrillation and for 4 weeks after conver-sion to sinus rhythm. Anticoagulation should be considered in the patient with atrial fibrillation and congestive heart failure. However, patients with this degree of cardiomyopathy should not attempt pregnancy because of their poor prognosis.

Cardioversion appears safe for the fetus. The presence of an artificial pacemaker similarly does not affect the course of preg-nancy.

Anticoagulation during pregnancy of patients with prosthetic heart valves

Goals of Therapy

To prevent valvular thrombosis or arterial thromboembolism.

Management Protocol

1. Sodium heparin, 2500–5000 units intravenously, followed by 1000 units/hour via infusion pump *or* sodium heparin, 8000–14,000 units every 12 hours, subcutaneously. (Use heparin with a concentration of at least 20,000 units/mL. Use insulin U-100 syringes.)

2. Adjust dose to achieve aPTT 1.5–2.0 times control at midinterval (6 hours after the heparin is injected). This corresponds to a heparin plasma concentration of 0.2–0.4 IU/mL plasma.

3. Withhold heparin when labor begins or prior to cesarean delivery. Check aPTT.

4. If the aPTT is prolonged prior to delivery, delay if possible. If delay not possible, administer protamine sulfate. Immediately following I.V. heparin injection, 1.0 mg protamine sulfate will neutralize 100 units of heparin. After 30 minutes, only one-half the aforementioned protamine dose is used. Several hours after subcutaneous injection, begin with small doses (5–10 mg) and titrate according to aPTT response. (In some laboratories, a protamine titration test may be available.)

5. Resume heparin 6–12 hours following vaginal delivery or 12–24 hours following cesarean delivery. Use an intravenous continuous infusion of heparin, and titrate the dose so that the patient is fully anticoagulated (the aPTT is 1.5–2 times the control).

6. Begin oral anticoagulant and adjust the dose so that the prothrombin time INR is 3.0–4.5. This corresponds to a prothrombin time ratio of 1.6–1.8 when rabbit brain thromboplastin is used. Discontinue heparin infusion when the prothrombin time is therapeutic for at least 4 days after beginning oral anticoagulants.

7. When switching from intravenous to subcutaneous doses, give one-half of the total 24-hour intravenous dose subcutaneously, every 12 hours.

Critical Laboratory Tests

aPTT (or heparin assay).

Consultation

Hematology, cardiology.

―――――

SUGGESTED READING

de Swiet M. Pregnancy and heart valve replacement. Inter J Cardiol 1984;5:741–743.

Eckstein H, Jack B. Breast feeding and anticoagulant therapy. Lancet 1970;1:672–673.

Ginsberg JS, Kowalchuk G, Hirsh J, Brill-Edwards P, Burrows R. Heparin therapy during pregnancy: Risks to the fetus and mother. Arch Int Med 1989;149:2233–2236.

Iturbe-Alessio I, Fonseca MDC, Mutchinik O, et al. Risk of anticoagulant therapy in pregnant women with artificial heart valves. New Engl J Med 1986;315:1390–1393.

Jaffe R, Gruber A, Fejgin M, Altaras M, Ben-Aderet N. Pregnant with an artificial pacemaker. Obstet Gynecol Survey 1987;42:137–139.

Nageotte MP, Freeman RK, Garite TJ, et al. Anticoagulation in pregnancy. Am J Obstet Gynecol 1982;141:472.

Oakley C. Valve prostheses and pregnancy [Editorial]. Br Heart J 1987;58:303–305.

Pavankumar P, Venugopal P, Kaul U, Iyer KS, et al. Closed mitral valvotomy during pregnancy: a twenty year experience. Scan J Thor Cardiovasc Surg 1988;22:11–15.

Phelps SJ, Cochran EC, Gonzalez-Ruiz A, Tolley EA, Hammond KD, Sibai BM. The influence of gestational age and preeclampsia on the presence and magnitude of serum endogenous digoxin-like immunoreactive substance(s). Am J Obstet Gynecol 1988;158:34–39.

Rotmensch HH, Rotmensch S, Elkayam U. Management of cardiac arrhythmias during pregnancy: current concepts. Drugs 1987;33:623–633.

Rubin PC. Beta-blockers in pregnancy. New Engl J Med 1981;305(22):1323–1326.

Salazar E, Zajarias A, Gutierrez N, Iturbe I. The problem of cardiac valve prostheses, anticoagulants, and pregnant. Circulation 1984;70(suppl I):169–177.

CHAPTER EIGHT

Thromboembolic Disease

DEEP VENOUS THROMBOSIS

GENERAL CONSIDERATIONS

Deep venous thrombosis (DVT) is an intravascular clot located in the deep veins of the leg or pelvis. In the course of pregnancy 0.18%–0.29% of deliveries are complicated by DVT. If untreated, 15%–25% of patients with DVT develop pulmonary embolism, compared with 5% in treated patients. The mortality rate from this disorder relates to the development of pulmonary emboli. Well-known etiologies for DVT are stasis, venous injury, and alterations in coagulation. Predisposing factors for this disorder are as follows: pregnancy, postpartum state, postcesarean, prolonged bed rest, fractured pelvis, prior DVT/pulmonary embolus (PE), and maternal obesity. If a patient has sustained a prior DVT, the likelihood of recurrence without treatment is 10%–22%.

PRESENTATION

The patient typically presents with signs or symptoms of pain, tenderness, edema, altered limb color, and/or a palpable cord.

Clinical findings may also include a positive Homans' sign. This is positive if pain is obtained on dorsiflexion of the foot. In a patient with suspected DVT, a Lowenberg test may be performed. A positive test is recorded if pain occurs distal to a blood pressure cuff rapidly inflated to 180 mm Hg. If swelling is suspected, there must be a 2-cm difference in the circumferences between the affected and normal limb to be significant.

DIAGNOSTIC STUDIES

If DVT is suspected, appropriate diagnostic studies such as ascending venography and ultrasonography/Doppler should be undertaken. During pregnancy and lactation, 125 I fibrinogen scanning is contraindicated.

Ascending venography is the diagnostic mainstay of DVT diagnosis in pregnancy. Radiation exposure to the fetus is well below the minimum accepted level considered to be teratogenic. Positive identification of DVT is a well-defined filling defect in more than one radiographic view. Suggestive signs of DVT include abrupt termination, absence of opacification, or diversion of flow.

An alternative technique is real-time ultrasound and Doppler. These techniques are 90% effective in detecting venous thrombosis in the popliteal, femoral, and iliac veins (Table 8-1). A reduction or absence of Doppler shift suggests a partial or complete venous occlusion. In cases of suspected pelvic or ovarian vein thrombosis, magnetic resonance imaging (MRI) may be more helpful.

CLINICAL MANAGEMENT AND GOALS OF THERAPY

When DVT is diagnosed, the patient should be hospitalized. Management is outlined in the protocol at the conclusion of the chapter.

After a period of continuous intravenous heparin infusion, therapeutic subcutaneous heparin injection for the remainder of pregnancy and coumadin anticoagulation postpartum is recommended. Sodium heparin (10,000–14,000 U) is injected subcutaneously twice a day to achieve an aPTT level of 1.5–2 times

TABLE 8-1

Symptoms and signs in 327 patients with pulmonary emboli

Symptoms	Percent	Signs	Percent
Chest Pain	88	Respirations above	92
Pleuritic	74	16/min	
Nonpleuritic	14	Rales	58
Dyspnea	84	S_2P increased	53
Apprehension	59	Pulse above 100/min	44
Cough	53	Temperature above	43
Hemoptysis	30	37.8°C	
Sweats	27	Diaphoresis	36
Syncope	13	Gallop	34
		Phlebitis	32
		Edema	24
		Murmur	23
		Cyanosis	19

(Reproduced by permission from Bell WR, Simon TL, DeMets DL. The clinical features of submassive and massive pulmonary emboli. Am J Med 1977;62:355.)

control six hours after injection. Occasionally, higher or more frequent doses are necessary. Anticoagulation should be continued for 6–12 weeks postpartum; during this time, coumadin may be used. Because of the occurrence of occasional idiopathic thrombocytopenia, it is prudent to monitor platelet count occasionally during long-term heparin therapy.

PULMONARY EMBOLUS

GENERAL CONSIDERATIONS

A pulmonary embolus (PE) is a complete or partial occlusion of a pulmonary vessel due to an intravascular clot arising in a separate location in the body. During the course of pregnancy, the incidence of pulmonary embolus is less than that encountered with DVT. However, the mortality associated with PE is related to whether the DVT has been treated. In untreated DVT, the maternal mortality rate with PE is 12%–15%. The mortality rate in treated DVT patients is 0.7%. Most cases of pulmonary emboli arise in the deep veins of the upper legs or the pelvis. Fatal PE secondary to calf thrombosis is essentially unknown. Predisposing factors for PE are similar to those of DVT.

PRESENTATION

The patient with a pulmonary embolus may have one or more of the predisposing factors listed previously under DVT. The most common signs and symptoms are dyspnea, tachypnea, and pleuritic chest pain. Other signs and symptoms specific to PE are outlined in Table 8-2.

LABORATORY AND DIAGNOSTIC STUDIES

Arterial blood gases are used to assist in the diagnosis of pulmonary embolus. A PaO_2 of 85 mm Hg or higher is reassuring but does not exclude a PE.

The EKG may be helpful in providing evidence of pulmonary embolus. The most common findings are a tachycardia and/or ST-T wave changes. Not uncommonly, the EKG will be normal. Signs of acute cor pulmonale such as $S_1Q_3T_3$ EKG pattern or P pulmonale can occasionally be seen.

In 70% of patients, the chest x-ray is abnormal. X-ray findings include hemidiaphragm elevation, atelectasis, pleural effusion, and infiltrates. Focal oligemia (an area of increased radiolucency and decreased vascular markings) is seen in 2%–3% of patients. A negative chest x-ray does not exclude a pulmonary embolus.

A perfusion lung scan is the most clinically useful technique to confirm the diagnosis of pulmonary embolus. A normal study virtually excludes the diagnosis of pulmonary embolus. Ventilation scans complement perfusion lung scans. Scans are inter-

TABLE 8-2

Comparison of various techniques for diagnosis of DVT
with venography

Diagnostic Study	Sensitivity (%)	Specificity (%)
Doppler Ultrasound		
Proximal veins	85–95	90
Calf veins	50 (maximum)	50 (maximum)
Plethysmography		
Nonpregnant:		
Proximal veins	95	98
Calf veins	<30	—
Pregnant, third trimester	—*	36
Iodine-125 fibrinogen: distal to midthigh	—	92
Thermography	—	75–80
Radionuclide venography: proximal veins (thigh, pelvis)	>90	>95
Indium-111 platelet imaging	90–95	95–100

*Lack of available data.

preted as showing low, moderate, or high probability of pulmonary embolus (Table 8-3). Because false positive diagnoses are not uncommon and may occasionally occur even with a high probability scan, algorithms have been developed that incorporate V/Q scan result with clinical findings (Figure 8-1).

The definitive technique for diagnosing pulmonary embolus is pulmonary arteriography. This procedure is indicated when lung scanning is indeterminate, does not correlate with clinical suspicion or when the heparin risks are high for the patient (Figure 8-1). In addition, pulmonary arteriography is indicated prior to thrombolytic therapy or vena cava plication. The morbidity and mortality rates for the procedure are 4%–5% and 0.2%–0.3%, respectively. Serious complications are most commonly seen in patients with preexisting pulmonary hypertension.

TABLE 8-3

Ventilation-perfusion lung scans: frequency of embolism by arteriography*

Interpretation	Scan Patterns	Frequency (%)
Normal	Normal perfusion	0
Low probability	Matching defects Small subsegmental defects with mismatch	<10
	(Q defects smaller than chest roentgenogram abnormalities)	
Intermediate probability	Single segmental defect with mismatch Multiple segmental defects with mismatch and match	20–30
	(Q defects same size as chest roentgenogram abnormalities)	
High probability	Multiple segmental or lobar defects with mismatch	90
	(Q defects larger than chest roentgenogram abnormalities)	

*When perfusion scans are done without ventilation studies, the frequencies are lower.

(Adapted from Biello DR, Mattar AG, McKnight RC, et al. Ventilation-perfusion studies in suspected pulmonary embolism. Am J Roentgenol 1979;133:1033.)

CLINICAL MANAGEMENT AND GOALS OF THERAPY

The clinical goals of therapy and management of the patient with a pulmonary embolus are illustrated in the concluding management protocol. The peripartum management of the anticoagulated patient is illustrated in Table 8-4.

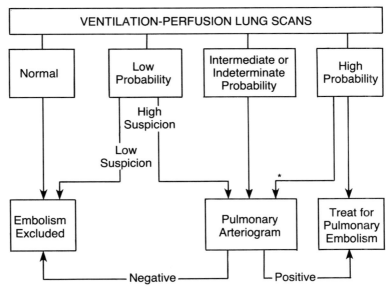

SUSPICION OF PULMONARY EMBOLISM

VENTILATION-PERFUSION LUNG SCANS

| Normal | Low Probability | Intermediate or Indeterminate Probability | High Probability |

High Suspicion

Low Suspicion

| Embolism Excluded | Pulmonary Arteriogram | Treat for Pulmonary Embolism |

Negative ——— Positive

*Contraindications to anticoagulant therapy.

FIGURE 8-1

Ventilation-perfusion lung scanning in the evaluation of the patient suspected of having pulmonary embolism.

TABLE 8-4

Intrapartum and perioperative management of the anticoagulated pregnant patient

1. Continuous heparin infusion to maintain a heparin level of 0.1–0.2 units/mL is recommended in patients with a recent PE, mechanical heart valve, or iliofemoral thrombosis.

2. In the low-risk, hemodynamically stable patient, heparin can be discontinued and restarted 4–6 hours after delivery or surgery.

3. In cases of urgent cesarean, heparin can be reversed with protamine in a dose 1 mg/100 units of heparin (if heparin was given I.V.). No single dose should exceed 50 mg. For patients having received subcutaneous therapeutic heparin, a 10–15 mg dose of protamine generally suffices.

4. Coumadin can be reversed with maternal and neonatal vitamin K in association with 2–4 units of fresh-frozen plasma.

Deep venous thrombosis in pregnancy

Goals of Therapy

Promotion of thrombus resolution.

Prevention of thrombus extension and recurrence.

Management Protocol

1. Immediately begin therapy, based on strong clinical suspicion, pending complete diagnostic work-up.
2. Administer heparin (5000 U I.V.), followed by 1000–2000 U/h via infusion pump.
3. Adjust heparin infusion to achieve aPTT 1.5–2 times that of control.
4. Maintain full anticoagulation for 7 days.
5. Continue anticoagulation with adjusted-dose subcutaneous heparin, initially 8000–12,000 U twice or three times daily (antepartum or postpartum) or oral anticoagulation (only if postpartum) until 6 weeks postpartum.
6. Implement bed rest, elastic hose, and extremity elevation if source of embolus is the leg.

Critical Laboratory Tests

aPTT, complete blood count (CBC) with platelet count.

Consultation

Hematology.

Pulmonary embolism in pregnancy

Goals of Therapy

1. Maintenance of oxygenation and cardiac output.
2. Promotion of thrombus resolution.
3. Prevention of thrombus extension and recurrence.

Management Protocol

1. Immediately begin therapy, based on strong clinical suspicion, pending complete diagnostic work-up.
2. Administer O_2 via mask, 6 L/min.
3. Administer heparin (5000–10,000 U I.V.), followed by 1000–2000 U/h via infusion pump.
4. Adjust heparin infusion to achieve aPTT 1.5–2 times that of control.
5. Maintain full anticoagulation for 7–10 days.
6. Continue anticoagulation with adjusted-dose subcutaneous heparin, initially 8000–12,000 U twice or three times daily (antepartum or postpartum) or oral anticoagulation (only if postpartum) until 6 weeks postpartum.
7. Implement bed rest, elastic hose, and extremity elevation if source of embolus is the leg.

Critical Laboratory Tests

ABG, aPTT, complete blood count (CBC) with platelet count, chest x-ray, electrocardiogram (EKG), invasive or noninvasive diagnostic tests, as indicated.

Consultation

Pulmonary medicine, hematology.

SUGGESTED READING

Bell WR, Simon TL, DeMets DL. The clinical features of submassive and massive pulmonary emboli. Am J Med 1977;62:355–360.

Change MKB, Harvey D, DeSwiet M. Follow-up study of children whose mothers were treated with warfarin during pregnancy. Br J Obstet Gynaecol 1984;91:70–73.

Franks AL, Atrash HK, Lawson HW, et al. Obstetrical pulmonary embolism mortality, United States, 1970–85. Am J Public Health 1990;80:720.

Ginsberg JS, Hirsh J, Turner C, et al. Risks to the fetus of anticoagulant therapy during pregnancy. Thrombo Haemomst 1989;61:197.

Rutherford SE, Phelan JP. Clinical management of thromboembolic disorders in pregnancy. Critical Care Clinics 1991;7(4):809–828.

Rutherford SE, Phelan JP. Deep venous thrombosis and pulmonary embolus. In: Clark SL, Cotton DB, Hankins GDV, Phelan JP, eds. Critical Care Obstetrics, 2nd ed. Boston: Blackwell Scientific Publications, Inc., 1991:105–179.

Sors H, Safran D, et al. An analysis of the diagnostic methods for acute pulmonary embolism. Intensive Care Med 1984;10:81–84.

Standing Advisory Committee for Haematology of the Royal College of Pathologists. Drug interaction with coumarin derivative anticoagulants. Br Med J 1982;185:274–275.

Tengborn L, Bergqvist D, Matzsch T, et al. Recurrent thromboembolism in pregnancy and puerperium: is there a need for thromboprophylaxis? Am J Obstet Gynecol 1989;160:90.

CHAPTER NINE

Disseminated Intravascular Coagulopathy Associated with Pregnancy

DISSEMINATED INTRAVASCULAR COAGULOPATHY

Disseminated intravascular coagulopathy (DIC) is said to exist whenever intravascular activation of clotting components results in excess consumption of at least the soluble coagulation components. DIC is an intermediary manifestation of multiple diseases and not a distinct, clinical entity (Table 9-1).

DIC is best viewed as a continuum within which a multitude of symptoms occur. These symptoms are predictive of the laboratory findings. For example, clotting cascade activation does not occur without concurrent plasmin generation. Should the intravascular clotting process dominate and the secondary fibrinogenolysis be minimal, as is common with malignancy, the clinical presentation will be thrombosis. Should secondary fibrinogenolysis dominate and fibrin-fibrinogen degradation products circulate at high concentration, the clinical presentation will be hemorrhage. On occasion, thrombosis and hemorrhage occur simultaneously. Finally, DIC may exist without clinical evidence and be detectable only by specific laboratory evaluation. So-called

---

TABLE 9-1

Conditions associated with DIC

   I. Obstetrical accidents
      A. Abruptio placenta
      B. Amniotic fluid embolus
      C. Dead fetus syndrome
      D. Saline abortion
  II. Septicemia
      A. Gram-negative (endotoxin)
      B. Gram-positive (mucopolysaccharides)
 III. Intravascular hemolysis
      A. Multiple transfusions (banked whole blood)
      B. Hemolytic transfusion reaction
  IV. Vascular disorders
   V. Acid-base imbalance

---

chronic, compensated DIC places the patient at increased risk for either thrombosis or hemorrhage.

PATHOPHYSIOLOGY OF DIC

DIC represents a failure of the normal checks and balances, which results in systemic rather than focal generation of thrombin and plasmin. Figure 9-1 illustrates many of the mechanisms by which a number of unrelated disorders might trigger excess coagulation. Under normal circumstances, endothelial disruption stimulates platelet activation, degranulation, and activation of the intrinsic clotting cascade. Fibrin monomer polymerizes as insoluble fibrin. Plasminogen bound to fibrin begins controlled degradation of fibrin. Any free plasmin is rapidly deactivated. The excess plasmin generated degrades fibrinogen as it circulates.

The breakdown products of fibrin and fibrinogen, known as "fibrin split products" (FSP), bind soluble fibrin monomer and

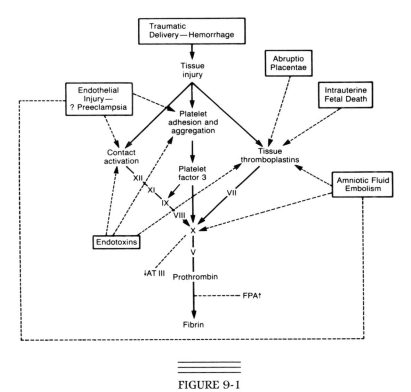

FIGURE 9-1

Obstetric disorders that initiate DIC. The processes illustrated are in many ways hypothetical.

prevent polymerization. These FSP are the basis of paracoagulation tests such as protamine sulfate and ethanol gelation. In addition to fibrin and fibrinogen, high levels of plasmin may inactivate factors V, VIII, IX, and XI, adrenocorticotropic hormone (ACTH), growth hormone, insulin, complement, and other plasma proteins. Even the platelet-mediated primary phase of coagulation can be inhibited by FSP. Fibrin monomer, which does polymerize, is filtered out within the microvasculature. These fibrin plugs restrict blood flow. The resulting tissue hypoxia· produces ischemic necrosis within multiple organs. Endothelial damage enhances platelet activation and alters vessel responsiveness to endogenous vasoactive substances. Thrombocytopenia results from increases in both consumption and clearance (because of FSP coating). Contact between fibrin and red blood cells (RBC) within the obstructed microvasculature produces hemolysis; the subsequent release of material from the RBC propagates the DIC cycle. Should the underlying disorder also activate factor XII (as is the case with endotoxins), the kinin system will be initiated. Excess bradykinin produces hypotension, increased vascular permeability, and other common clinical manifestations of the DIC syndrome. Finally, plasmin activates the first and third complement components, which trigger cell lysis, immunoadherence, and other immune phenomena. Clearly, once established, DIC can become self-perpetuating.

DIAGNOSIS OF DIC

Hemorrhage and/or thrombosis associated with one of the clinical conditions listed in Table 9-1 is strongly suggestive of DIC. A patient hemorrhaging secondary to acute DIC has multiple hemostatic defects, as well as clinical bleeding (e.g., melena, hematuria, epistaxis, hemoptysis, oozing from puncture wounds, purpura, or petechiae). Shock secondary to acute DIC is often out of proportion to the observed blood loss because of bradykinin generation. Renal failure is common.

In contrast to acute DIC, the diagnosis of chronic compensated DIC hinges on laboratory tests. Patients with chronic DIC (e.g., due to malignancy or intrauterine fetal demise) are well compensated and rarely bleed dramatically. They are more likely to suffer minor mucosal bleeding, hematuria, epistaxis, and/or easy bruisability. However, their clotting mechanism is only tenuously preserved and is likely to fail should another stress be imposed. Thromboembolic phenomena are also common in malignancy.

Antithrombin III (AT III), the major in vivo inhibitor of thrombin generation and of thrombin, is presently the most sensitive laboratory parameter for the diagnosis of DIC. Abnormal consumption of this inhibitor by either thrombin or another activated serine protein must occur if DIC is present. The concentration of AT III declines when consumption exceeds production. It loses some sensitivity in patients who have either a malignancy or diabetes where AT III can behave as an acute phase reactant. In contrast to malignancy, pregnancy actually increases the predictive value of a low AT III. During normal pregnancy, plasma AT III activity is, for the most part, unchanged. However, activity decreases dramatically during systemic illnesses coincidental to pregnancy, such as pyelonephritis, viral infection, and bacterial pneumonia, whereas a decline is unusual in nongravid subjects in the absence of overwhelming sepsis. Thus, pregnancy is associated with a reduction in the AT III "reserve."

Laboratory confirmation of DIC should usually be obtained prior to initiating pharmacologic therapy. Table 9-2 lists those parameters that are frequently abnormal. Over 50% of patients with acute DIC have a prolongation of the prothrombin time (PT) and partial thromboplastin time (PTT). In the remainder, these values are either normal or shortened. The latter is more often associated with chronic DIC, and its significance is unclear. Fifteen percent of patients with acute DIC have normal FSP levels, and about 10% have negative paracoagulation tests. It is possible that the FSP are degraded past the point detectable by commercially available kits. In addition, the actual FSP titer may have little clinical relevance because of altered renal clearance.

TABLE 9-2
Laboratory abnormalities in DIC

1. Antithrombin III consumption
2. Elevated fibrinopeptide A
3. Abnormal prothrombin time
4. Abnormal partial thromboplastin time
5. Abnormal platelet count
6. Elevated fibrinogen–fibrin split products
7. Schistocytosis
8. Leukocytosis
9. Positive protamine sulfate test
10. Abnormal clot retraction

THERAPY

The morbidity and mortality of DIC result both from the coagulopathy and the underlying illness that precipitated it. The primary therapeutic goal is treatment of the underlying disorder, accompanied by aggressive support of blood volume and pressure. Hypoxic ischemia secondary to hypotension and hypoperfusion exacerbate the cycle by damaging the vascular endothelium and must be corrected; otherwise, it will lead to multiple organ failure. Underreplacement of blood and clotting factors is likely the single most common therapeutic error. An approach applicable to most patients with DIC associated with pregnancy is outlined in Table 9-3. The initial three steps constitute adequate therapy in the vast majority of obstetric-related DIC syndromes. Patients with mild wound oozing associated with labora-

---

TABLE 9-3
Suggested therapy for acute DIC

I. Treat or remove the triggering event
   A. Antibiotics (when indicated)
   B. Evacuate the uterus (when indicated)
   C. Drain pus
II. Volume replacement and expansion (crystalloid, plasmanate, albumin)
III. Component therapy
   A. Fresh-frozen plasma/cryoprecipitate
   B. Prothrombin complex
   C. Platelets
   D. Packed red cells (in the face of hemorrhage)
IV. Support cardiorespiratory system to maintain cardiac output and oxygenation
V. Anticoagulant therapy*
   A. Low-dose heparin
   B. AT III concentrates (if unavailable, fresh frozen plasma)

*Use of this agent is controversial and is uncommonly indicated in DIC.

---

tory abnormalities may, on occasion, benefit from component replacement (platelets, cryoprecipitate, or fresh-frozen plasma). There is no good evidence to support the old adage regarding "adding fuel to the fire" if the underlying cause of DIC has been treated and the cycle of activation broken. If the hemorrhage is not severe, observe the patient for a period of time after treatment of the underlying disease to assess response to treatment before initiating component therapy. This permits an adequate laboratory evaluation and (one would hope) a pinpointing of the clotting defect(s).

In the past, anticoagulation of the obstetric patient with acute DIC has been synonymous with large quantities of heparin. When effective, the results are dramatic; when ill timed, anticoagulation can be fatal. The AT III activity at the time of anticoagulation may be one cause of the variable response. Heparin is ineffective if AT III is deficient. If possible, AT III activity should be determined during the observational period if heparin therapy is contemplated. The obstetric patient with DIC will rarely require anticoagulant therapy.

A low dose of heparin is often as effective as a large dose for the treatment of acute DIC if the AT III activity exceeds 70%. Low-dose heparin minimizes the risk of exacerbating preexisting hemorrhage. A reasonable approach is to administer subcutaneous heparin (2500–5000 units) every 8–12 hours. The response to therapy is evaluated using both clinical and laboratory parameters. The AT III concentrates have also been used successfully alone to treat acute DIC secondary to obstetric complications.

After undertaking each of the three steps outlined, a rare patient may continue to bleed secondary to residual fibrinogenolysis. This is one instance in obstetrics when an antifibrinolytic agent may be of value for the treatment of DIC.

SUGGESTED READING

Jimenez JM, Pritchard JA. Pathogenesis and treatment of coagulation defects resulting from fetal death. Obstet Gynecol 1968;32:449.

Pritchard JA, Cunningham FG, Mason RA. Coagulation changes in

eclampsia: their frequency and pathogenesis. Am J Obstet
Gynecol 1976;124:855.

Transfusion Alert. NIH Publication No. 89-2974a, May 1989.

Weiner CP, Bonsib S. Relationship between renal histology and
plasma antithrombin III activity in women with early onset
preeclampsia. Am J Perinatol 1990;7:139.

CHAPTER TEN

Obstetric Hemorrhage and Hypovolemic Shock

PATHOPHYSIOLOGY OF HYPOVOLEMIC SHOCK

Shock can be defined as a disparity between the circulating blood volume and the capacity of the vascular bed. It is a complex pathophysiologic process initiated by altered hemodynamic function and resulting in poor tissue perfusion. In hemorrhage shock, the disparity is a result of blood loss, which sequentially leads to hypotension, decreased tissue perfusion, cellular hypoxia, organ damage, and finally death. Hemorrhage shock is a leading cause of obstetric death in the United States (see Table 10-1).

Shock evolves through several pathophysiologic stages as body mechanisms combat the acute blood volume loss. Blood flow to the capillary beds of various organs is controlled by arterioles, resistance vessels that in turn are controlled by the central nervous system. On the other hand, 70% of the total blood volume is contained in venules, capacitance vessels controlled by humoral factors.

Early in the course of massive hemorrhage, there are decreases in mean arterial pressure, cardiac output, central venous pressure and pulmonary capillary wedge pressure (PCWP), stroke volume and work, and oxygen consumption, as well as

TABLE 10-1

Maternal mortality in the United States 1980–1985

Cause	Percent
Embolism	20
Hypertensive disease	15
Ectopic pregnancy	12
Hemorrhage	11
Cerebrovascular accident	10
Anesthetic complications	8
Abortion complications	6
Cardiomyopathy	5
Infection	4
Hydatidiform mole	1
Other	8

(Adapted from Rochat RW, Koonin LM, Atrash HK, et al. Maternal mortality in the United States: report for the Maternal Mortality Collaborative. Reprinted with permission from the American College of Obstetricians and Gynecologists. Obstet Gynecol 1988;72:91.)

increases in arteriovenous oxygen content difference. Catecholamine release also causes a generalized increase in venular tone, resulting in an autotransfusion from the capacitance reservoir. These changes are accompanied by compensatory increases in heart rate, systemic and pulmonary vascular resistance, and myocardial contractility. In addition, redistribution of cardiac output and blood volume occurs via selective arteriolar constriction mediated by the central nervous system, which results in diminished perfusion to the kidneys, gut, skin, and uterus, with relative maintenance of blood flow to the heart and brain. In the pregnant patient, such redistribution may result in fetal hypoxia and distress even before the mother becomes overtly hypotensive; in such situations, the uterus has become, from a teleologic viewpoint, relatively unimportant. Regardless of the absolute maternal blood pressure, significant maternal shock is highly unlikely in the presence of a reassuring fetal heart rate tracing.

Although initial O_2 extraction by maternal tissue is increased, continued maldistribution of blood flow results in local tissue hypoxia and metabolic acidosis. If not promptly corrected, such shunting of blood from the renal and splanchnic beds may result in acute tubular necrosis, and it may contribute to pulmonary capillary endothelial damage and adult respiratory distress syndrome (ARDS), even if resuscitation is eventually successful. As the blood volume deficit approaches 25%, such compensatory mechanisms become inadequate to maintain cardiac output and arterial pressure. At this point, small additional losses of blood result in rapid clinical deterioration, producing a vicious cycle of cellular death and vasoconstriction, leading to organ ischemia, loss of capillary membrane integrity, and additional loss of intravascular fluid volume.

Increased platelet aggregation also is found in hypovolemic shock. Aggregated platelets release vasoactive substances; the vasoactive substance release causes small vessel occlusion and impaired microcirculatory perfusion. These platelet aggregates can embolize to the lungs and be a factor contributing to respiratory failure, which is often seen following prolonged shock.

Pregnancy-associated hypovolemia prepares the mother for a blood volume loss of up to 1000 mL. Actual measurements show that the average blood loss after normal spontaneous vaginal delivery is over 600 mL. Following a postpartum blood loss of less than 1000 mL, the parturient's vital signs may not reflect acute blood loss (i.e., hypotension and tachycardia). Following a normal spontaneous vaginal delivery, a first-day postpartum hematocrit usually is not altered significantly from the admission value.

MANAGEMENT OF HYPOVOLEMIC SHOCK IN PREGNANCY

A frequent cause of death of a patient in shock is inadequate respiratory exchange. The duration of relative tissue hypoxia is important in the accumulation of by-products of anaerobic metabolism. Thus, increasing the partial pressure of oxygen across the pulmonary capillary membrane by giving 6–8 L of oxygen per minute by mask may forestall the onset of tissue hypoxia and is a logical first priority. If the airway is not patent or the tidal volume inadequate, the clinician should not hesitate to perform endotracheal intubation and institute positive-pressure ventilation in order to achieve adequate oxygenation.

Protracted shock appears to cause secondary changes in the microcirculation; these changes affect circulating blood volume. In early shock, there is a tendency to draw fluid from the interstitial space and into the capillary bed. However, as the shock state progresses, damage to the capillary endothelium occurs and is manifested by an increase in capillary permeability, which further accentuates the loss of intravascular volume. This deficit is reflected clinically by the disproportionately large volume of fluid necessary to resuscitate patients in severe shock; sometimes, the amount of fluid required for resuscitation is two to three times the amount indicated by calculation of blood loss volume. Thus, replacement of intracellular fluid with crystalloid administration may be considered the primary therapeutic goal.

Fluid resuscitation in young, previously healthy patients can be accomplished safely with modest volumes of either colloid or crystalloid fluid and with little risk of pulmonary edema. The use of crystalloid versus colloid solution for initial resuscitation of patients in hypovolemic shock remains a controversy. Blood and component therapy is discussed in detail in Chapter 30.

Vasopressors are not used in the treatment of hypovolemic shock except as a last resort in decompensated shock following adequate volume replacement.

After the patient's oxygenation and expansion of intravascular volume have been accomplished and her condition is beginning to stabilize, it is essential for the health care team to evaluate the patient's response to therapy, to diagnose the basic condition that resulted in circulatory shock, and to consider the fetal condition. Serial evaluation of vital signs, urine output, acid-base, blood chemistry, and coagulation status aid in this assessment; pulmonary artery catheterization is rarely of benefit. Following massive blood loss and replacement, a coagulopathy may occur; it may be secondary to a relative dilution of clotting factors, ischemia-induced activation of the coagulation cascade, or both.

During volume resuscitation, an aggressive search for the origin of hemorrhage is essential. Atony, lacerations, or varying forms of retained placenta should be addressed simultaneously with the treatment of hypovolemia.

Hypovolemic shock

Goals of Therapy

1. Maintain the following:
   A. Systolic pressure $\geq$90 mm Hg.
   B. Urine output $\geq$25 mL/h.
   C. Normal mental status.
2. Eliminate source of hemorrhage.
3. Avoid overzealous volume replacement that may contribute to pulmonary edema.

Management Protocol

1. Establish two large-bore intravenous lines.
2. Place patients in Trendelenburg's position.
3. Rapidly infuse 5% dextrose in lactated Ringer's solution while blood products are obtained.
4. Infuse fresh whole blood or packed red blood cells, as available.
5. Infuse platelets and FFP only as indicated by documented deficiencies in platelets (<50,000/mL) or clotting parameters (fibrinogen, PT, PTT).
6. Search for and eliminate source of hemorrhage.
7. Use invasive hemodynamic monitoring if patient fails to respond to clinically adequate volume replacement.

Critical Laboratory Tests

Complete blood count (CBC), platelet count, fibrinogen, PT, PTT, arterial blood gases.

Postpartum hemorrhage

Management Protocol

(To be undertaken simultaneously with management of hypovolemic shock.)
1. Examine uterus to rule out atony.
2. Examine vagina and cervix to rule out lacerations. Repair if present.
3. Explore uterus and perform curettage to rule out retained placenta.
4. For uterine atony:
   A. Firm bimanual compression.
   B. Oxytocin infusion, 40 units in 1 L of D_5RL.
   C. 15-methyl prostaglandin F_{2a}, 0.25–0.50 mg I.M., may be repeated.
   D. Bilateral uterine artery ligation.
   E. Bilateral hypogastric artery ligation (if patient clinically stable and future childbearing of great importance).
   F. Hysterectomy.

SUGGESTED READING

Clark SL, Phelan JP, Yeh S-Y, et al. Hypogastric artery ligation for control of obstetric hemorrhage. Obstet Gynecol 1985;66:353.

Clark SL, Yeh S-Y, Phelan JP, et al. Emergency hysterectomy for the control of obstetric hemorrhage. Obstet Gynecol 1984;64:376.

Consensus conference. Fresh-frozen plasma. AMA 1985;253:551.

Counts RB, Haisch C, Simon TL, et al. Hemostasis in massively transfused trauma patients. Ann Surg 1979;190:91.

Hayashi RH, Castillo MS, Noah ML. Management of severe postpartum hemorrhage with a prostaglandin F_2 analogue. Obstet Gynecol 1984;63:806.

O'Leary JL, O'Leary JA. Uterine artery ligation for control of post cesarean section hemorrhage. Obstet Gynecol 1974;43:849.

Rackow EC, Falk JL, Fein IA. Fluid resuscitation in circulatory shock: a comparison of the cardiorespiratory effects of albumin, hetastarch, and saline solutions in patients with hypovolemic and septic shock. Crit Care Med 1983;11:839.

Slater G, Vladek BA, Bassin R, et al. Sequential changes in the distribution of cardiac output in various stages of experimental hemorrhage shock. Surgery 1973;73:714.

Takagi S. The effects of intramyometrial injection of prostaglandin F_2 on severe postpartum hemorrhage. Prostaglandins 1976;12:565.

CHAPTER ELEVEN

Sickle-Cell Crisis

Pregnancies complicated by sickle hemoglobinopathies are associated with significantly increased maternal, as well as perinatal, morbidity and mortality. This group of disorders is characterized by chronic anemia, a heightened susceptibility to infection, and intermittent episodes of vascular occlusion by abnormal erythrocytes. The usually acute, painful, recurring vaso-occlusive episodes are known as a "sickle-cell crisis." The clinical severity and frequency of these episodes among gravid patients are highly variable. Although painful sickle-cell (SC) crisis occurs infrequently, this complication may occur as an obstetric emergency at any time during pregnancy, labor and delivery, and the puerperium.

CLINICAL PRESENTATION

Crises can be divided into two major groups: vaso-occlusive and hematologic. During gestation, most crises are vaso-occlusive, occur in the latter half of pregnancy, and produce recurring sudden attacks of pain which most often involve the abdomen, chest, vertebrae, and extremities. For each patient, the probability of having a sickle-cell crisis increases significantly with the number of prior crisis episodes. Clinical manifestations usually follow a characteristic repetitive pattern from one crisis to the next. No organ system or area of the body is immune to attack. Some pregnant patients have generalized pain, while others exhibit more localized syndromes. These may involve the obstructed microcirculations of bone or joints, the chest and lungs, the intra-abdominal organs such as the liver and the kidneys, or the central nervous system, either alone or in combination.

Hematologic crises are characterized by sudden anemia and reticulocytopenia. They are infrequent in pregnancy and more characteristic of the pediatric age group. Marked pallor without significant icterus is the outstanding clinical feature of various forms of hematologic crisis. Affected patients generally are weak, have pale conjunctivae, and also may show evidence of cardiac failure. The most common type of hematologic crisis is the aplastic crisis, which is self-limited and usually associated with infection. Other hematologic crises include hemolytic (as associated either with hereditary spherocytosis or glucose-6-phosphate dehydrogenase deficiency), megaloblastic secondary to folate depletion, and splenic sequestration (confined most often to childhood). Acute splenic sequestration crisis, characterized by acute splenic enlargement, worsening anemia with or without thrombocytopenia, and frequently by signs of hypovolemia, probably are not uncommon in adults with sickle-cell disease and sickle thalassemia, but they may be underdiagnosed or misdiagnosed as splenic infarction.

PATHOPHYSIOLOGY

In the presence of low oxygen, molecules of hemoglobin S (Hgb S) aggregate in small numbers in a process referred to as "nucleation." Hydrophobic bonds involving several areas of the sickle hemoglobin molecule lead to the formation of strands of polymerized hemoglobin. Rapidly thereafter, the multistranded fibers form well-ordered spherulitic arrays called "polymer domains" in a process referred to as "gelation." Thus, the affected red cell evolves into the characteristic half-moon sickled shape. Other intermediate processes are considered to be involved in the progression or regression of gelation events into crises. Sickle-cell hemoglobin gelation is enhanced by increased Hgb S concentration, temperature, or 2,3-diphosphoglycerate levels and decreased by lowered pH or oxygenation. Small changes in pH, temperature, intracellular Hgb S concentrations, or components of the coagulation-anticoagulation system can have significant impact on a gravida's potential to develop a sickle-cell crisis.

Repetitive cycles of gelation during the red-cell life cycle adversely affect the cell membrane, producing potassium and water loss, calcium accumulation, membrane fragmentation, loss of surface area, a relative increase in intracellular hemoglobin concentration, and ultimately membrane rigidity and the irreversibly sickled cell. Consequently, there is a significant increase in blood viscosity, with resistance to flow beginning at the terminal arterioles rather than in the capillary beds. SC crisis is an acute, exaggerated expression of this continuous process rather than discrete episodes of vascular occlusion. The occlusion of small vessels leads to ischemia or infarction, which produces pain.

Viral and bacterial infections, fever, acid-base imbalance, dehydration, trauma, blood loss, anesthesia, severe emotional disturbance, strenuous physical activity, exposure to cold, antivenom injections, alcohol intoxication, extreme fatigue, air travel, and drug overdose can initiate a vaso-occlusive crisis.

DIAGNOSIS

Most women with hemoglobinopathies are known to have the condition before they become pregnant. For undetected disease, however, the most accurate diagnostic test is hemoglobin electrophoresis at an alkaline pH. The obstetrician must determine whether a possible painful crisis is a vaso-occlusive episode, a crisis associated with an infection, malingering, or a surgical or obstetric complication. The diagnosis is one of exclusion and may become clear only after a failed trial of conservative management.

As many as one-third of adult vaso-occlusive crises are associated with apparent or occult infection. Particularly common in young patients is pneumococcal infection of the lung and meninges, which, if present, are the cause of death in up to two-thirds of children younger than 5 years of age with sickle-cell disease. Gram-negative sepsis with *Escherichia coli* and salmonella replace the pneumococcus during pregnancy and the reproductive years as the major offending organisms. Mycoplasma can also cause pneumonia in these patients. The most frequently encountered types of infection are pneumonia, urinary tract infection, puerperal endomyometritis, and oseteomyelitis.

Although the total white blood cell count and the number of segmented leukocytes usually increase during infection as well as during vaso-occlusive crisis, only with a significant bacterial infection is there a consistently increased band level above 1000 mm^3. Leukocyte alkaline phosphatase activity has been reported to be greatly increased following bacterial infection, compared with a normal range for vaso-occlusive crisis in the absence of an infection. Serum lactate dehydrogenases are also elevated, especially isoenzymes 1 and 2 (alpha-hydroxybutyrate dehydrogenase) in the steady state of sickle-cell disease. These isoenzyme levels rise significantly during vaso-occlusive episodes in proportion to the severity of the crisis. If the patient's own baseline value is available for comparison, it may be possible to differentiate between true infarctive crisis and some other condition by analyzing isoenzymes 1 and 2.

Platelet counts and coagulation factors are not helpful in differential diagnosis but may be useful for overall clinical management. Augmented platelet activity and turnover, hypercoagulability, and hyperviscosity characterize crises and are phenomena secondary to an acute-phase protein reaction to both vascular stasis and infection. Renal and liver function testing, serum testing for human immunodeficiency virus (HIV) and hepatitis B surface antigen, and an ultrasound of the gallbladder may be useful, especially when right-upper-quadrant pain complicates the clinical presentation. If indicated, biliary scintigraphy using iminodiacetic acid derivatives can be performed; if normal, it has high negative predictive value that the cystic duct is patent, and unnecessary surgery can be obviated. Finally, magnetic resonance imaging (MRI) may facilitate differentiation between acute and chronic marrow infarcts and serve as a guide to direct and monitor therapy.

TREATMENT

There is no specific therapy for the acute or chronic complications; the only general modalities available are supportive care and the judicious use of transfusions. Our understanding of the features that precipitate painful sickle-cell crisis provide the rationale for therapy with fluids to reduce intracellular hemoglobin concentration, correct acidosis when present, reduce fever, and increase the oxygen concentration of inspired air. It also forms the basis for modern attempts at drug therapy to prevent or mitigate the sickling process.

There are special concerns for pregnant patients with painful vaso-occlusive crisis. Basic goals of therapy at any time during gestation and the puerperium include managing pain, alleviating dehydration, and treating intercurrent infections and other complications. In severe cases, the clinician must be aware of the possibility of acute renal or pulmonary failure. A potentially important therapy is some form of partial exchange transfusion to decrease the amount of Hgb S in the circulation (Table 11-1).

TABLE 11-1

Manual partial exchange transfusion guidelines

---

1. Measure maternal Hg A level and hematocrit (Hct).
2. Type and cross-match 6 units packed Hb AA red cells.
3. Start I.V. in the right arm. Give 1 L of Ringer's lactate or normal saline, infusing 200–400 mL in first hour.
4. Phlebotomize 500 mL blood from opposite arm over 30 minutes.
5. Give 2 units (150–300 mL/unit) of buffy-coat-poor washed packed red cells (under pressure and warmed) over next 2 hours. These units should be AA hemoglobin.
6. Wait 2–4 hours and repeat procedure.
7. If the next morning Hct ≥35% and Hgb A ≥50% and symptoms resolved, discharge; if Hct ≤34%, repeat the exchange transfusion.

Sickle cell crisis

Goals of Therapy

1. Relief of symptoms.
2. Minimize maternal and fetal morbidity/mortality.

Management Protocol

1. Hospitalize. Administer mild sedation and analgesia.
2. Monitor the fetal heart rate carefully if gestational age is sufficient to consider intervention for fetal well-being.
3. Vigorously hydrate with warm fluids if there are no signs of congestive heart failure, infusing 1 L of Ringer's lactate solution or normal saline over a 2-hour period and continuing fluid replacement at 125–175 mL/h based on maternal size and such clinical conditions.
4. Record fluid intake and output.
5. Administer acetaminophen if mild analgesia is needed, acetaminophen with codeine for moderate pain, or intravenous morphine or butorphanol for severe pain. In severe crisis pain situation, continuous morphine administration by standard intravenous infusion or by patient-controlled administration pump should be considered.
6. If physical findings and laboratory test results suggest a crisis-associated infection, obtain appropriate cultures and begin antibiotics immediately. Otherwise, prophylactic antibiotic use is discouraged.
7. If the pregnant gravida in crisis is in labor, has evidence of a respiratory infection or a partial pressure of oxygen less than 70 mm Hg, or a hemoglobin saturation <94%, begin oxygen at 6–8 L/min by mask. Hyperoxia should be avoided in order to avert acute suppression of erythropoiesis.
8. Institute partial exchange transfusion. Several considerations apply:
   A. Continuous automated erythrocytophoresis utilizing an IBM 2997 Cell Separator is optimal. Closely monitor withdrawal and return rates to protect the patient and her fetus from volume overload or hypovolemia. This is particularly important for the patient in crisis who also has congestive heart failure or acute renal failure. Six units of packed red cells are exchanged by this process, generally with rapid alleviation of crisis pain, as well as a decrease in Hgb S concentration, blood viscosity, and sickling.
   B. A partial exchange transfusion using a manual protocol may also be performed (See Table 11-1).

C. A simple manual transfusion is helpful when the patient's initial packed red cell volume is dangerously low (hematocrit <15% or hemoglobin <6 g/dL).

9. At the conclusion of blood transfusion therapy, measure the complete blood count as well as the Hgb A concentration (which should be greater than 50%).

Critical Laboratory Tests

Arterial blood gas or SaO_2 by pulse oximetry, complete blood count with differential count, chemistry panel, lactic dehydrogenase isoenzymes 1 and 2, hemoglobin electrophoresis, type and cross-match of 6 units of packed red blood cells, HIV/hepatitis screen. Consider chest x-ray, electrocardiogram, or pulmonary function tests if clinically indicated.

Consultation

Hematology.
Anesthesiology.

SUGGESTED READING

American College of Obstetricians and Gynecologists. Hemoglobinopathies in pregnancy. ACOG Technical Bulletin. Washington, DC: ACOG, 1987.

Cunningham FG, Pritchard JA, Mason R. Pregnancy and sickle hemoglobinopathy: results with and without prophylactic transfusions. Obstet Gynecol 1983;62:419.

Dean J, Schechter AN. Sickle-cell anemia: molecular and cellular bases of therapeutic approaches. N Engl J Med 1978; 299:752,804–863.

Koshy M, Burd L, Wallace D, et al. Prophylactic red-cell transfusions in pregnant patients with sickle cell disease. N Engl J Med 1988;310:1447.

Morrison JD, Douvas SG, Martin JN Jr. Erythrocytophoresis in pregnant patients with sickle hemoglobinopathies. Am J Obstet Gynecol 1984;149:912.

Morrison JC, Whybrew WD, Bucovaz ET. Use of partial exchange transfusion preoperatively in patients with sickle hemoglobinopathies. Am J Obstet Gynecol 1978;132:59.

CHAPTER TWELVE

Complications of Beta-Sympathomimetic Tocolytic Agents

METABOLIC EFFECTS

Parenteral administration of beta-agonists results in an acute rise in the plasma glucose concentration mediated by direct stimulation of the pancreas to secrete glucagon, which in turn causes gluconeogenesis and glycogenolysis. With a continuous infusion of either ritodrine or terbutaline, peak glucose concentrations are achieved 3–4 hours into the infusion and fall toward preinfusion levels by 24 hours of tocolytic therapy. In the absence of either overt or gestational diabetes mellitus, it is rare to achieve a glucose concentration in excess of 200 mg/dL.

Terbutaline, even when used in the relatively low concentration range of 2.5–17.5 μg/min, results in significantly more women with a serum glucose level exceeding 140 mg/dL than occurs with intravenous ritodrine. The effects of long-term oral agents on maternal glucose hemostasis appear to depend on the drug used. No increase in maternal serum glucose concentration occurred in women exposed to chronic ritodrine administration. Chronic oral terbutaline tocolytic therapy may, however, be associated with maternal glucose intolerance.

Beta-agonists must be used with extreme caution, if at all, in patients with diabetes. If the physician elects to proceed with beta-agonist in this high-risk setting, a continuous intravenous insulin infusion with hourly serum glucose determinations and strict attention to fluid balance are suggested.

Significant and rapid falls in serum potassium concentrations occur following intravenous administration of ritodrine and terbutaline. Low serum potassium concentrations, generally 0.6–1.0 mEq below the preinfusion level, have been reported approximately 3 hours into the beta-agonist infusion in conjunction with the highest plasma glucose and insulin concentrations. Such hypokalemia tends to normalize over time. Since total body potassium is not decreased by beta-agonist therapy, opinions regarding replacement therapy for the low serum potassium levels are divided. No adverse effects of beta-agonist-induced hypokalemia have been documented. We currently withhold replacement therapy in the absence of a serum potassium concentration <2.0 mEq/L, cardiac arrhythmias, or the administration of a diuretic.

Promptly upon beta-agonist infusion, arginine vasopressin (AVP) and renin are both released. Renin and angiotension, potent vasoconstrictors, effect a marked increase in renal resistance and a concomitant fall in renal plasma flow. Concurrently, renal tubular sodium reabsorption increases and carries with it an obligatory flow of water. Any remaining free water then is subject to reabsorption under the influence of AVP in the distal collecting tubules.

By giving women treated with these drugs free water, as opposed to balanced salt solutions, the physician can reduce the amount of fluid retained. The administration of beta-sympathomimetic tocolytic agents in either 0.25% normal saline or 5% dextrose in water, combined with hourly intake and output surveillance, is recommended.

CARDIOPULMONARY EFFECTS

Cardiopulmonary complications of beta-sympathomimetic therapy include tachycardia, hypotension, arrhythmias, myocardial ischemia, and pulmonary edema. The importance of these derangements cannot be overstated as they have been associated with several maternal deaths. Although beta-1 receptor stimulation of the heart is important in the pathogenesis of many of the complications seen with these agents, the pregnant state and its attendant complications (such as labor, anemia, and multiple gestation) are probably equally important. In pregnant women exposed to these medications, cardiac output demands may be increased by over 300% when compared with basal nonpregnant levels.

The most pronounced cardiopulmonary effects are seen shortly after initiation of therapy; thereafter, most of the measured hemodynamic variables and parameters return towards the baseline measurements obtained prior to treatment. Usual findings include an increase in maternal heart rate, a decrease in diastolic blood pressure, and no change or a modest elevation in systolic blood pressure. Cardiac output is uniformly elevated, the increase approaching 60% shortly after institution of the drug. With continuation of therapy, the cardiac output stabilizes at approximately 35%–40% above the preinfusion level. The ventricular ejection fraction and fractional shortening both increase, and the left ventricular end-systolic dimensions decrease. Long-term treatment with beta-agonists may lead to slow but progressive increases in the PCWP and deterioration of left ventricular function.

PULMONARY EDEMA

Pulmonary edema is the most frequently reported serious complication of beta-agonist therapies occurring in 3%–9% of the women receiving these agents. Pulmonary edema was a key clinical presentation in 11 of the 14 maternal deaths occurring in conjunction with beta-agonist tocolytic therapy.

Volume overload appears to be etiologic in the development of pulmonary edema in one-quarter of cases. One of every 10 women developing pulmonary edema while undergoing beta-agonist tocolytic therapy has also received a concomitant blood transfusion; thus, transfusion should be considered a risk factor for the development of pulmonary edema.

Multifetal gestations have complicated over 19% of the reports of beta-agonist-associated pulmonary edema (Table 12-1).

TABLE 12-1

Potential precipitants of pulmonary edema in 93 women in
conjunction with tocolytic therapy

	Number	Percentage (%)
Infection	27	29.0
Volume overload	22	23.7
Twins	18	19.4
No factor identified	18	19.4
Multiagent therapy	12	12.9
Blood transfusion	9	9.7
Heart disease	9	9.7
Myopathy	4	—
Valvular	2	—
Ischemia	3	—
Preeclampsia	5	5.4

Women with twin gestations are at increased risk of premature
labor and, hence, exposure to the complications of beta-sympathomimetic agents; thus, these patients' frequent association
with pulmonary edema may reflect an ascertainment artifact.
Alternatively, increased volume expansion associated with multiple gestations may be of primary importance.

Heart failure can occur solely on the basis of tacyhcardia,
resulting in decreased diastolic filling and systolic ejection times.
The titration of these drugs to the heart rate, with the goal of
limiting maternal tachycardia to 140 beats per minute (bpm) or
less has apparently served as an excellent safeguard against this
mechanism of heart failure. Rate-related myocardial ischemia
has been reported in three women who developed pulmonary
edema, and cardiac valvular lesions were found in two such
women. Selection of an alternative first-line tocolytic agent
would appear to be reasonable for any woman with either valvular or ischemic heart disease.

The final mechanism of heart failure that might account for pulmonary edema in conjunction with the use of the beta-agonist is abnormal myocardial contractility. A direct effect of catecholamines on the myocardium has been known for many years. To date, at least four women developing pulmonary edema in conjunction with tocolytic therapy have done so on the basis of a presumed cardiomyopathy or myocarditis.

There is no evidence to incriminate the beta-agonist per se as being responsible for an increase in pulmonary vascular permeability. By comparison, 29% of patients developing pulmonary edema have had a clinically obvious infection in conjunction with the tocolytic therapy. Historically, most cases of pulmonary edema have occurred in the setting of prolonged tocolysis for refractory preterm labor, a scenario that may represent silent chorioamnionitis. It is reasonable to hypothesize that seeding of the maternal bloodstream with either the bacteria or their by-products may result in small alterations in the permeability of these women's lungs. Extrapolating from animal data, even small alterations of permeability of the lungs can result in significant accumulation of interstitial water when concomitantly exposed to beta-agonist therapy. With overt clinical infection and concurrent use of beta-agonist tocolytics, the risk of pulmonary edema is 21%.

Pulmonary edema is an endpoint and can be reached by several paths. Currently, the majority of evidence points toward either infection or volume overload as the leading contributors/mechanisms of lung injury during beta-agonist therapy. Congestive heart failure in the setting of valvular heart disease, anemia, twins, severe hypertension, or overly vigorous transfusion therapy can also lead to pulmonary edema.

THERAPY

Irrespective of the mechanism of pulmonary edema, initial therapy should consist of oxygen, the upright position, furosemide, and discontinuation of the beta-agonist. The clinical status can be monitored by arterial blood gas determinations or by pulse oximetry. If prompt improvement is not achieved, invasive hemodynamic monitoring should be instituted and used to guide further therapy.

─────

ISCHEMIA

Up to 20% of women treated with ritodrine complain of chest pain. Ischemic changes have frequently been found in patients with chest pain, and electrocardiogram (EKG) changes consistent with ischemia have occurred in patients both with and without symptoms. Ischemia, occurring when the myocardial oxygen demand exceeds supply, can progress to myocardial infarction or serve as a focus for dangerous arrhythmias. The combination of pregnancy, premature labor, and beta-agonist therapy is in many ways similar to an exercise stress test and can serve to identify underlying myocardial disease (Figure 12-1). Heart rate and contractility both increase with beta-agonists therapy, thereby increasing myocardial oxygen consumption. Cardiac oxygen availability, however, may actually be compromised by the fall in mean arterial pressure and a shortened diastolic filling time, both serving to reduce flow to the myocardium.

At six hours of intravenous ritodrine therapy, up to 78% of asymptomatic women have nonspecific ST- and T-wave changes consistent with ischemia. Interestingly, these changes are less apparent at 24 hours of therapy. Because tachyphylaxis is a well-documented occurrence with ritodrine therapy, the initial EKG changes simply may have reflected the faster heart rate and not ischemia, or alternatively, ischemia that resolved as the heart rate normalized. Symptoms and EKG changes have also been documented in patients on oral therapy.

In the setting of significant chest pain or substernal tightness, especially if with concurrent EKG changes, evaluation of the women's creatine kinase isoenzymes may be indicated. Following a normal labor and delivery, approximately 10% of women will demonstrate a significant elevation of the MB fraction of creatine kinase (CK). Additionally, women in premature labor have also been shown to have an elevation of the CK-MB fraction 10% of the time. It is known that the CK isoenzymes can pass from the fetus into the maternal circulation. Accordingly, the use of these isoenzymes to indicate myocardial injury

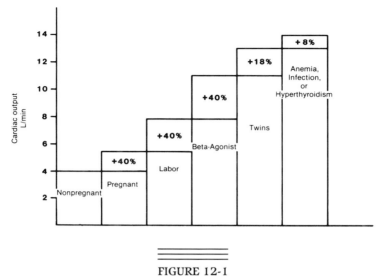

FIGURE 12-1

Cumulative effects of pregnancy and various pregnancy complications on cardiac output.

and necrosis is much less specific in the gravid woman than in her nonpregnant counterpart.

Documented ischemic cardiac disease is a contraindication to beta-sympathomimetic therapy. Routine EKGs prior to or during therapy are unnecessary, but EKGs become mandatory, along with a thorough physical examination and discontinuation of the drug, immediately upon the patient's observation of any symptoms of chest pain or discomfort.

ARRHYTHMIAS

In addition to pulmonary edema, cardiac arrhythmias, including supraventricular tachycardia, atrial fibrillation, and premature ventricular contractions, have occurred during beta-sympathomimetic therapy. Women with the Lown-Ganong-Levine or Wolff-Parkinson-White syndromes seem particularly prone to reentrant phenomenon and supraventricular tachycardia. These arrhythmias usually respond simply by stopping the beta-agonist. A thorough search should be made for known precipitating events, including hypokalemia, hypoxemia, and myocardial ischemia.

Sympathomimetic-associated pulmonary edema

Goals of Therapy

1. Relief of symptoms.
2. Maintenance of adequate oxygenation (Pao_2 > 60 mm Hg or Sao_2 > 90%).
3. Diuresis of excess fluid.
4. Avoid problem by avoiding fluid overload and infusing D_5W, as opposed to isotonic crystalloid solutions.

Management Protocol

1. Discontinue sympathomimetic agent.
2. O_2 by mask.
3. Furosemide 20–40 mg I.V.
4. Morphine sulfate 10 mg I.V.
5. Foley catheter for hourly output determinations.
6. Insert pulmonary artery catheter if clinical response to steps 1–4 is not prompt. Additional hemodynamic manipulations (preload optimization [5–14 mm Hg] or inotropic support) as indicated by hemodynamic indices.

Laboratory Tests

Arterial blood gas, chest x-ray, serum electrolytes, electrocardiogram.

Monitoring Techniques

1. Pulse oximetry.
2. Foley catheter.
3. Pulmonary artery (PA) catheter.

Consultation

Pulmonary medicine, cardiology, respiratory therapy.

SUGGESTED READING

Benedetti TJ. Maternal complications of parenteral B-sympathomimetic therapy for premature labor. Am J Obstet Gynecol 1983;145:1–6.

The Canadian Preterm Labor Investigators Group. Treatment of preterm labor with the beta-adrenergic agonist ritodrine. N Engl J Med 1992;327:308–312.

Finley J, Katz M, Rojas-Perez M, Roberts JM, Creasy RK, Schiller NB. Cardiovascular consequences of B-agonist tocolysis: an echocardiographic study. Obstet Gynecol 1984;64:787–791.

Hadi HA, Abdulla AM, Fadel HE, Stefadouros MA, Metheny WP. Cardiovascular effects of ritodrine tocolysis: a new noninvasive method to measure pulmonary capillary pressure during pregnancy. Obstet Gynecol 1987;70:608–612.

Hatjis CG, Swain M. Systemic tocolysis for premature labor is associated with an increased incidence of pulmonary edema in the presence of maternal infection. Am J Obstet Gynecol 1988;159:723–728.

Hauth JC, Hankins GD, Kuehl T, Pierson WP. Ritodrine hydrochloride infusion in pregnant baboons. I. Biophysical effects. Am J Obstet Gynecol 1983;146:916–924.

Young DC, Toofanian A, Leveno KJ. Potassium and glucose concentrations without treatment during ritodrine tocolysis. Am J Obstet Gynecol 1983;145:105–106.

CHAPTER THIRTEEN

Complications of Pregnancy-Induced Hypertension

Hypertensive disease in pregnancy is the second most common cause of maternal mortality in advanced gestations. Pathological changes may commonly affect the maternal cardiovascular, renal, hematologic, neurologic, and hepatic systems. Equally important are the effects on the uteroplacental unit, resulting in fetal and neonatal complications (see Table 13-1).

Severe preeclampsia is diagnosed when any of the following occur in a patient with preeclampsia:

1. Blood pressure of at least 160/110 mm Hg on two occasions at least six hours apart.
2. 5 g of protein excreted in a 24-hour urine specimen, or persistent 3–4+ proteinuria on a semiquantitative assay.
3. Oliguria, less than 400–500 mL of urine output over 24 hours.
4. Significant cerebral or visual disturbances such as altered consciousness, headaches, scotomata, or blurred vision.
5. Pulmonary edema or cyanosis.
6. Epigastric or right-upper-quadrant pains.
7. Impaired liver function of unclear etiology.
8. Thrombocytopenia.
9. Certain cases of severe fetal growth retardation.

TABLE 13-1
Complications of severe pregnancy-induced hypertension

Cardiovascular	Severe hypertension, pulmonary edema
Renal	Oliguria, renal failure
Hematologic	Hemolysis, thrombocytopenia, DIC*
Neurologic	Eclampsia, cerebral edema, cerebral hemorrhage, amaurosis
Hepatic	Hepatocellular dysfunction, hepatic rupture
Uteroplacental	Abruption, IUGR†, fetal distress, fetal death

*DIC = disseminated intravascular coagulopathy.
†IUGR = intrauterine growth retardation.

The development of these severe manifestations of the disease necessitates careful evaluation and consideration of delivery.

FLUID THERAPY

Fluid management in severe pregnancy-induced hypertension (PIH) consists of crystalloid infusions of normal saline of lactated Ringer's solution, at a rate of 100–125 mL/h. Additional fluid volumes, in the order of 1000–1500 mL, may be required prior to use of epidural anesthesia or vasodilator therapy in order to prevent maternal hypotension and fetal distress.

ANTISEIZURE PROPHYLAXIS

Magnesium sulfate ($MgSO_4 7H_2O$ USP) has long been standard therapy in preeclampsia-eclampsia in the United States.
    Plasma magnesium levels maintained at 4–7 mEq/L are felt

to be therapeutic in preventing eclamptic seizures. Patellar reflexes usually are lost at 8–10 mEq/L, and respiratory arrest may occur at 13 mEq/L. An intravenous loading dose of 4–6 g, followed by an infusion of 2–3 g/h will generally achieve therapeutic and nontoxic levels in patients with good urine output. Urine output, patellar reflexes, respiratory rates, or serum magnesium levels should be closely monitored, especially in those patients who have renal dysfunction. Calcium gluconate (10 mL of 10% solution), oxygen therapy, and the ability to perform endotracheal intubation should be available in the event of magnesium toxicity.

ANTIHYPERTENSIVE THERAPY

Careful control of hypertension must be achieved in order to prevent maternal cerebral vascular accident. Medical intervention is usually recommended when the diastolic blood pressure exceeds 110 mm Hg; the level at which acute intervention for isolated severe systolic pressure elevation is not as well established.

Hydralazine hydrochloride (Apresoline) has long been the gold standard of antihypertensive therapy in obstetrics in the United States because of extensive clinical experience with this agent. Hydralazine reduces vascular resistance via direct relaxation of arteriolar smooth muscle, affecting precapillary resistance vessels more than postcapillary capacitance vessels. The use of this agent results in a fall in maternal blood pressure with no change in intervillous blood flow and an increase in umbilical vein blood flow.

An initial intravenous dose of 5 mg is recommended, followed by observation of hemodynamic effects. If appropriate change in blood pressure is not achieved, 5–10-mg doses may be administered intravenously at 20-minute intervals to a total acute dose of 30–40 mg. Hypertension refractory to the preceding approach warrants consideration of central hemodynamic monitoring and the use of the more potent antihypertensive agents.

Labetalol is a combined alpha- and beta-adrenoceptor antagonist that may be used to induce a controlled, rapid decrease in blood pressure via decreased systemic vascular resistance (SVR) in patients with severe hypertension. Labetalol may exert a positive effect on early fetal lung maturation in patients with severe hypertension who are remote from term. An initial dose of 10 mg is given, followed by progressively increasing doses (20, 40, 80 mg) every 10 minutes, to a total dose of 300 mg. A constant intravenous infusion may be started at 1–2 mg/min until therapeutic goals are achieved, then decreased to 0.5 mg/min or completely stopped. The use of labetalol has been associated with increased uteroplacental perfusion and decreased uterine vascular resistance.

Nitroglycerin relaxes predominantly venous, but also arterial, vascular smooth muscle. It has been shown to decrease preload at low doses and afterload in high doses. It is a rapidly acting potent antihypertensive agent with a very short hemodynamic half-life. Nitroglycerin is administered via an infusion pump at an initial rate of 10 μg/min and titrated to the desired pressures by doubling the dose every 5 minutes. Methemoglobinemia may result from high-dose (>7 μg/kg/min) intravenous infusion.

Sodium nitroprusside is another useful and potent antihypertensive agent. A dilute solution may be started at 0.25 μg/kg/min and titrated to the desired effect through an infusion pump by increasing the dose by 0.25 μg/kg/min every 5 minutes. Arterial blood gases should be monitored to watch for developing metabolic acidosis which may be an early sign of cyanide toxicity, and central hemodynamic monitoring with arterial line and possibly pulmonary artery catheter is generally indicated. Treatment time should be limited because of the potential for fetal cyanide toxicity. Correction of hypovolemia prior to initiation of nitroprusside infusion is essential in order to avoid abrupt and often profound drops in blood pressure.

Nifedipine is a calcium channel blocker, which lowers blood pressure primarily by relaxing arterial smooth muscle. An initial oral dose of 10 mg is administered, which may be repeated after 30 minutes if necessary, for the acute management of severe hypertension; 10–20 mg may then be administered orally every 3 to 6 hours as needed. Care must be given when nifedipine is administered to patients receiving concomitant magnesium sulfate because of the possibility of an exaggerated hypotensive response.

TABLE 13-2

Hemodynamic findings in severe PIH

Common Central Hemodynamic Findings in Severe Preeclampsia

1. Cardiac output is variable.
2. Mean arterial pressure (MAP) is elevated. Systemic vascular resistance (SVR) is normal (early) or elevated (late).
3. Central venous pressure (CVP) is usually low to normal and may not correlate with pulmonary capillary wedge pressure (PCWP).
4. Pulmonary hypertension is not present.
5. PCWP may be low, normal, or high.
6. Oliguria may not reflect volume depletion.
7. Ventricular function is usually hyperdynamic, but it may be depressed in the presence of marked elevation in SVR.
8. Colloid osmotic pressure (COP) is usually low.

(Reproduced with permission from Clark SL, Cotton DB. Clinical indications for pulmonary artery catheterization in the patient with severe preeclampsia. Am J Obstet Gynecol 1988;158:453–458.)

HEMODYNAMIC MONITORING

Common central hemodynamic findings in severe preeclampsia are summarized in Table 13-2. Current indications for the use of a pulmonary artery catheter in preeclamptic women are listed in Table 13-3. Routine use of pulmonary artery catheter in uncomplicated severe preeclampsia is not recommended.

PULMONARY EDEMA

The etiology of pulmonary edema in preeclamptic patients appears to be multifactorial. Reduction of COP, alteration of capil-

TABLE 13-3
Indications for possible use of pulmonary artery catheter in PIH

Complications related to central volume status (pulmonary edema or persistent oliguria).

Intractable severe hypertension unresponsive to hydralazine, requiring nitroglycerin or nitroprusside.

Induction of conduction anesthesia in hemodynamically unstable patients.

lary membrane permeability, and elevated pulmonary vascular hydrostatic pressures all lead to extravasation of fluids into the interstitial and alveolar spaces, resulting in pulmonary edema. Each of the mechanisms, singly or in combination, has been demonstrated in patients with PIH and pulmonary edema.

Initial management of pulmonary edema includes oxygen administration and fluid restriction. A pulse oximeter should be placed, if available, so that oxygen saturation may be continuously monitored. Many authorities recommend placement of a pulmonary artery catheter in severe preeclamptic patients who develop pulmonary edema of uncertain origin in order to distinguish between fluid overload, left ventricular dysfunction, and nonhydrostatic pulmonary edema, each of which may require different approaches to therapy.

Furosemide administered in a 10- to 40-mg dose intravenously over one to two minutes represents the first line of conventional therapy for fluid overload pulmonary edema. If adequate diuresis does not commence within one hour, an 80-mg dose may be administered slowly to achieve diuresis. In severe cases of pulmonary edema, a diuresis of 2–3 L needs to be achieved before oxygenation begins to improve. The degree of diuresis appropriate for these hemodynamically complex patients may be clarified by complete hemodynamic evaluation, using parameters derived by a pulmonary artery catheter. An alternative approach to preload reduction involves the administration of intravenous nitroglycerin. While hydrostatic derangements may be corrected quickly, rapid improvement in arterial oxygenation may not be seen. Afterload reduction with arterial vasodilators such as hydralazine or sodium nitroprusside may be necessary for the treatment of pulmonary edema secondary to left ventricular failure associated with increased systemic vascular resistance. Continuous arterial blood pressure monitoring is often helpful in this setting because of the potent activity of some arteriodilating agents.

When hypoxemia persists despite initial treatment, mechanical ventilation my be required. In all cases, close monitoring of the patient's respiratory status with frequent arterial blood gases should be performed. Fluid balance is maintained by careful monitoring of intake and output. Serum electrolytes should be closely monitored, especially in patients receiving diuretics.

OLIGURIA

Three different hemodynamic subsets of preeclamptic-eclamptic patients with persistent oliguria have been described. The first group has a low PCWP, hyperdynamic left ventricular function, and mild to moderately increased SVR. These patients responded to further volume replacement. This is the most common clinical scenario, and it is felt to be secondary to intravascular volume depletion.

The second group is characterized by normal or increased PCWP, normal CO, and normal SVR, accompanied by intense uroconcentration. The pathophysiologic basis of oliguria in this group is thought to be secondary to intrinsic renal arterial spasm out of proportion to systemic vasospasm. Low–dose dopamine ($1–5$ μg/kg/min) has been shown to produce a significant rise in urine output in severe preeclamptic patients in this hemodynamic subgroup.

The third group of oliguric patients has markedly elevated PCWPs and SVR, with depressed ventricular function. These patients respond to aggressive afterload reduction and diuresis. Oliguria in this subgroup may be the first sign of incipient pulmonary edema. Central hemodynamic assessment will allow the clinician to distinguish the preceding subgroups and tailor therapy accordingly. In patients with preeclampsia, urinary diagnostic indices such as urine:plasma ratios of creatinine, urea nitrogen, and

osmolality may be clinically misleading if applied to fluid management. Patients often may have urinary diagnostic indices consistent with prerenal dehydration, but PCWP consistent with
euvolemia.

If urine output falls below 25 mL per hour over two consecutive hours, a management plan should be instituted. The cause of
oliguria is prerenal in most instances. A fluid challenge of 500–
1000 mL of normal saline or lactated Ringer's solution may be
administered over 30 minutes. If urine output does not respond
to such fluid challenge and the patient is remote from delivery,
pulmonary artery catheterization is indicated if further hemodynamic manipulation is contemplated in an effort to resolve the
oliguria. Repetitive fluid challenges are to be avoided in the absence of invasive monitoring, as pulmonary edema can evolve
quickly in this setting. In the presence of oliguria, delivery is, of
course, indicated.

HELLP SYNDROME

HELLP syndrome is a variant of severe preeclampsia affecting
4%–12% of patients with preeclampsia-eclampsia. HELLP syndrome is characterized by various combinations of *h*emolysis,
*e*levated *l*iver enzymes, and *l*ow *p*latelets. Unlike most forms of
preeclampsia, HELLP syndrome is not primarily a disease of
primigravidas, the incidence among multigravidas being almost
twice that seen in primigravid patients.

Ten to twenty percent of patients with HELLP syndrome do
not meet the standard blood pressure criteria for preeclampsia.

The clinical signs and symptoms of patients with HELLP
syndrome are commonly related to the impact of vasospasm on
the maternal liver. These include malaise, nausea (with or without vomiting), and epigastric pain. Right-upper-quadrant or
epigastric tenderness is commonly seen.

A peripheral smear may demonstrate burr cells and/or
schistocytes with polychromasia, consistent with microangiopathic hemolytic anemia. Hemolysis can sometimes also be demonstrated by an elevated haptoglobin or unconjugated bilirubin

level. Though some degree of hemolysis may be noted, significant anemia is uncommon.

Thrombocytopenia is defined as a platelet count of less than 100,000–150,000/mL. The decline in platelets in patients with HELLP syndrome is believed to be due to increased peripheral destruction. However, thrombocytopenia is generally not accompanied by additional clotting abnormalities unless the picture is complicated by placental abruption or prolonged fetal demise.

Significant elevation of alkaline phosphatase is seen in normal pregnancy; elevation of serum glutamic oxaloacetic transaminase (SGOT) and/or serum glutamic pyruvic transaminase (SGPT), however, indicate hepatic pathology. In HELLP syndrome, the SGOT and SGPT are rarely in excess of 1000 IU/L; values in excess of this level suggest hepatic rupture or other hepatic disorders, such as hepatitis. Laboratory abnormalities usually return to normal within a short time after delivery; however, it is not unusual to see transient worsening of both thrombocytopenia and hepatic function in the first 24–48 hours postpartum.

HELLP syndrome can be a "great masquerader," and both clinical presentation and laboratory findings associated with this syndrome may suggest an array of clinical diagnoses. Because of the numerous misdiagnoses associated with this syndrome and because a delay in diagnosis may be life threatening, HELLP syndrome must be considered in any pregnant woman in the third trimester with thrombocytopenia, elevated serum transaminase levels, or epigastric pain.

Complications associated with HELLP syndrome include placental abruption, acute renal failure, hepatic hematoma with rupture, and ascites. Placental abruption in HELLP syndrome patients occurs at a rate 29 times that seen in the general obstetrical population. The reported incidence ranges from 7% to 20%.

Platelet transfusion in preeclamptic patients with thrombocytopenia is not necessary if the platelet count exceeds 10,000/mL in a nonsurgical patient. If cesarean delivery is contemplated, a platelet count of at least 50,000/mL is desirable. One way to manage such patients is to prepare 10 units of platelet concentrate and to infuse 5 units in the operating room just prior to the incision. The remaining units are infused during the operative procedure. Exchange plasmapheresis with fresh-frozen plasma has been used to treat hemolysis and thrombocytopenia that did not resolve following delivery and standard medical treatment. It cannot be overemphasized that ultimate clinical success depends on prompt delivery.

Hepatic infarction may lead to intrahepatic hemorrhage and development of a subcapsular hematoma which may rupture into the peritoneal space and result in shock and death. Subcapsular hematomas usually develop on the anterior and superior aspects of the liver. The maternal and fetal prognosis of liver rupture are poor, with a 59% maternal and 62% fetal mortality rate reported. When the diagnosis of liver hematoma is made in the postpartum period, conservative management with blood transfusion and serial ultrasonography may be reasonable.

Liver rupture with intraperitoneal hemorrhage, when suspected, requires laparotomy. Hemostasis may be achieved by compression, simple suture, topical coagulant agents, arterial embolization, omental pedicles, ligation of the hepatic artery, or lobectomy, depending on the extent of the hepatic damage. Temporary control of bleeding may be achieved by packing the rupture site or by application of a gravity suit.

NEUROLOGIC COMPLICATIONS

Cerebral hemorrhage, cerebral edema, temporary blindness (amaurosis), and eclamptic seizures are separate but related neurologic conditions that may occur in preeclampsia. Cerebral hemorrhage and cerebral edema are two major causes of maternal mortality in preeclampsia. Intracranial hemorrhage is generally secondary to severe hypertension and/or hemostatic compromise.

Cerebral edema is defined as increased water content of one or more of the intracranial fluid compartments of the brain. Signs of diffuse cerebral edema may be found in eclamptic women, on computed tomography (CT). Cerebral edema may develop when the forces affecting the Starling equilibrium are disturbed. The three most important factors include increased intravascular pressure, damage to vascular endothelium, and reduced plasma COP. Miller's classification of cerebral edema includes:

1. Vasogenic edema with breakdown of the blood-brain barrier, secondary to vascular damage.
2. Cytotoxic edema, secondary to damage to the cellular sodium pump.
3. Hydrostatic edema, from increased intravascular pressure.
4. Interstitial edema, related to acute obstructive hydrocephalus.
5. Hypoosmotic edema, in which intravascular free water decreases plasma osmolality.

In PIH, cerebral edema may occur secondary to anoxia associated with eclamptic seizures, or it may be secondary to loss of cerebral autoregulation as a result of severe hypertension.

Cerebral edema is diagnosed on CT scan by the appearance of areas with low density or low radiographic absorption coefficient. Magnetic resonance imaging (MRI) has also been useful in providing an index of water content in select areas of the brain.

Amaurosis may complicate 1%–3% of cases of preeclampsia. Such blindness may be central, as a result of occipital lake edema or infarction, or peripheral, secondary to macular edema or hemorrhage.

The precise cause of seizures in preeclampsia remains unknown. Hypertensive encephalopathy, as well as vasospasm, hemorrhage, ischemia, and edema of the cerebral hemisphere have been proposed as etiologic factors. Thrombotic and hemorrhagic lesions have been identified on autopsy of preeclamptic women.

Eclamptic seizures usually occur without a preceding aura, although many patients will manifest some form of apprehension, excitability, or hyperreflexia prior to the onset of seizure. Once a seizure occurs, it is usually a forerunner of more convulsions unless anticonvulsant therapy is initiated. Eclamptic seizures occur prior to the delivery in roughly 80% of patients. In the remainder, convulsions occur postpartum, and they have been reported up to 23 days following delivery. Where eclampsia occurs more than 24 hours postpartum, however, a thorough search for other potential causes of seizures is mandatory.

As a rule, a maternal seizure results in fetal bradycardia. Although the fetal heart rate pattern usually returns to normal following the seizure, appropriate steps should be taken to enhance maternal-fetal well-being, including maintenance of maternal airway, oxygen administration, and maternal lateral repositioning. Maternal recovery following eclampsia is generally complete. The standard therapy for the management of eclampsia is: 1) magnesium sulfate and 2) delivery of the fetus. We administer 4–6 g of magnesium sulfate intravenously over 20 minutes and initiate an intravenous infusion at 2–3 g/h. If control of seizures is not successful after the initial intravenous bolus, a second 2-g bolus of magnesium sulfate may be administered. No more than a total of 8 g of magnesium sulfate are recommended at the outset of treatment. Seizures refractory to standard magnesium sulfate regimens may by treated with a slow 100-mg intravenous dose of thiopental sodium (Pentothal) or 1–10 mg of diazepam. Alternatively, sodium amobarbital (up to 250 mg) may be administered intravenously. Eclamptic patients with repetitive seizures despite therapeutic magnesium levels warrant CT evaluation of the brain.

Contemporary maternal mortality rates for patients with eclampsia range from 0 to 14% (Table 13-4).

The perinatal mortality rate among eclamptic ranges from 14% to 27% and is most commonly secondary to placental abruption, prematurity, and perinatal asphyxia. Antenatal deaths account for 62% of the overall perinatal mortality.

TABLE 13-4
Cause of death in 86 eclamptic patients

Cause of Death	Number	%
Cerebrovascular accident	62	72
Respiratory failure	10	12
Postpartum hemorrhage	5	5
Consumption coagulopathy	3	4
Acute renal failure	1	1
Ruptured liver	1	1
Septic shock	1	1
Other	3	3

General therapeutic principles in the treatment of cerebral edema include correction of hypoxemia and hypercarbia, avoidance of volatile anesthetic agents, control of body temperature, and control of blood pressure.

Assisted hyperventilation reduces intracranial hypertension and the formation of cerebral edema. Partial pressure of carbon dioxide (Pco_2) levels are maintained between 27 mm Hg and 30 mm Hg. Hyperbaric oxygenation therapy, considered experimental in the control of cerebral edema, is aimed at maintaining a partial pressure of oxygen (Po_2) level of 1000 mm Hg, using an ambient pressure of 2.0–2.5 atmospheres to effect cerebral vasoconstriction.

The administration of hypertonic solutions such as mannitol increases serum osmolality and draws water from the brain into the vascular compartment, thus reducing brain tissue water and volume. A 20% solution of mannitol is given as a 0.5–1 g/kg dose over 10 minutes or as a continuous infusion of 5 g/h. The serum osmolality is maintained in a range between 305 and 315 mosm.

Steroid therapy (dexamethasone, betamethasone, methylprednisolone) is thought to be most effective in the treatment of focal chronic cerebral edema, which may occur in association with a tumor or abscess, and is less beneficial in cases of diffuse cerebral edema.

PIH hypertensive crisis

Goals of Therapy

1. Diastolic BP <110 mm Hg.
2. Systolic BP <180–200 mm Hg.

Management Protocol

1. Assure adequate intravascular volume. Consider 500–1000 cc NS fluid load.
2. Hydralazine hydrochloride 5 mg I.V., followed by 10 mg I.V. as often as every 20 minutes to achieve blood pressure goals.

or

Labetalol 10 mg I.V. followed by progressively increasing doses (20,40, 80 mg) every 10 minutes to achieve blood pressure goals or to total dose of 300 mg.

3. If hydralazine or labetalol is ineffective, place arterial line and possibly pulmonary artery catheter, and consider nitroglycerine or nitroprusside. Nitroglycerine: 10 mg/min, doubling dose every 5 minutes to achieve blood pressure goals. Nitroprusside: 0.25 mg/kg/min, increasing by same dose every 5 minutes to achieve blood pressure goals.

4. Fetal monitoring.

5. Initiate delivery.

Critical Laboratory Tests

Hematocrit and red blood cell morphology, platelet count, aspartate aminotransferase (AST), alanine aminotransferase (ALT).

SUGGESTED READING

The American College of Obstetricians and Gynecologists. Management of preeclampsia. ACOG Technical Bulletin. February 1986;91:1–5.

Benedetti TJ, Kates R, Williams V. Hemodynamic observations in severe preeclampsia complicated by pulmonary edema. Am J Obstet Gynecol 1985;152:330–334.

Chesley LC, Annitto JE, Cosgrove RA. The remote prognosis of eclamptic women. Am J Obstet Gynecol 1976;124:446–459.

Clark SL, Cotton DB. Clinical indications for pulmonary artery catheterization in the patient with severe preeclampsia. Am J Obstet Gynecol 1988;158:453–458.

Clark SL, Cotton DB, Lee W, et al. Central hemodynamic observations in normal third trimester pregnancy. Am J Obstet Gynecol 1989;161:1439–1442.

Clark SL, Divon Y, Phelan JP. Preeclampsia/eclampsia: Hemodynamic and neurologic correlations. Obstet Gynecol 1985;66:337–340.

Clark SL, Greenspoon JS, Aldahl D, Phelan JP. Severe preeclampsia with persistent oliguria: management of hemodynamic subsets. Am J Obstet Gynecol 1986;154:490–494.

Cotton DB, Gonik B, Dorman KR. Cardiovascular alterations in severe pregnancy-induced hypertension: acute effects of intravenous magnesium sulfate. Am J Obstet Gynecol 1984;148:162–165.

Cotton DB, Gonik B, Dorman K, Harrist R. Cardiovascular alterations in severe pregnancy-induced hypertension: relationship of central venous pressure to pulmonary capillary wedge pressure. Am J Obstet Gynecol 1985;151:762–764.

Cotton DB, Jones MM, Longmire S, Dorman KF, Tessem J, Joyce TH. Role of intravenous nitroglycerin in the treatment of severe pregnancy-induced hypertension complicated by pulmonary edema. Am J Obstet Gynecol 1986;154:91–93.

Cotton DB, Longmire S, Jones MM, Dorman KF, Tessem J, Joyce TH. Cardiovascular alterations in severe pregnancy-induced hypertension: effects of intravenous nitroglycerin coupled with blood volume expansion. Am J Obstet Gynecol 1986;154:1053–1059.

Cunningham FG, Pritchard JA. Hematologic considerations of pregnancy-induced hypertension. Sem Perinatol 1978;2:29–38.

Downing I, Shepherd GL, Lewis PJ. Kinetics of prostacyclin synthetase in umbilical artery microsomes from normal and preeclamptic pregnancies. Br J Clin Pharmacol 1982;13:195–198.

Easterling TR, Benedetti TJ. Preeclampsia: A hyperdynamic disease model. Am J Obstet Gynecol 1989;160:1447–1453.

Friedman SA. Preeclampsia: a review of the role of prostaglandins. Obstet Gynecol 1988;71:122–137.

Gant NF, Daley GL, Chand S, Whalley PJ, MacDonald PC. A study of angiotensin II pressor response throughout primigravid pregnancy. J Clin Invest 1973;52:2682–2689.

Gutsche B. The experts opine: is epidural block for labor and delivery and for cesarean section a safe form of analgesia in severe preeclampsia or eclampsia? Surv Anesth 1986;30:304–311.

Hankins GDV, Wendell GD, Cunningham FG, Leveno KJ. Longitudinal evaluation of hemodynamic changes in eclampsia. Am J Obstet Gynecol 1984;150:506–512.

Herbert WNP, Brenner WE. Improving survival with liver rupture complicating pregnancy. Am J Obstet Gynecol 1982;142:530–534.

Kirshon B, Lee W, Mauer MB, Cotton DB. Effects of low-dose dopamine therapy in the oliguric patient with preeclampsia. Am J Obstet Gynecol 1988;159:604–607.

Krane NK. Acute renal failure in pregnancy. Arch Intern Med 1988;148:2347–2357.

Lee W, Gonik B, Cotton DB. Urinary diagnostic indices in preeclampsia-associated oliguria: correlation with invasive hemodynamic monitoring. Am J Obstet Gynecol 198;156:100–103.

Mabie WC, Gonzalez AR, Sibai BM, Amon E. A comparative trial of labetalol and hydralazine in the acute management of severe hypertension complicating pregnancy. Obstet Gynecol 1987;70:328–333.

Pritchard JA. The use of magnesium sulfate in preeclampsia-eclampsia. J Reprod Med 1979;23:107–114.

Pritchard JA, Cunningham FG, Pritchard SA. The Parkland Memorial Hospital protocol for treatment of eclampsia: evaluation of 245 cases. Am J Obstet Gynecol 1984;148:951–963.

Redman CWG, Beilin LJ, Bonner J. Renal function in preeclampsia. J Clin Path 1976;10:96.

Rodgers GM, Taylor RN, Roberts JM. Preeclampsia is associated with a serum factor cytotoxic to human endothelial cells. Am J Obstet Gynecol 1988;159:908–914.

Romero R, Lockwood C, Oyarzun E, Hobbins JCJ. Toxemia: New concepts in an old disease. Sem Perinatal 1988;12:302–323.

Romero R, Mazor M, Lockwood CJ, et al. Clinical significance, prevalence, and natural history of thrombocytopenia in pregnancy-induced hypertension. Am J Perinatol 1989;6:32–38.

Sibai BM. Pitfalls in diagnosis and management of preeclampsia. Am J Obstet Gynecol 1988;159:1–5.

Sibai BM, Mabie BC, Harvey CJ, Gonzalez AR. Pulmonary edema in severe preeclampsia-eclampsia: analysis of thirty-seven consecutive cases. Am J Obstet Gynecol 1987;156:1174–1179.

Sibai BM, Schneider JM, Morrison JC, et al. The late postpartum eclampsia controversy. Obstet Gynecol 1980;55:74–78.

Sibai BM, Spinnato JA, Watson DL, Hill GA, Anderson GD. Pregnancy outcome in 303 cases with severe preeclampsia. Obstet Gynecol 1984;64:319–325.

Sibai BM, Spinnato JA, Watson DL, Lewis JA, Anderson GD. Eclampsia: IV. Neurological findings and future outcome. Am J Obstet Gynecol 1985;152:184–192.

Sibai BM, Taslimi MM, El-Nazer A, Amon E, Mabie BC, Ryan GM. Maternal-perinatal outcome associated with the syndrome of hemolysis, elevated liver enzymes, and low platelets in severe preeclampsia-eclampsia. Am J Obstet Gynecol 1986;1515:501–509.

Villar MA, Sibai BM. Clinical significance of elevated mean arterial blood pressure in second trimester and threshold increase in systolic or diastolic blood pressure during third trimester. Am J Obstet Gynecol 1989;160:419.

Weiner CP. The mechanism of reduced arterial antithrombin activity in women with preeclampsia. Obstet Gynecol 1988;72:847–849.

CHAPTER FOURTEEN

Septic Shock in Obstetrics

Septic shock in obstetrics is an uncommon event. The incidence of bacteremia, in general, appears to be quite low (approximately 8%–10%). More striking is the fact that patients with bacteremia rarely develop septic shock. Ledger and colleagues identified only a 4% rate of shock in pregnant patients with bacteremia. Obstetrical conditions that have been identified as predisposing to the development of septic shock are listed in Table 14-1.

Fortunately, mortality, which in other medical and surgical specialty fields is extremely high in the face of septic shock, tends to be an infrequent event in obstetrics and gynecology. The incidence of death from sepsis is estimated at 0%–3% in obstetric patients, as compared with 10%–81% in nonobstetric patients.

PATHOPHYSIOLOGY OF SEPTIC SHOCK

Septic shock is a generic term describing vascular collapse secondary to infection caused by a wide variety of microorganisms. For the most part, gram-negative sepsis has been the model used

TABLE 14-1

Bacterial infections associated with septic shock and found in the obstetric patient

	Incidence (%)
Chorioamnionitis	0.5–1
Postpartum endometritis	
Cesarean section	0.5–85
Vaginal delivery	< 10
Urinary tract infections	1–4
Pyelonephritis	1–4
Septic abortion	1–2
Necrotizing fasciitis (postoperative)	< 1
Toxic shock syndrome	< 1

to study this phenomenon in experimental animals. Endotoxin, a complex lipopolysaccharide present in the cell wall of aerobic gram-negative bacteria, appears to be the critical factor in producing the pathophysiologic derangements associated with septic shock. Endotoxin is released from the bacterium at the time of the organism's death.

In patients with gram-positive sepsis, shock also can develop and appears to be closely related to the release of an exotoxin. From a clinical perspective, alterations induced by either of these substances are the same. However, some investigators have suggested that, with regard to these various bacterial toxins, differences may exist at the cellular level. This may be particularly important in the obstetric patient, where mixed polymicrobial infections are identified most often. Although gram-negative coliforms make up a significant portion of the organisms recovered in obstetrical bacteremic subjects, other organisms, including aerobic and anaerobic streptococci, *Bacteroides fragilis,* and *Gardnerella vaginalis,* are found frequently.

The series of events initiated by bacteremia or endotoxins is presented schematically in Figure 14–1. Activation of the comple-

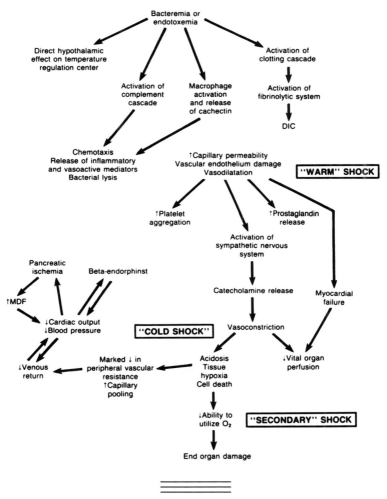

FIGURE 14-1

Pathophysiology of septic shock. (DIC = disseminated intravascular coagulopathy.)

ment cascade plays a central role in this regard. Macrophage-mediated release of the cytokine cachectin is also critical to the progression of this pathologic process. Leukocyte migration and interaction with the organisms result in a release of vasoactive substances such as histamine, serotonin, and bradykinin. These substances, in turn, increase capillary permeability, induce endothelial damage, and promote vasodilation. Phagocytosis and killing of gram-negative bacteria by leukocytes potentiate two further events: an increased release of endotoxin and exposure to the systemic circulation of intracellular toxins such as superoxide free radicals, lysosomes, and hydrogen peroxide. Direct effects of endotoxin and bacterial immunologic complexes are thought also to play an important role in tissue injury. Neutropenia and thrombocytopenia appear to result from endotoxin adherence and sequestration. Immune complex precipitants have been identified within the lung vasculature, and they are thought to be the etiologic basis for the development of adult respiratory distress syndrome (ARDS). Likewise, focal areas of acute tubular necrosis seen in the kidney have been associated with the deposition of inflammatory infiltrates.

Intact reflex responses to these local initial events via sympathetic activation may produce profound vasoconstriction in some organ systems; this vasoconstriction results in a reduction in tissue perfusion. Further capillary leakage also continues and leads to increasing intravascular fluid loss. In addition, cellular hypoxia and acidosis disrupt the ability of individual cells to utilize available oxygen. Marked reductions in peripheral vascular resistance now appear, with extensive capillary pooling of blood. In all likelihood, these pathophysiologic patterns do not follow in series but rather are occurring simultaneously and represent a heterogeneous response, depending on the organ system involved.

The aforementioned events lead to continuing decreases in tissue perfusion and cardiac output. This classic complex is usually referred to as "secondary" or "irreversible shock." A central feature of this stage of shock is the finding of profound myocardial depression, related to the systemic release of a myocardial depressant factor. Subsequent multiple end-organ failures are invariably followed by coma and death.

PREGNANCY AND SEPTIC SHOCK

The peripartum host may be different from the traditional septic shock host in the presence of different microbiologic pathogens and the presentation and course of septic shock. In the experimental animal model, using endotoxin-induced septic shock, Beller and coworkers compared pregnant and nonpregnant responses to fixed doses of lipopolysaccharide. The pregnant animals had a much more pronounced metabolic acidosis than did the controls and had an earlier cardiovascular collapse. Although the pathophysiologic basis for this observation remains speculative, the results suggest that the gravida should be considered a compromised host.

In the experimental model, the fetus and the neonate are much more resistant to the direct deleterious effects of endotoxin than is the mother. Bech-Jansen et al. demonstrated that the fetus and the neonate were capable of tolerating endotoxin doses 10 times those proving to be lethal to the adult pregnant sheep. The investigators hypothesized that these altered effects related to the immature status of the fetus's (and newborn's) vasoactive response. Conversely, Morishima et al. demonstrated profound asphyxia and rapid deterioration in the fetus when a pregnant baboon was administered endotoxin. These effects were thought to result primarily from maternal factors such as hypotension and increased myometrial activity, both of which contribute to a reduction in placental perfusion.

CLINICAL PRESENTATION

From a clinical perspective, septic shock can be classified into three relatively distinct clinical phases: 1) early ("warm") shock, 2) late ("cold") shock, and 3) secondary ("irreversible") shock. The clinical characteristics of each of these phases is shown in Table 14-2. Each of these phases represents a continued downward progression in the course of this disease state.

Laboratory findings are quite variable during the early stages of septic shock. The white blood cell count may be depressed at

TABLE 14-2

Presenting features of septic shock

Early (Warm) Shock

Altered mental status

Peripheral vasodilation (warm skin, flushing)

Tachypnea or shortness of breath

Tachycardia

Temperature instability

Hypotension

Increased cardiac output and decreased peripheral resistance

Late (Cold) Shock

Peripheral vasoconstriction (cool, clammy skin)

Oliguria

Cyanosis

ARDS

Decreased cardiac output and decreased peripheral resistance

Secondary (Irreversible) Shock

Obtundation

Anuria

Hypoglycemia

DIC

Decreased cardiac output and decreased peripheral resistance

Myocardial failure

first; soon afterward, a marked leukocytosis is usually evident. Although there is a transient increase in blood glucose level secondary to catecholamine release and tissue underutilization, hypoglycemia may prevail later when a reduction in gluconeogenesis occurs secondary to hepatic dysfunction. Early evidence of disseminated intravascular coagulation (DIC) may be represented by a decreased platelet count, decreased fibrinogen, elevated fibrin split products, and elevated thrombin time.

Initial arterial blood gases may show a transient respiratory alkalosis. These parameters later reflect an increasing metabolic acidosis, because tissue hypoxia and lactic acid levels increase. Overt evidence of prolonged cellular hypoxia and dysfunction include profound metabolic acidosis, electrolyte imbalances, and DIC. If these symptoms are left unabated, rapid progression to irreversible shock is the rule.

TREATMENT OF SEPTIC SHOCK

Initial intervention in the patient with septic shock should be directed at the following general goals: 1) improvement in functional circulating intravascular volume, 2) establishment and maintenance of an adequate airway to facilitate management of respiratory failure, 3) initiation of diagnostic evaluations to determine the septic focus, and 4) institution of empiric antimicrobial therapy to eradicate the most likely pathogens. If the patient is pregnant, priorities should be directed toward maternal well-being, even in the face of the potential deleterious effects of septic shock on the fetus. Because fetal compromise results primarily from maternal cardiovascular decompensation, improvements in the maternal status will have positive effects on the fetal condition. Furthermore, attempts at delivery of the fetus in a hemodynamically compromised mother may lead to increased risks of fetal distress and the need for more aggressive obstetrical management. In a mother who is already partially decompensated, such iatrogenic insults may produce disastrous results. (This, of course, presumes that the fetal compartment is not the source of sepsis. Under such circumstances, therapy would include attempts at initiating delivery while stabilizing the mother.)

VOLUME EXPANSION

The mainstay of the acute management of septic shock involves volume expansion to correct absolute or relative hypovolemia. Such therapy is always needed and correlates closely with improvement in cardiac output, oxygen delivery, and survival. At times, considerable quantities of fluid are needed because of profound vasodilation, increased capillary permeability, and extravasation of fluid into the extravascular space. The best means of monitoring this crucial component of therapy is with the use of a flow-directed pulmonary artery catheter. The optimal range for the PCWP is 14–16 mm Hg, a point at which ventricular performance is generally optimal, according to the Starling law.

VASOACTIVE DRUG THERAPY

At times, fluid resuscitation proves inadequate in restoring optimal cardiovascular function. Under these circumstances, the use of vasoactive agents is indicated. The most useful agent in this regard is dopamine hydrochloride, a drug with dose-dependent alpha- and beta-adrenergic effects. In very low doses (<5 μg/kg/min), a selective dopaminergic increase in mesenteric and renal blood flow occurs. As the dosage is increased, the predominant effect is to increase myocardial contractility and cardiac output without increasing myocardial oxygen consumption. With doses exceeding 10 μg/kg/min, alpha effects predominate, with marked vasoconstriction and a further reduction in tissue perfusion. Dopamine is administered as a continuous infusion, starting at 2–5 μg/kg/min and titrated according to clinical and hemodynamic responses. Of the various other pressor agents available, most produce a cardiac output increase at the expense of rather significant vasoconstriction. Maintenance of cardiac output is an important goal in the therapy of septic shock; however, because of untoward vasoconstriction, their indications in septic shock are limited to patients in whom blood pressure cannot be supported by dopamine. An exception to this limitation is dobutamine, an inotropic agent that may have fewer chronotropic effects. Of note is the recent demonstration by Rolbin et al. that dopamine decreases uterine blood flow in hypotensive pregnant sheep. Therefore, dopamine and the other vasoactive agents may lead to a compromise in the fetal status while improving the maternal condition. These considerations clearly support the need for external fetal monitoring in the gestationally viable fetus during resuscitation attempts with vasopressor therapy.

OXYGENATION

In the patient with septic shock, peripheral tissue utilization of oxygen is frequently reduced. Two possible mechanisms are thought to play a pivotal role in this phenomenon. First, there is evidence to suggest that cellular dysfunction during later stages of septic shock can lead to underextraction of delivered oxygen. Second, microvascular shunting of blood may decrease local availability of oxygen. An indirect measurement of poor tissue extraction of oxygen is the finding of a high mixed-venous oxygen saturation or the determination of a reduction in the arteriovenous oxygen content difference. Actual peripheral oxygen consumption can be calculated by using the Fick equation; the normal indexed nonpregnant range is 120–140 mL O_2/min/m^2. Clinical improvement in the patient's condition should be reflected in an increase or normalization of peripheral oxygen consumption.

ANTIMICROBIAL THERAPY

In concert with attempts at restoring normal cardiovascular function, the clinician should determine the etiology of sepsis. Because the course of septic shock can be short and fulminant, such a workup must be carried out without delay and empiric antimicrobial therapy started. In most cases, the diagnostic workup should include the microbiologic evaluation of specimens from sputum, blood, urine, amniotic fluid, endometrial cavity, and wound. In patients thought to have chorioamnionitis, transabdominal amniocentesis or cultures taken from a free-flowing internal pressure transducer catheter may be useful.

Empiric therapy in the obstetric patient should include coverage for a wide variety of both aerobic and anaerobic bacteria (both gram-negative and gram-positive). Parenteral therapy that includes a combination of aqueous penicillin (3,000,000 units every 4 hours), an aminoglycoside (80–120 mg every 8 hours), and clindamycin phosphate (600 mg every 6 hours or 900 mg every 8 hours) is recommended. In patients who previously received cephalosporin therapy, additional coverage specifically directed against enterococci may be warranted. In addition, if *Staphylococcus aureus* is a suspected pathogen, a semisynthetic penicillin may be substituted for aqueous penicillin. Because nephrotoxicity is a well-established complication of aminoglycoside usage (and these patients may already have renal compromise), monitoring of peak (6–10 μg/mL) and trough (<2 μg/mL) aminoglycoside levels should be routine. When available, culture results and organism sensitivities should be used to guide more selectively the subsequent antimicrobial therapy.

SURGICAL THERAPY

In a life-threatening condition such as septic shock, extirpation of infected tissues may be needed to ensure survival. In patients with septic abortion, attempts at evacuating the uterus should begin promptly after initiating antibiotics and stabilizing the patient. Septic shock in association with chorioamnionitis in a gestationally viable fetus is treated best by expeditious evacuation of the uterus; this can be accomplished by the vaginal route if maternal hemodynamic parameters are stable and delivery is imminent. Under certain circumstances, after initial maternal resuscitation, a cesarean section may be appropriate, given the increased chance of survival of the fetus and the uncertain risks to the mother if the nidus for infection is not removed rapidly. In the postpartum patient, hysterectomy may be needed if microabscess formation is identified within myometrial tissues or if there is clinical evidence of deterioration in the patient's condition despite appropriate antibiotic therapy. When the diagnosis of septic pelvic thrombophlebitis is entertained, treatment with heparin in combination with broad-spectrum antibiotics is appropriate. If this treatment proves unsuccessful, a surgical approach may be necessary.

Additional measures that require the attention of the clinician include management of electrolyte imbalances, correction of metabolic acidosis, stabilization of coagulation defects, and monitoring of renal function. If the serum glucose levels are depressed, some clinicians advocate the administration of glucose in combination with insulin to improve tissue uptake of the substrate.

Laboratory coagulation abnormalities often tend to reflect a generalized DIC. Aggressive correction of these defects should be pursued. If platelets fall below 10,000–20,000/mm^3, platelet transfusion to prevent spontaneous hemorrhage may be indicated.

Renal function is monitored best with an indwelling catheter and serial creatinine and blood urea nitrogen (BUN) determinations. Serum creatinine concentrations rise at a rate of 0.5–1.5 mg/dL/day. Provided irreversible acute tubular necrosis has not occurred, correction of the hemodynamic and perfusion deficits should result in restoration of renal function.

CONTROVERSIAL TREATMENT MODALITIES

Corticosteroids reduce mortality in animals with experimental septic shock. However, controlled perspective studies in humans have demonstrated no benefit.

Preliminary studies have shown that the use of antibodies specifically directed against endotoxin has reduced mortality in human septic shock patients. Lachman et al. administered antilipopolysaccharide immunoglobulin to obstetric and gynecologic patients in septic shock. In the treated patients, a reduction in both morbidity and mortality was observed. Similarly, monoclonal antibodies directed against the cytokine cachectin have been shown to ameliorate endotoxin–induced shock in the animal model. These new immunoregulatory modalities, when used in combination with conventional antimicrobial agents, show promise in the treatment of septic shock, but have not been approved in the United States.

Beta–endorphins are a group of polypeptides present in the central nervous system. Recent work has suggested that there is a release of this opiatelike substance in the presence of septic shock. After release, this peptide is thought to produce a profound blood pressure reduction, which can be reversed by using narcotic antagonists such as naloxone. It is interesting to note that beta-endorphin levels have been shown to increase progressively throughout gestation. This specific pregnancy-related effect on septic shock remains to be elucidated.

Septic shock

Goals of Therapy

1. Systolic BP >90 mm Hg.
2. Urine output >25 mL/h.
3. Cardiac output >4 L/min.
4. Arterial Po_2 >60 mm Hg.
5. Normal mental status.
6. Eradication of source of infection.

Management Protocol

1. Rapid volume expansion with D_5RL (1000–2000 mL, followed by 150 to 200 mL/h).
2. Administer O_2 to maintain Po_2 >60 mm Hg.
3. Initiate empiric antibiotic therapy: Gentamicin 1.5 mg/kg, then 1 mg/kg I.V. every 8 hours. Clindamycin 900 mg I.V. every 9 hours. Penicillin 3,000,000 units I.V. every 4 hours.
4. Search for surgically correctable origin of infection (abscess, appendicitis, etc.).
5. Use pulmonary artery catheterization if no clinical response to initial volume loading. Optimize preload, with PCWP of 14–15 mm Hg.
6. After optimal preload achieved, begin dopamine if necessary (starting dose 2–5 μg/kg/min), titrated to hemodynamic and clinical response.
7. Consider digitalization or other inotropic support if invasive monitoring parameters—left ventricular stroke work index (LVSWI)—indicated myocardial failure.
8. Control overt hyperthermia with acetaminophen or cooling blanket.

Critical Laboratory Tests

Complete blood count (CBC), platelet count, urinalysis, fibrinogen, prothrombin time, partial thromboplastin time, fibrin split products, electrolytes, blood urea nitrogen (BUN), creatinine, SGPT, SGOT, arterial blood gas, urine and blood cultures, other cultures as clinically indicated, serum lactate, chest x-ray, pelvic/abdominal computed tomography scan or magnetic resonance imaging (MRI) if abscess suspected. Monitor mixed venous oxygen saturation or arterial-venous O_2 content difference.

Consultation

Infectious disease.

Anaphylactic shock in pregnancy

Goals of Therapy

1. Maintain airway and oxygenation.
2. Support blood pressure.
3. Eliminate exposure to inciting agent.
4. Decrease release of vasoactive substances.
5. Monitor fetus, if viable ex utero.

Management Protocol

1. Maintain airway. Intubation or tracheostomy if necessary.
2. Administer oxygen.
3. Epinephrine, 0.5 mg (5 mL of 1:10,000 solution) I.V. or endotracheal q 5–10 minutes (severe reactions). Epinephrine 0.5 mg (0.5 mL of 1:1000 solution) subcutaneous, q 20–30 minutes (mild reactions).
4. Volume expand with normal saline.
5. Hydrocortisone sodium succinate 500 mg, I.V. q 6 hours.
6. Diphenhydramine hydrochloride 50 mg I.V. or P.O.

7. Delay absorbtion (if possible):
   A. For oral antigen, Ipecac 30 cc P.O. then activated charcoal.
   B. For parenteral antigen, venous torniquet proximal to injection site.
8. Support blood pressure as necessary with volume and dopamine.
9. Careful fetal heart rate monitoring if viability has been achieved.

SUGGESTED READING

Beller FK, Schmidt EH, Holzgreve W, et al. Septicemia during pregnancy: a study in different species of experimental animals. Am J Obstet Gynecol 1985;151:967.

Bryan CS, Reynolds KL, Moore EE. Bacteremia in obstetrics and gynecology. Obster Gynecol 1984;64:155.

Kaufman BS, Rackow EC, Falk JL. The relationship between oxygen delivery and consumption during fluid resuscitation of hypovolemic and septic shock. Chest 1984;85:33.

Ledger WJ, Norman M, Gee C, et al. Bacteremia on an obstetric-gynecologic service. Am J Obstet Gynecol 1975;121:205.

Lee W, Clark SL, Cotton DB, et al. Septic shock during pregnancy. Obstet Gynecol 1984;159:410.

Marksad AK, Ona CJ, Stuart RC, et al. Myocardial depression in septic shock: physiologic and metabolic effect of a plasma factor on an isolated heart. Circ Shock [Suppl] 1979;1:35.

Monif GRG, Baer H. Polymicrobial bacteremia in obstetric patients. Obstet Gynecol 1976;48:167.

Packman MI, Rackow EG. Optimum left heart filling pressure during fluid resuscitation of patients with hypovolemic and septic shock. Crit Care Med 1983;11:165.

Parillo JE. Pathogenetic mechanisms of septic shock. N Engl J Med 1993;328:1471.

CHAPTER FIFTEEN

Thyroid Storm in Pregnancy

THYROID FUNCTION TESTS

Most of the pregnancy-induced changes in thyroid physiology are stimulated by hyperestrogenemia. High estrogen levels cause secretion of thyroxine-binding globulin (TBG) enriched with sialic acid, a modification that prolongs its survival in vivo. This results in an increase in TBG and, as a direct consequence, a decrease in triiodothyronine (T_3) resin uptake and an increase in serum levels of thyroxine (T_4) and T_3 (Table 15-1). Total serum levels of T_4 begin to rise during the first trimester and ultimately increase to 9–16 mg%, compared with 5–12 mg% in nonpregnant, euthyroid women. In early pregnancy, when chorionic gonadotropin levels reach their peak, serum levels of free T_4 also increase, and those of thyroid-stimulating hormone (TSH) decrease. For most of pregnancy, however, serum levels of free T_4, free T_3, and TSH are within the normal, nonpregnant range; thus, overt hyperthyroidism does not occur.

It is not generally practical for the clinician to measure either TBG or T_4 in its metabolically active free state. Consequently, T_3 resin uptake is measured to provide an indirect assessment of TBG and to allow the calculation of the free T_4 index. The free

TABLE 15-1
Effects of pregnancy and hyperthyroidism on tests commonly used to evaluate thyroid function

Test	Normal Pregnancy	Hyperthyroidism
TBG	Increased	No change
Total T_4	Increased	Increased
Free T_4	No change	Increased
Total T_3	Increased	Increased
Free T_3	No change	Increased
Thyroid radioiodine uptake	Increased	Increased
T_3	Decreased	Increased
FT_4I^*	No change	No change
$FT_3I^\dagger$	No change	No change

$^*FT_4I$ = Total thyroxine $\times \dfrac{\text{Patient's } RT_3U^\ddagger}{\text{Mean normal } RT_3U \text{ value}}$.

$^\dagger FT_3I$ = Total triiodothyronine $\times \dfrac{\text{Patient's } RT_3U^\ddagger}{\text{Mean normal } RT_3U \text{ value}}$.

$^\ddagger RT_3U$ = Resin T_3 uptake.

T_4 index represents the product of total serum T_4 and T_3 resin uptake and provides a reliable estimate of free T_4 in pregnancy.

CARDIAC FUNCTION IN SEVERE HYPERTHYROIDISM

Frequently observed hemodynamic findings in most hyperthyroid patients include an increase in stroke volume, an increase in pulse rate, and cardiac indices of 5–7 L/min/m². Peripheral circulation is characterized by reduced systemic vascular resistance, reduced circulatory time, and increased blood volume.

Electrocardiogram (EKG) changes in umcomplicated hyperthyroidism have been studied by several investigators. EKG changes consistent with left ventricular hypertrophy were found in 21% of patients and atrial fibrillation in 15%. Less frequent findings include first-degree atrial-ventricular (A-V) block, atrial flutter, Wolff-Parkinson-White syndrome, shortened QT_c interval, increased QRS duration, and complete right bundle branch block. The chest x-ray is normal in uncomplicated hyperthyroidism, and an enlargement of the heart usually signifies congestive heart failure.

Studies of myocardial contractility in long-standing untreated or partially treated hyperthyroidism have shown a significant impairment. The classic work in dogs showed congestive heart failure in 25% of the animals after being treated for 8 months with T_4. Further, although the left ventricular ejection fraction (LVEF) was significantly greater at rest in the hyperthyroid state as compared with the euthyroid state in the same patients, there was a significant decrease in LVEF during exercise. While administration of propranolol during exercise did not correct the decrease in LVEF, these changes were reversible, but often persisted for several weeks after establishment of a biochemical euthyroid state. During pregnancy, cardiac decompensation is most likely to occur in uncontrolled patients who have long histories of Graves' disease and poor compliance and who are in stressful situations such as anemia, infection, and pregnancy-induced hypertension.

Treatment of patients with hyperthyroidism and cardiac compromise requires a careful assessment of the effect of beta-blocking agents prior to their institution. Beta-adrenergic blockade must be used with extreme caution in congestive heart failure since adrenergic stimulation of the heart is one of the major compensating mechanisms in preventing cardiac decompensation. Furthermore, their negative inotropic effect may directly depress myocardial contractility. However, propranolol is effective in controlling atrial fibrillation and severe sinus tachycardia. Because congestive heart failure in pregnancy is often rate-related, propranolol may be used to control the supraventricular rate with careful cardiac monitoring. The use of verapamil in such situations has also been suggested.

━━━━━

THYROID STORM

This is a rare situation in pregnancy, estimated to occur in 2% of pregnancies complicated by thyrotoxicosis. Most cases have occurred either in untreated patients at the time of delivery or during an intercurrent stressful situation. Thyroid storm is a life-threatening condition in which the symptoms of thyrotoxicosis are greatly exacerbated. Acute surgical emergencies, induction of anesthesia, infections, myocardial infarction, diabetic ketoacidosis, and pulmonary embolism are the most common precipitating factors.

The clinical diagnosis (Table 15-2) is suspected in the presence of severe hypermetabolic symptoms (fever over 100°F) and central nervous system (CNS) changes, including irritability, agitation, tremor, or alterations in mental state varying from disorientation to frank psychosis and coma. Cardiovascular manifestations are common and include tachycardia, atrial fibrillation, and congestive heart failure. Nausea, vomiting, and diarrhea are frequent gastrointestinal manifestations, sometimes accompanied by jaundice. The skin is warn and flushed. To consider thyroid storm as a clinical diagnosis, both fever and CNS manifestations must be present. On occasion, thyroid storm may be the first manifestation of thyrotoxicosis. The mortality is significant, especially in patients with severe intercurrent disease.

Laboratory abnormalities include leukocytosis, elevations in hepatic enzymes, and occasionally hypercalcemia. An elevation in both FT_4I and FT_3I are almost always present, although their absolute values many not be different when compared with uncomplicated hyperthyroidism. In general, there is poor correlation between serum concentration of thyroid hormones and the clinical severity of thyrotoxicosis.

Management of thyroid storm includes general and specific measures. The patient should be admitted to the intensive care unit, and the physician should begin a diligent search for a precipitating illness. Intravenous fluids and electrolytes, cardiac monitor, cooling measures, and oxygen therapy are the first steps, along with routine laboratory tests and blood and urine cultures. Spinal fluid examination should be obtained if an underlying neurological disease is suspected. Broad-spectrum antibi-

TABLE 15-2
Clinical manifestations of thyroid storm

Hypermetabolic

Fever > 100°F
Perspiration
Warm skin

Cardiovascular

Tachycardia
Arrhythmias
Congestive heart failure

Central Nervous System

Agitation
Disorientation
Tremor
Delirium
Psychosis
Stupor
Coma

Gastrointestinal

Abdominal pain
Vomiting
Diarrhea
Jaundice

otic therapy should be started until culture results are available. Temperature control measures include a cooling blanket or sponge bath with tepid water and alcohol. Salicylates are not recommended because they may increase free hormone concentrations by inhibiting binding of thyroid hormone to thyroxine-binding proteins. Acetaminophen may be given rectally every 3 to 4 hours. Antithyroid drugs are available only in oral form; therefore, a nasogastric tube is placed if the patient is unable to swallow. Intravenous fluids should be given in quantities sufficient to maintain blood pressure and urine output at acceptable levels. In patients with significant cardiovascular compromise, invasive monitoring of cardiovascular function is recommended.

Once the general measures have been implemented, specific therapy to reduce synthesis and release of thyroid hormones should begin. The goal of antithyroid treatment is to achieve suppression of thyroid action at the tissue level as soon as possible. Several drugs are used simultaneously.

Propylthiouracil (PTU) is the antithyroid drug of choice for thyroid crisis, given in a loading dose of up to 1000 mg orally or via nasogastric tube, followed by 150–300 mg every 6 hours. PTU has the additional beneficial effect of blocking the peripheral conversion of T_4 to T_3. Methimazole in equivalent amounts (1:10 ratio) may be given instead of PTU if the patient is allergic to PTU or if PTU is not available.

Iodides acutely inhibit thyroid hormone secretion; they are given orally as Lugol's solution, 30–60 drops daily in divided doses, or in the form of sodium iodide, 1000 mg I.V. every 8–12 hours. Iodides should be given one hour after the initial dose of PTU or methimazole to avoid the buildup of hormone stores within the gland.

Propranolol is effective in controlling tachycardia. It also blocks the peripheral conversion of T_4 to T_3. Intravenously administered at a rate of 1 mg/min, it is titrated to reduce the heart rate to 100–120 bpm; the effect lasts for about 3 to 4 hours. It may also be given orally or by nasogastric tube, 40–80 mg every 4 to 6 hours. The clinical response is usually rapid, with improvement in tachycardia, fever, tremor, and restlessness.

Adrenal glucocorticoid agents may also be used in the treatment of thyroid storm. Although in the past, these agents were used empirically for treatment of "adrenal exhaustion," they also have a specific role in inhibiting peripheral tissue conversion of

T_4 to T_3. Hydrocortisone, 300 mg/day or equivalent amounts of prednisone (60 mg) or dexamethasone (8 mg) daily are administered in divided doses.

Removal of circulating hormones by plasmapheresis and peritoneal dialysis, although reported to be effective, should be reserved for patients who fail to respond to conventional therapy.

After initial clinical improvement, iodine and glucocorticoids may be discontinued; antithyroid drugs are continued until the patient becomes euthyroid. Ablative therapy with radioactive iodine or surgery is indicated in all patients after an episode of thyroid crisis. In pregnancy, ablative therapy should be postponed until after delivery. In the occasional patient who develops thyroid crisis in the early part of pregnancy, subtotal thyroidectomy in the second trimester is an acceptable therapeutic alternative.

Thyroid storm in pregnancy

Goals of Therapy

1. Control of synthesis and release of thyroid hormone.
2. Reversal of peripheral effects of hyperthyroidism.
3. Prevention or treatment of hypotension, extreme hyperthermia, severe tachycardia, cardiac dysrhythmias, or congestive heart failure.
4. Identification and treatment of precipitating factors.

Management Protocol

1. Transfer to intensive care unit.
2. Judicious hydration with crystalloid solution.
3. Cooling blanket.
4. Acetaminophen 325 mg rectally every 3 hours.
5. Electrocardiographic monitoring.
6. Sodium iodine 0.5:1 g I.V. every 8 hours.
7. Propylthiouracil 1000 mg orally, then 300 mg every 6 hours.
8. Propranolol 1 mg/min I.V. titrated to achieve maternal heart rate of 100–120

or

Propranolol 40–80 mg orally every 4 hours.

9. Hydrocortisone 100 mg I.V. every 8 hours.
10. Search for precipitating cause, especially infection. Treat with broad-spectrum antibiotics (pending culture).

Critical Laboratory Tests

Complete blood count (CBC), electrolytes, blood and urine cultures, thyroid function tests.

Consultation

Medical endocrinology.
Intensivist.
Cardiologist.

SUGGESTED READING

American College of Obstetricians and Gynecologists. Thyroid disease in pregnancy. ACOG Technical Bulletin. Washington, DC: ACOG, 1993.

Burrow GN: The management of thyrotoxicosis during pregnancy. N Engl J Med 1985;313:562.

Davis LE, Lucas MJ, Hankins GDV, Roark ML, Cunningham FG. Thyrotoxicosis complicating pregnancy. Am J Obstet Gynecol 1989;160:63.

Forfar JC, Caldwell GC. Hyperthyroid heart disease. Clin Endocr Metab 1985;14:491.

Forfar JC, Sawers JSA, Muir HC, et al. Left ventricular function in hyperthyroidism: evidence for a reversible myocardiopathy. N Engl J Med 1982;307:1165.

Matsuura N, Konishi J, Fujieda K, et al. TSH-recptor antibodies in mothers with Graves' disease and outcome in their offspring. Lancet 1988;1:14.

Mackin JF, Canary JJ, Pittman CS. Thyroid storm and its management. N Engl J Med 1974;291:1396.

Mori M, Amino N, Tamaki H, Miyai K, Tanizawa O. Morning sickness and thyroid function in normal pregnancy. Obstet Gynecol 1988;72:355.

Piatnek-Leunissen D, Olson RE. Cardiac failure in the dog as a consequence of exogenous hyperthyroidism. Circ Research 1967;20:242.

Singer PA, Mestman JH. Thyroid storm need not be lethal. Contemp OB/GYN, 1983;135.

Tamaki H, Amino N, Aozasa M, Mori M, Iwatani Y, Tachi J, Nose O, Tanizawa O, Miyai K. Universal predictive criteria for neonatal overt thyrotoxicosis requiring treatment. Am J Perinat 1988;5:152.

CHAPTER SIXTEEN

Diabetic Ketoacidosis
in Pregnancy

Diabetic ketoacidosis (DKA) is an acute emergency with fetal loss rates reported in excess of 50%. This complication accounted for most maternal deaths attributable to diabetes in the preinsulin era. Current maternal loss rates are 1% or less, but no substantial reduction in the maternal mortality rate has occurred in the past 25 years. Newly diagnosed diabetes often occurs in women previously not identified as being diabetic presenting in pregnancy with DKA following treatment with beta–agonist tocolytics. Ketoacidosis has also been reported in women with uncomplicated gestational diabetes who were given these agents for preterm labor inhibition. This chapter reviews the pathophysiology of DKA and discusses management approaches to correct fluid imbalance, restore glucose homeostasis, and monitor maternal and fetal condition.

PATHOPHYSIOLOGY

Ketoacidosis results from a relative or absolute lack of circulating insulin in the face of an excess of glucose counterregulatory hormones. Rarely does DKA develop solely due to an insufficient amount of injected insulin; instead, it is associated with an identifiable stress factor, often an infection.

The balance between circulating insulin and glucagon is critical in maintaining normal glucose, amino acid, and lipid homeostasis. Insulin promotes glucose uptake in fat, liver, and skeletal muscle. Adipocytes are stimulated to store free fatty acids, and lipolysis is inhibited. Gluconeogenesis and glycogenolysis are inhibited in the liver. Insulin is also necessary for utilization of free fatty acids in peripheral tissues.

Glucagon augments hepatic ketone production and increases glucose output by inducing glycogenolysis and gluconeogenesis. The stimulation of ketosis is vital to the understanding of the development of DKA. Enhancement of hepatic ketone production by 300%, independent of free fatty acids (FFA) availability, occurs in conditions of glucagon excess.

Catecholamines and cortisol are excreted during conditions of stress, dehydration, and acidosis; the same conditions present during DKA. Epinephrine and norepinephrine stimulate fatty acid release and glycogenolysis. Additionally, the sensitivity of both liver and other tissues to insulin is blunted due to stimulation of the cellular beta-receptors. Free cortisol also enhances ketone production. Regulation of glucose, amino acid, and lipid metabolism is finely balanced by the cellular effects of these hormones.

With falling insulin:glucagon ratios, hyperglycemia and ketosis occur. Oxidative metabolism of ketone bodies yields increased amounts of β-hydroxybutyrate and acetoacetate, the two most prominent ketoacids. These moderately strong acids decrease the pH, and breathing rates increase (Kussmaul respirations), producing a compensatory respiratory alkalosis. Ketone utilization is impaired by the relative lack of insulin, and the body's major source for bicarbonate regeneration is damped. Gluconeogenesis accelerates, driven by glucose counterregulatory hormones, adding to the already elevated circulating levels of glucose while depleting the amino acid stores of the liver.

Concomitant with these metabolic changes, there is a massive shift in fluid and electrolyte balance. These changes are a direct result of the increased osmotic load of solutes presenting to the kidney. Water is excreted proportionate to the elevation in osmotic pressure, causing concomitant loss of electrolytes. As fluid is lost from within the vascular tree, cardiac output and blood pressure fall, leading to vascular collapse and shock. Potassium is lost, along with sodium, due to the osmotic diuresis. Additional potassium may be lost because of the vomiting usually present with acidosis. Intracellular potassium is forced out of cells by the acidosis in exchange for hydrogen ions; thus, serum potassium may appear normal or elevated initially, while total body potassium is actually depleted.

Insulin resistance is encountered due to the relatively large amount of glucagon and other counterregulatory hormones. Shock or coma, with accompanying vascular collapse, further increases the secretion of these compounds.

Fetal loss during episodes of DKA is probably due to a combination of factors. Alterations in maternal fluid and electrolyte balance affect fetal homeostasis. Maternal hypovolemia decreases cardiac output and decreases uterine blood flow. Circulating maternal fatty acids cross to the fetus, as do lactate and glucose. Miodovnik et al. describe ketonemic–induced hypoxia and lactic acidemia in lamb fetuses of hyperglycemic, hyperketotic pregnant ewes. These combined effects favor a reduction in fetal oxygenation and the clearance of metabolic acids.

The sequence of pathophysiologic events generating DKA is shown in Figure 16-1. Therapy seeks to disrupt this cycle, restore intravascular volume, lower serum glucose, correct severe acid-base balance disturbances, and eliminate circulating ketone bodies.

DIAGNOSIS

Though nonspecific, the signs and symptoms of DKA often present a reasonably clear picture that suggests the proper diagnosis. Malaise, headache, dry mouth, weight loss, nausea, and vomiting in the presence of polyuria, polydipsia, and shortness of

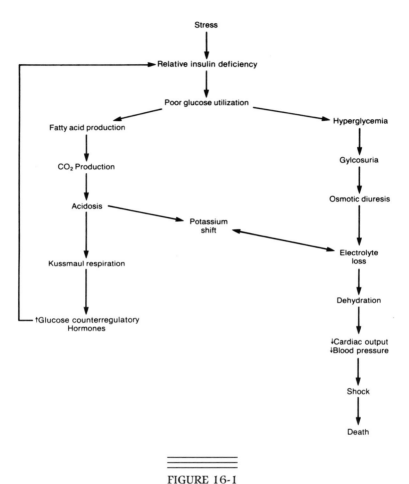

FIGURE 16-1
Sequence of events generating DKA.

breath are usual complaints. Occasionally, there is generalized abdominal pain with elevation of liver transaminase, suggesting abdominal disease. Blood glucose is elevated, but it may be only moderately so during pregnancy; DKA may develop in pregnant patients with serum glucose less than 200 μg%. Ketonemia, measured by the nitroprusside method, is strong in undiluted sera. Acidosis, measured by arterial blood gas determination, shows a pH of less than 7.30. There is an anion gap [$NA - (Cl + HCO_3) \leq 12$ mEq/L]. The reduction in HCO_3 is proportionate to the increased concentration of β-hydroxybutyrate and acetoacetate; thus, the anion gap is equal to the decrease in bicarbonate concentration. If shock is present, lactate is increased, and the metabolic picture is more complex.

Fluid shifts are large in DKA, with water loss in excess of electrolytes due to the osmotic diuresis. Prerenal azotemia is common, with elevation of blood urea nitrogen (BUN) and creatinine. Water deficits are often 100 mL H_2O/kg body weight; occasionally, they may be as high as 150 mL H_2O/kg body weight. This represents total body water deficits of 4–10 L.

Ketone production, triggered by glucagon excess, favors β-hydroxybutyrate formation. Rarely, ketosis is caused exclusively by this compound. Production of acetone, which is very volatile, yields the characteristic fruity breath of DKA. With the administration of insulin, the concentration of β-hydroxybutyrate rapidly declines, but that of acetoacetate remains unchanged. This preferential fall in β-hydroxybutyrate is thought to be due to the decreased production with cessation of lipolysis and enhanced conversion to acetoacetate. Indeed, the concentration of acetoacetate may actually rise. Because nitroprusside measures only acetone and acetoacetate, ketosis may appear to increase after treatment.

Patients thought to be diabetic may have other causes for coma. Alcoholic ketoacidosis, due to accumulation of acetoacetate, dehydration, and malnourishment, generally is associated with normal blood glucose, and ketosis is usually mild to moderate. Hypoglycemic coma is associated with low blood glucose. Lactic acidosis produces acidosis with a large anion gap, but ketone bodies are usually absent or are present in only trace amounts. Serum lactate levels, however, are elevated in this condition, but are usually normal in DKA. Nonketotic, hyperosmolar coma is rarely seen in patients of childbearing age. Dehydration in this condition is profound, and serum glucose is markedly elevated, often over 1000 mg/dL. Ketonemia and ketoacidosis, however, are not present.

———

TREATMENT

The benchmarks of therapy for DKA involve correcting the metabolic and fluid deficits imposed by hyperglycemia and ketosis. Comatose patients should be given a challenge of 25 mL of 50% glucose after a serum glucose is drawn. A protocol for management of pregnant patients with DKA is outlined at the conclusion of this chapter. Serum glucose, ketones, electrolytes and bicarbonate, creatinine, and BUN should be obtained immediately. An arterial blood gas will aid in analyzing the degree of acidosis present. An intravenous line should be placed immediately to rehydrate the patient whose fluid deficits often exceed 6 L and occasionally reach 10–12 L.

Fluid replacement is perhaps of more initial importance than the institution of insulin therapy. Severe dehydration is the cause of obtundation and impaired renal function. Ketoacids are concentrated by the fluid deficit induced from the osmotic diuresis of hyperglycemia. Because patients have lost more water than salt, hypotonic solutions should be used. An initial infusion of a liter of 0.45 or 0.9 normal saline, given over the first hour, is recommended. Infusion of similar solutions at a rate of 250–500 mL/h should follow until at least 75% of the fluid deficit has been corrected. Generally 6–8 L of fluid over the ensuing 24 hours is required, depending upon the patient's state of dehydration.

As insulin is given and blood glucose falls below 250 mg%, fluid replacement should be continued with 5% glucose solutions. Five percent dextrose in water (D_5W) or 5% dextrose, with one-half the normal saline ($D_51/2NS$), are well suited. Avoid lactate-containing solutions, as this could theoretically contribute to the acid load of the patient.

Potassium replacement can begin once renal competence is established. It is usually not necessary to monitor urine flow with an indwelling catheter, as this is a potential cause of infection. Total potassium lost by vomiting and passive osmotic diuresis usually is in the range of 5–10 mEq/kg of body weight. The acidosis displaces some of the intracellular potassium to the extracellular compartment so that measured serum potassium may not reflect the true level of deficiency. Correction of the acidosis allows potassium to reenter the cell, and serum potassium falls. Replace potassium with potassium chloride (KCl) solution added to the intravenous fluids at a concentration of no more than 40 mEq/L. Reevaluation of the potassium concentration every 24 hours is important because significant fluctuations occur with correction of fluid and acid–base balance. Insulin also promotes cellular phosphate utilization. Although complications of hypophosphatemia in patients with DKA are very rare, some authorities advocate the use of potassium phosphate solution in maintenance intravenous fluids.

Bicarbonate replacement is rarely indicated and is not necessary unless the arterial pH is <7.10. If the pH is below 7.10, correction with a single ampule of bicarbonate (44 mEq sodium bicarbonate) is usually sufficient. Sodium bicarbonate should be administered in a liter of 0.45 normal saline rather than injected from the ampule. If the pH fails to correct to 7.10, it may be necessary to administer another ampule. Rapid correction of the acid–base balance with bicarbonate can lead to overcorrection, with an iatrogenic metabolic alkalosis, or to a paradoxical fall in cerebrospinal fluid pH. This is caused by the rapid diffusion of volatile carbon dioxide across the blood–brain barrier, while less volatile bicarbonate crosses much more slowly. The resultant effect is a worsening cerebral acidosis and increased obtundation despite correction of systemic pH.

Patients with DKA are insulin resistant, and the degree of hyperglycemia encountered may be surprisingly low. Insulin therapy should be instituted after initial blood work is drawn and hydration begun. Regular insulin, given intravenously, is the method of choice. Subcutaneous injection of regular insulin can be employed if the patient is not in circulatory collapse (decreased peripheral perfusion occurs with both acidosis and dehydration). An initial priming dose of 0.1 units of regular insulin/kg body weight, intravenous push, can be given while an infusion is being mixed. An infusion of 8–10 units per hour is usually necessary to overcome the insulin resistance and to begin lowering blood sugar. Intravenous insulin infusions can be piggybacked into the intravenous site for precise control of insulin administration. Serum glucose should be monitored every one to two hours to measure the effectiveness of treatment. If serum glucose does not respond within 2 hours with a decrease of at least 25%, the rate of insulin infusion should be doubled. Once the blood glucose level falls to 250 mg/dL, fluid replacement should be switched to a solution containing 5% glucose. The insulin infusion rate should be cut in half at this time, and hourly glucose determinations should be made. When blood glucose declines below 150 mg/dL, a basal rate of one to two units per hour is usually sufficient to maintain homeostasis.

Once the acidosis and dehydration is corrected and glucose levels are below 150 mg/dL, the patient may be given an appropriate diet and restarted on a subcutaneous insulin dose of intermediate and short-acting insulin. Table 16-1 shows a rule of thumb for calculating the dose for those individuals not previously on a split dose of insulin before the DKA episode.

The underlying cause of DKA should not be neglected. Correction of the metabolic derangements can only be successful if the underlying cause is treated. A thorough search for infection should be made within the first 30 minutes of treatment. Skin and soft tissues should be inspected for infection, urine should be microscopically analyzed and cultured, and the lungs should be carefully auscultated and sputum samples obtained if relevant. If an underlying infection is discovered, it should be treated rapidly while fluid and insulin are being given.

The fetus should be carefully monitored if it has attained a potentially viable gestational age. Delivery of a compromised fetus should be delayed unless the mother is metabolically stable. If signs of fetal distress persist after correction of major maternal deficits, intervention may be considered. Correction of the maternal deficiencies generally rapidly corrects the metabolic deficits of the fetus as well. Hence, all efforts should be directed toward adjusting maternal acid–base and fluid balance. Electronic fetal heart rate monitoring is recommended, but intervention for fetal distress should be tempered by assessment of the maternal condition.

Beta-mimetic tocolytic therapy for patients with DKA is contraindicated. These agents antagonize insulin action and can actually induce DKA in pregnant women. For most diabetic women and for all patients in DKA, magnesium sulfate ($MgSO_4$) is the tocolytic agent of choice. Loading doses of $MgSO_4$ should be 4-g I.V. push, and a maintenance infusion of at least 2 g/h. Occasionally, higher infusion rates are necessary to maintain therapeutic drug levels. Infusion rates as high as 6 g/h may be necessary.

TABLE 16-1

Guideline for dosage calculation

Priming dose: 0.1 unit regular insulation/kg body weight, given I.V.

Initial I.V. infusion dose: 0.1 unit regular insulin/kg of body weight, per hour.

Preparation of IV Infusion

1. Place 100 units regular insulin/L $\frac{1}{2}$ N saline (1 unit regular insulin/mL).
2. Run and discard first 50–100 mL of solution through the infusion system. This saturates insulin binding sites on the plastic tubing.
3. Begin infusion at initial I.V. dose.
4. Decrease infusion rate hourly by one-half when BG* reaches 250 mg/dL. Switch I.V. fluids to $D_5 \frac{1}{2}$ N saline at this time.
5. When patient is eating, switch to depot insulin (see below). Taper I.V. insulin infusion over next 4–6 hours, then discontinue.

Calculation of Subcutaneous Insulin Dose

Total daily dose: 0.5–0.8 units per kg of body weight, per 24 h, (use 0.5 units/kg if < 20 wks; 0.8 if ≥ 30 wks).

1. $\frac{2}{3}$ total dose in A.M.

   $\frac{2}{3}$ of A.M. dose as NPH or lente.

   $\frac{1}{3}$ of A.M. dose as regular.

2. $\frac{1}{3}$ total dose in P.M.

   $\frac{1}{2}$ of P.M. dose as regular before dinner.

   $\frac{1}{2}$ of P.M. dose as NPH or lente at 10 P.M.

*BG = blood glucose.

Diabetic ketoacidosis in pregnancy

Goals of Therapy

1. Rehydration.
2. Restoration of electrolyte homeostasis.
3. Correction of acidemia.
4. Normalization of serum glucose.
5. Elimination of underlying cause.
6. Return of maternal-fetal homeostasis.

Management Protocol

1. Infuse 0.9 saline, 1000 mL over first hour, 1000 mL over subsequent 2 hours, 250 mL/h thereafter.
2. Change I.V. solution to D_5NS as serum glucose falls below 250 mg/dL.
3. Add KCl 20 to 40 mEq/L to I.V. fluids after adequate urine output is established.
4. A. Administer regular insulin 0.1 U/kg I.V. push.
   B. Begin an infusion of 5–10 U/h.
   C. Double infusion rate if serum glucose has not decreased by 25% in 2 hours.
   D. Reduce infusion to 1–2 U/h as serum glucose falls below 150 mg/dL.
5. Administer sodium bicarbonate 44 mEq I.V. in 1000 mL 0.45 NS for arterial pH <7.10.
6. Search for underlying cause, such as infection.

Critical Laboratory Tests

Serum electrolytes, glucose, arterial blood gas, complete blood count (CBC), bicarbonate, blood urea nitrogen (BUN), ketones.

Consultation

Internal medicine.

SUGGESTED READING

Drury MI, Greene AT, Stronge JM. Pregnancy complicated by clinical diabetes mellitus: a study of 600 pregnancies. Obstet Gynecol 1977;49:519.

Foster DW, McGarry JD. The metabolic derangements and treatment of diabetic ketoacidosis. N Engl J Med 1975;308:159.

Gabbe SG, Mestman JH, Hibbard LT. Maternal mortality in diabetes mellitus: An 18-year survey. Obstet Gynecol 1976;48:549.

Genuth SM. Constant intravenous insulin infusion in diabetic ketoacidosis. JAMA 1973;223:1348.

Lipshitz J, Vinik AI. The effects of hexoprenoline, a β_2-sympathomimetic drug, on maternal glucose, insulin, glucagon, and free fatty acid levels. Am J Obstet Gynecol 1978;130:761.

Lobue C, Goodlin RC. Treatment of fetal distress during diabetic ketoacidosis. J Reprod Med 1978;20:101.

CHAPTER SEVENTEEN

Adult Respiratory Distress Syndrome

Adult respiratory distress syndrome (ARDS) is a diagnosis that includes both primary lung epithelial injuries initiated via the airways and endothelial injuries initiated via the pulmonary vasculature. The injuries result in increased pulmonary capillary permeability, loss of lung volume, and shunting with resultant arterial hypoxemia. Physiologic criteria required for the diagnosis of ARDS are listed in Table 17-1. In pregnant patients, diffuse sepsis, viral pneumonia, hemorrhagic shock, and aspiration of gastric contents are the most common single-agent causes of ARDS. Over 70% of patients, however, will have some combination of sepsis, shock, trauma, fluid overload, or aspiration as the etiology of the injury. Multiplicity of cause is, in fact, the rule with acute and severe lung injury.

Regardless of the initial inciting agent, a cascade is initiated which results in increased pulmonary capillary permeability and extravasation of fluid from the vasculature into the interstitium of the lung and the alveolus itself. With inhaled irritants, such as noxious chemicals or gastric aspiration, the initial injury is to the alveolar epithelial lining and, if severe, sequentially to vascular endothelial cells. The complement system, polymorphonuclear

TABLE 17-1

Physiologic criteria for the diagnosis of the adult respiratory distress syndrome

P_{O_2}	<50 with F_{IO_2} >0.6
Pulmonary capillary wedge	≤12 mm Hg
Total respiratory compliance (usually 20–30 mL/cm)	<50 mL/cm
Functional residual capacity reduced	
Shunt (Q_S/Q_T)	>30%
Dead space (V_D/V_T)	>60%
Alveolar-arterial gradient on 100% oxygen	≥350 mm Hg

leukocytes (PMNs), macrophages, platelets, and the endothelium all may play important roles in perpetuating the injury after it is initiated.

CLINICAL COURSE

The course of ARDS can be divided into four distinct histologic and clinical phases:

PHASE 1

The initial injury is accompanied by minimal or no physical findings other than spontaneous hyperventilation and respiratory allealosis. Arterial oxygenation is usually adequate.

PHASE 2

The latent period is characterized by minor auscultatory and radiographic evidence of pulmonary disease, decreased lung compliance, and increased intrapulmonary shunting of blood. Histologically, these two stages are characterized by progressive formation of alveolar and interstitial edema and movement of red blood cells and inflammatory cells into the interstitium. Damage to type I alveolar cells occurs, and hyaline membrane formation begins.

PHASE 3

Manifest from 24 to 72 hours after the initial onset, phase 3 is characterized by acute respiratory failure, with marked dyspnea, tachypnea, and hypoxemia. Further loss of lung volume results in worsening of both pulmonary compliance and intrapulmonary shunting. Chest radiographs demonstrate bilateral lung involvement, and auscultation reveals diffuse abnormalities. Intubation, assisted ventilation, and high inspired oxygen concentrations are often required to sustain life. The alveolar septum in phase 3 is 5–10 times thicker than normal and is infiltrated by leukocytes, plasma cells, and histiocytes. Hyaline membranes begin to organize, with proliferation of fibroblasts and infiltration of inflammatory cells. Type II alveolar cells proliferate and cover the previously denuded basement membrane. It is believed that, if the patient survives, type II alveolar cells can differentiate into type I cells.

PHASE 4

The pathologic and physiologic derangements are essentially irreversible. Intrapulmonary shunts in excess of 30% result in severe refractory hypoxemia. The marked increase in dead space, often exceeding 60% of tidal volume, leads to hypercapnia and an inability to ventilate, as well as an inability to oxygenate the patient. Metabolic and respiratory acidosis result in myocardial irritability and dysfunction; this dysfunction often leads to a terminal myocardial arrest. Intraalveolar fibrosis and fibroblastic infiltration of the alveolar septum combine to form massive tissue plates that completely mask the original architecture of the lung parenchyma.

———

CLINICAL MANAGEMENT

Optimal treatment of acute pulmonary failure in association with pregnancy entails preventing the development of end-stage disease by early and aggressive treatment. The cause of lung failure must be identified and corrected as quickly as possible. Therapy should not compound or worsen the initial injury (i.e., injudicious use of blood, fluid, or oxygen therapy). There should be no hesitancy to proceed with intubation and assisted ventilation if the patient is in respiratory failure or if respiratory failure appears to be imminent. Guidelines for the diagnosis of respiratory failure are presented in Table 17-2. Similarly, invasive hemodynamic monitoring should be considered early to avoid any iatrogenic worsening of the pulmonary injury and to better assess therapeutic manipulations.

———

OXYGEN DELIVERY

Oxygen delivery is directly proportional to cardiac output; if cardiac output falls by 50%, so does oxygen delivery. Conversely, doubling cardiac output will double oxygen delivery. Secondly, the overwhelming majority of oxygen transported in blood is bound to hemoglobin and is not in solution. Accordingly, oxygen delivery can be improved dramatically by correction of anemia; each gram of hemoglobin carries 1.35 mL of oxygen when 97% saturated and 1.25 mL when 90% saturated. Third, increasing the arterial pressure of oxygen (Pao_2) above 100 torr has very little effect on oxygen delivery. For each 100-torr increase in the Pao_2 above 100 mm Hg, an additional 0.3 mL of oxygen is carried in solution in each 100 mL of maternal blood. Because oxygen unequivocally contributes to further lung injury at high inspired concentrations, tissue oxygen delivery should be increased primarily by optimization of cardiac output and hemoglobin and only secondarily by increasing the inspired concentration of oxygen. Reasonable goals in caring for

TABLE 17-2

Guidelines for instituting ventilator therapy

	Normal	**Intubate**
Respiratory rate	12–20	>35
Vital capacity (mL/kg)	65–75	<15
FEV_1 (mL/kg)	50–60	<10
Inspiratory force (cm H_2O)	75–100	<25
Pao_2 (mm Hg)	100–75 (air)	<70 mask ($Fio_2 = 0.4$) <300 ($Fio_2 = 1.0$)
$Paco_2$ (mm Hg)	35–45	>55
V_D/V_T	0.35–0.40	>0.6

women with severe lung injury are to obtain a Pao_2 of 60 mm Hg, corresponding to a 90% hemoglobin saturation under unusual conditions.

SHUNT (Q_S/Q_T) ASSESSMENT

In severe lung injury, the loss of volume results in a fall in compliance and in ventilation–perfusion inequality and its resultant pulmonary veno-arterial shunt. A calculated veno-arterial shunt is a summation expression of the ventilation–perfusion relationships that exist in over 300 million alveolar capillary units. At rest, the normal shunt is 2%–5% of the cardiac output that results from the coronary, bronchial, and pleural circulations. A shunt of 10%–15% may exist as a manifestation of the pulmonary dysfunction associated with major trauma or surgery and is usually secondary to microatelectasis. A shunt of 25% or greater, despite adequate respiratory therapy, is strongly suggestive of ARDS.

Shunt can be estimated by analysis of an arterial blood sample and use of a nomogram, or it can be calculated using simultaneously obtained arterial and pulmonary artery blood samples. Use of blood obtained from a central venous line for shunt calculations is discouraged since it does not represent a true mixed venous specimen and leads to an average 20% underestimate of shunt. If a nomogram and a single arterial blood sample are used, the greatest accuracy in shunt estimate is achieved by having the patient breath 100% oxygen. Shunt calculation serves as a useful index of lung function over time, as well as for the assessment of benefits of acute changes of therapy. In acute lung injury and respiratory failure, shunt tends to mirror the cardiac output by rising and falling in parallel with the cardiac output. Accordingly, proper interpretation of the shunt fraction requires a knowledge of the cardiac output because a stable shunt in the face of increasing cardiac output represents improved lung function, whereas a stable shunt and falling cardiac output are ominous.

MECHANICAL VENTILATION

Mechanical ventilation in patients with acute respiratory failure requires a volume-cycled ventilator. Appropriate initial settings include a rate of 12 breaths/min, tidal volume of 15 mL/kg body weight, a sigh volume of 200–400 mL above tidal volume, a positive end-expiratory pressure (PEEP) of 5 cm of water, and 100% inspired oxygen. An arterial blood sample is analyzed in approximately 20 minutes and the ventilator adjusted to obtain a $Pa_{O_2} \geq 60$ mm Hg or a 90% hemoglobin saturation and a pressure of carbon dioxide (Pa_{CO_2}) of 35–45 mm Hg. The Pa_{O_2} is a reflection of oxygenation and is determined more by the shunt than by the inspired concentration of oxygen delivered. Adequacy of ventilation, however, is determined by the arterial pressure of carbon dioxide (Pa_{CO_2}) and should be normalized by changes in the ventilatory rate or in the tidal volume. Assessment of changes in shunt, mixed venous oxygen saturation, compliance, and cardiac output allow the clinician to decide whether an adjustment of tidal volume or of respiratory rate can best be used to adjust minute ventilation.

POSITIVE END-EXPIRATORY PRESSURE (PEEP)

With severe lung injury and high intrapulmonary shunt fractions, it may not be possible to oxygenate the patient adequately even on 100% oxygen. Criteria used as indications for the addition of PEEP include a static compliance of <40 mL/cm H_2O, a shunt fraction exceeding 20%, an alveolar–arterial oxygen gradient on 100% oxygen exceeding 400 mm Hg, or an inability to achieve a 90% hemoglobin saturation in arterial blood. PEEP is almost universally successful in decreasing shunt by recruiting collapsed alveoli. At low levels (5–15 cm H_2O), PEEP usually can be employed safely without invasive cardiovascular monitoring. At the higher levels, however, venous return to the right heart can be impaired and result in a fall in cardiac output. High levels of PEEP can also result in overdistention of alveoli, falling compliance, and barotrauma. PEEP should be adjusted, whether increasing or decreasing the level, in small increments (i.e., ≤5 cm H_2O), with the effect on the patient's status documented prior to any further adjustments. Additionally, the PEEP should not be discontinued when collecting hemodynamic information, such as pulmonary capillary wedge pressure (PCWP) measurements. Such sudden changes in PEEP can result in significant clinical deterioration of the patient.

FLUID THERAPY

Treatment of acute respiratory failure requires assiduously detailed attention to fluid balance because fluid overload further compromises the patient's pulmonary status and contributes to progression of the basal injury. Intake and output records are mandatory and should be supplemented with daily weights. A patient on mechanical ventilation retains an extra liter of fluid per day; 300 mL of the liter result from humidification of air, and 700 mL result from arginine vasopressin stimulation via increased intrathoracic pressure. Because ARDS is characterized by a pulmonary permeability lung defect and a tendency, even at normal pressures, to leak fluid into the interstitium, we strive to maintain the lowest PCWP possible while avoiding a fall in cardiac output.

PROPHYLACTIC ANTIBIOTICS

The routine use of prophylactic antibiotics in acute respiratory failure is not advised. In the critically ill patient, however, colonization with gram-negative bacteria is common, and many patients with acute respiratory failure do develop concurrent pulmonary infection. Antibiotic treatment is reserved for patients who develop clinical signs of bacterial suprainfection.

WEANING AND EXTUBATION

Weaning and extubation should not be attempted until all other organ system failures or compromises have been resolved lest the attempt fail and the patient sustain further pulmonary injuries. Because both high inspired oxygen concentrations and high levels of PEEP have associated complications, these variables should be the first tapered. Once the fraction of inspired oxygen (FIO_2) is reduced to 0.3 and the PEEP to 5 cm H_2O, lung mechanics should be tested at the bedside prior to further weaning. Using a Wright's spirometer, the forced vital capacity can be tested and should measure at least 15 mL/kg body weight. The patient should also be able to generate a negative pressure or inspiratory force of 20–25 cm H_2O and have a resting minute ventilation of less than 10 L. Intermittent mandatory ventilation (IMV) has proven very effective as a technique of weaning pregnant women. Once the FIO_2 is reduced to 0.3–0.4 and the PEEP to 5 cm of H_2O, decrease the number of ventilator-assisted breaths to one or two per minute and then extubate the patient.

Alternatively, trials on a T-piece can be used to assess the ability of the patient to be extubated. Using this approach, we prefer to maintain 5 cm of positive airway pressure in order to prevent loss of lung volume. If the patient maintains satisfactory blood gases, we proceed with extubation. Serial monitoring of blood gases is required postextubation, just as when intubated, and supplemental oxygen may be provided by face mask.

Adult respiratory distress syndrome (ARDS)

Goals of Therapy

1. To identify and climinate the causal agent.
2. To achieve:
   Pa_{O_2} >60 mm Hg or 90% hemoglobin saturation.
   Pv_{O_2} >30 mm Hg.
   Pa_{CO_2} 35–40 mm Hg.

Management Protocol

1. Identify that a lung injury has been sustained and eliminate the causal agent.
2. Assess pulmonary function:
   A. $Pa_{O_2} \div Fi_{O_2}$.
      >3 = good function.
      <3 = suspect injury.
   B. 100% oxygen × 2 minutes.
      Pa_{O_2} 400 mm Hg: probably hypoventilation. Aggressive pulmonary toilet and/or incentive spirometry.
      Pa_{O_2} 300–400 mm Hg: possible early ARDS. Aggressive pulmonary toilet; supplemental mask oxygen; monitor with pulse oximetry. Reevaluate immediately if there is any clinical, laboratory deterioration.
      Pa_{O_2} 300 mm Hg: probable ARDS. Intubate, ventilate.
3. Maximize oxygen delivery to tissue. Correct anemia, hypothermia, and alkalosis. Optimize cardiac output via pulmonary artery catheter guided hemodynamic manipulation.
4. Avoid therapeutic pitfalls:
   A. Fluid overload: daily weights, intake and output balance, invasive hemodynamic monitoring.
   B. Oxygen toxicity: use minimum Fi_{O_2} required to achieve a Pa_{O_2} of 60 mm Hg or a 90% hemoglobin saturation.
   C. Barotrauma: limit by use of "best" PEEP.

D. Iatrogenic lung injury: administration of colloid, mannitol, and hetastarch in the setting of a permeability lung injury should be avoided.

E. Nosocomial infections: sinus infections in intubated patients, urinary tract infections resulting from indwelling catheter, and phlebitis from peripheral and central lines should be identified. Central and peripheral intravenous lines should be changed every 72 hours.

Critical Laboratory Tests

Arterial blood gases, mixed venous blood gases, complete blood count (CBC), electrolytes, chest x-ray.

Consultation

Respiratory therapy, pulmonary medicine, intensivists.

SUGGESTED READING

Ashbaugh DG, Bigelow DB, Petty TL, et al. Acute respiratory distress in adults. Lancet 1967;2:319.

Cunningham FG, Lucas MJ, Hankins GDV. Pulmonary injury complicating antepartum pyelonephritis. Am J Obstet Gynecol 1987;156:797–807.

Pontoppidan H, Geffin B, Lowenstein E. Acute respiratory failure in the adult. N Engl J Med 1972;287:690.

Pontoppidan H, Geffin B, Lowenstein E. Acute respiratory failure in the adult. N Engl J Med 1972;287:799.

Rinaldo JE, Rogers RM. Acute respiratory distress syndrome. Changing concepts of lung injury and repair. N Engl J Med 1982;306:900.

CHAPTER EIGHTEEN

Severe Acute Asthma
in Pregnancy

Pregnancy may or may not affect the course of asthma in any individual patient. In the large retrospective studies published to date, roughly equal numbers of patients experienced improvement in their asthma, remained unchanged, or noted worsening disease. Over 40% of patients will require alterations in therapy at some time during gestation. The natural history of asthma during one pregnancy tends to be repeated in subsequent gestations. Approximately 10% of pregnant women with asthma experience exacerbations during labor and delivery.

Asthma can substantially alter pregnancy outcome. Several studies have reported significant increases in rates of abortion, preterm labor, low birth weight, intrauterine growth retardation, and neonatal hypoxia in asthmatic pregnant patients with an overall perinatal mortality rate double that of controls. With severe asthma (repetitive attacks, persistent symptoms, or status asthmaticus), the perinatal mortality rate approaches 28%.

Severe asthma during pregnancy is associated with a definite risk to the life of the mother. The mortality rate is over 40% when asthma has progressed to the point of requiring mechanical ventilation. Studies analyzing the causes of death in severe asthma have shown that most occur outside of a hospital and that the severity of the disease was usually not appreciated by the patient or the physician. Thus, it is essential that the obstetrician thoroughly evaluate and aggressively manage any pregnant woman presenting with reactive airway disease.

PATHOPHYSIOLOGY

Pathologic examination of the lung from patients who have died of status asthmaticus discloses several characteristic features. These include desquamation of the respiratory epithelium, bronchial smooth muscle hypertrophy, thickening of the basement membrane, and a dense, eosinophil-laden mucoid exudate. Other findings may include mucosal edema, mucus gland hypertrophy, vascular and lymphatic obstruction, and hyperinflated airways.

CLINICAL COURSE

The functional result of bronchospasm is airway obstruction with a concomitant decrease in airflow. As airways constrict, the work of breathing increases, and patients experience chest tightness, wheezing, or dyspnea. Subsequent alterations in oxygenation are primarily the result of ventilation/perfusion (V/Q) mismatching as the distribution of airway narrowing during an acute attack is uneven. With mild disease, initial hypoxia is well compensated for, as reflected by a normal arterial oxygen tension and decreased carbon dioxide, with resultant respiratory alkalosis. As airway narrowing worsens, V/Q defects increase, and hypoxemia ensues. With severe obstruction, ventilation becomes impaired enough to result in early CO_2 retention. Superimposed on hyperventilation, this may only be seen as an arterial CO_2 tension returning to the normal range. Finally, with critical obstruction, respiratory failure follows, characterized by hypoxemia, hypercarbia, and acidemia. At this extreme, O_2 consumption and cardiac work are increased, and the magnitude of pulmo-

TABLE 18-1

Clinical stages of asthma

Arterial Blood Gases

Stage	P_{O_2}	P_{CO_2}	pH	FEV, peak flow % predicted	Comment
I	Normal	↓	↑	65–80	Mild respiratory alkalosis
II	↓	↓	↑	50–64	Respiratory alkalosis
III	↓	Normal	Normal	35–49	Danger zone
IV	↓	↑	↓	35	Respiratory acidosis

nary hypertension is frequently severe. The clinical stages of asthma are outlined in Table 18-1.

While such changes in pulmonary function are generally reversible and well tolerated in the healthy nonpregnant individual, even the early stages of asthma may pose grave risk to the gravida and her fetus. Maternal factors responsible for this include 1) increased basal metabolic rate and O_2 consumption, 2) a decreased diffusing capacity, 3) decreased available buffer, and 4) pregnancy-induced alterations in lung volumes. Most importantly, as pregnancy progresses, functional residual capacity (FRC) decreases 10%–25% and frequently falls below the critical closing volume, a phenomenon much more likely to occur during the advanced stages of pregnancy. The smaller FRC and the increased effective shunt thus render the gravida more rapidly susceptible to the effects of hypoxia. Clinically, only 30 seconds of apnea are needed to drop maternal arterial O_2 tension to less than 60 mm Hg.

As the mother increases ventilation to maintain oxygen tension, respiratory alkalosis develops. Such maternal alkalosis may adversely affect the fetus before maternal oxygenation is compromised. Because the fetus may be in jeopardy before maternal disease becomes severe, the obstetrician should take an aggressive approach to the management of any pregnant woman presenting with asthma.

CLINICAL MANAGEMENT

Outpatient management of asthma in pregnancy must be undertaken cautiously, and we recommend liberal hospitalization in patients with acute disease. A patient's subjective impression of the severity of her asthma frequently does not accurately reflect objective measures of airway function or ventilation. Physical examination of the patient with asthma, while helpful in establishing the diagnosis, is also an inaccurate predictor of the severity of airway disease. Expiratory wheezing correlates with neither objective measures of airflow nor derangements in arterial blood gas analysis. Indeed, an increase in auscultated wheezing may indicate an increase in airflow, while the absence of wheezing may indicate critical airway narrowing and absent flow. Historical factors that should warn the physician of the possibility of rapid progression and potentially fatal airway obstruction include a recent history of status asthmaticus, prior use of corticosteroids, prolonged hospitalization, or a history of endotracheal intubation.

ARTERIAL BLOOD GASES

Care must be taken to interpret results in light of normal values for pregnancy. A normal maternal PaO_2 varies from 101 to 108 mm Hg early in pregnancy and falls to 90–100 mm Hg near term, secondary to an increased critical closing volume. These changes are responsible for the widened alveolar-arterial oxygen gradient $[P(A - a)O_2]$, which averages 20 mm Hg in the third trimester. The normal physiologic increase in minute ventilation during pregnancy is reflected by a $PaCO_2$ of 27–32 mm Hg and an increase in pH from 7.40 to 7.45. Consequently, a $PaCO_2$ greater than 35 mm Hg with a pH less than 7.35 in the presence of a falling PaO_2 should be considered respiratory failure in a pregnant asthmatic.

PULMONARY FUNCTION TESTS

Measurement of either the FEV_1 or the peak expiratory flow rate (PEFR) can help both to assess the severity of obstruction and to monitor the response to therapy. Clinically useful pulmonary function tests are not altered by pregnancy. Several investigations have shown that an FEV_1 of less than 1 L or 20% of predicted correlates with severe disease manifested by hypoxia, a poor response to therapy, and a high relapse rate. Unfortunately, bedside spirometry equipment is not commonly available. Peak flow rates, however, may now be measured with simple, hand-held spirometers that are operated entirely by the patient. Peak flow rates in acute asthma less than 100 L/min correlate well with severe obstruction. Pulmonary function tests should not be used to the exclusion of arterial blood gases in management of the pregnant asthmatic, however, because, in over 16% of acute asthmatics whose FEV_1 is 1.0 L or more, the PaO_2 is less than 60 mm Hg.

TREATMENT

Therapy should be directed toward correcting maternal hypoxia, relieving inflammation and bronchospasm, assuring adequate ventilation, and optimizing uteroplacental function (Figure 18-1 through Figure 18-6). The first step is administration of supplemental oxygen to the mother, with a goal of maintaining a PaO_2 greater than 65 mm Hg or an O_2 saturation of 95% or more. This can usually be achieved with a face mask and a fraction of inspired oxygen (FIO_2) of 35%–60%, without causing hypercarbia. The patient should be placed in a near-sitting position, with leftward tilt, especially if in the third trimester.

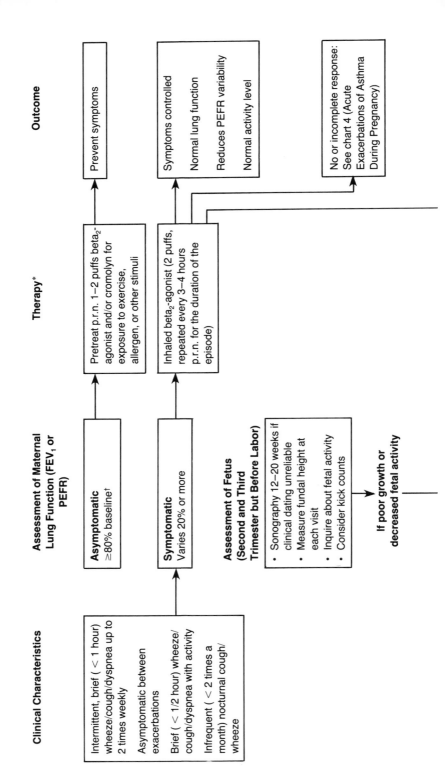

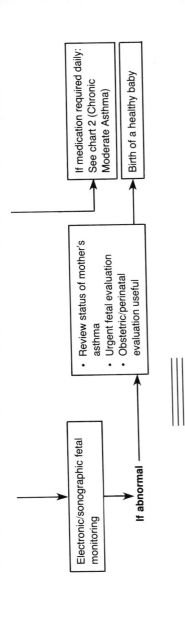

FIGURE 18-1

Management of asthma during pregnancy: chronic mild asthma. *All therapy must include patient education about prevention (including environmental control where appropriate) as well as control of symptoms. †PEFR percent baseline refers to the norm for the individual, established by the clinician. This may be percent predicted based on standardized norms or percent of patient's personal best.

191

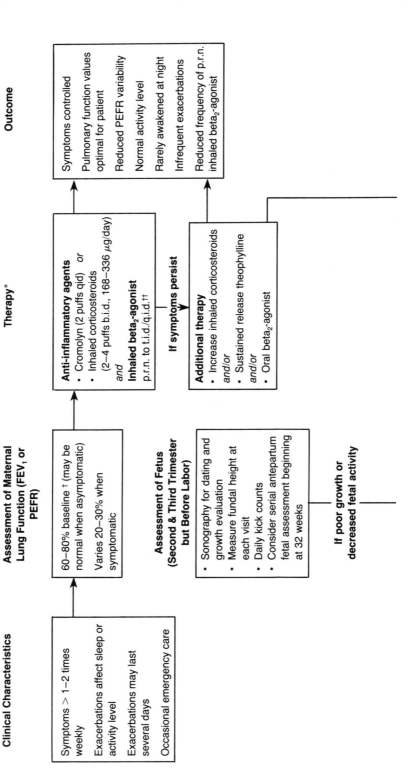

Clinical Characteristics

Symptoms > 1–2 times weekly

Exacerbations affect sleep or activity level

Exacerbations may last several days

Occasional emergency care

Assessment of Maternal Lung Function (FEV₁ or PEFR)

60–80% baseline † (may be normal when asymptomatic)

Varies 20–30% when symptomatic

Assessment of Fetus (Second & Third Trimester but Before Labor)

· Sonography for dating and growth evaluation
· Measure fundal height at each visit
· Daily kick counts
· Consider serial antepartum fetal assessment beginning at 32 weeks

If poor growth or decreased fetal activity

Therapy*

Anti-inflammatory agents
· Cromolyn (2 puffs qid) *or*
· Inhaled corticosteroids (2–4 puffs b.i.d., 168–336 μg/day) *or*
Inhaled beta₂-agonist
p.r.n. to t.i.d./q.i.d.††

If symptoms persist

Additional therapy
· Increase inhaled corticosteroids *and/or*
· Sustained release theophylline *and/or*
· Oral beta₂-agonist

Outcome

Symptoms controlled

Pulmonary function values optimal for patient

Reduced PEFR variability

Normal activity level

Rarely awakened at night

Infrequent exacerbations

Reduced frequency of p.r.n. inhaled beta₂-agonist

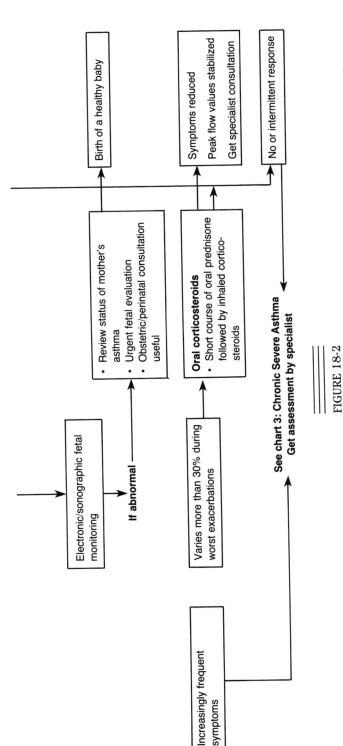

FIGURE 18-2

Management of asthma during pregnancy: chronic moderate asthma. *All therapy must include patient education about prevention (including environmental control where appropriate) as well as control of symptoms. †PEFR percent baseline refers to the norm for the individual, established by the clinician. This may be percent predicted based on standardized norms or percent of patient's personal best. ††If exceed 3–4 doses a day, consider additional therapy other than inhaled beta₂-agonist.

193

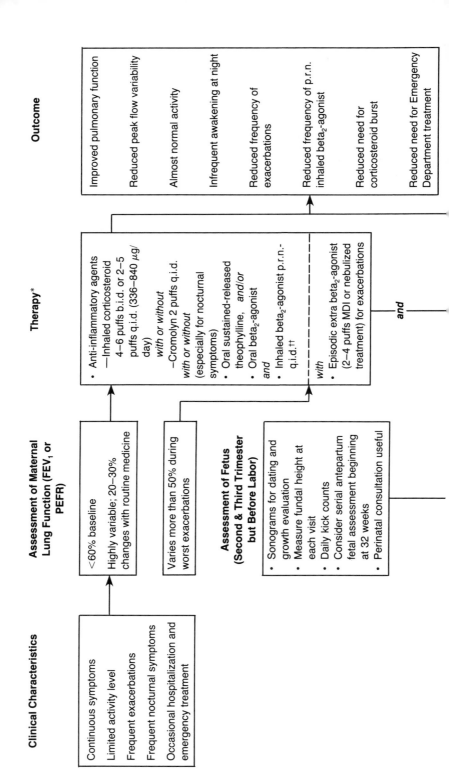

Clinical Characteristics

Continuous symptoms
Limited activity level
Frequent exacerbations
Frequent nocturnal symptoms
Occasional hospitalization and emergency treatment

Assessment of Maternal Lung Function (FEV_1 or PEFR)

<60% baseline

Highly variable; 20–30% changes with routine medicine

Varies more than 50% during worst exacerbations

Assessment of Fetus (Second & Third Trimester but Before Labor)

- Sonograms for dating and growth evaluation
- Measure fundal height at each visit
- Daily kick counts
- Consider serial antepartum fetal assessment beginning at 32 weeks
- Perinatal consultation useful

Therapy*

- Anti-inflammatory agents
  —Inhaled corticosteroid 4–6 puffs b.i.d. or 2–5 puffs q.i.d. (336–840 μg/day)
  with or without
  –Cromolyn 2 puffs q.i.d.
  with or without
  (especially for nocturnal symptoms)
- Oral sustained-released theophylline, *and/or*
- Oral beta$_2$-agonist

and

- Inhaled beta$_2$-agonist p.r.n. q.i.d.††

with

- Episodic extra beta$_2$-agonist (2–4 puffs MDI or nebulized treatment) for exacerbations

and

Outcome

Improved pulmonary function

Reduced peak flow variability

Almost normal activity

Infrequent awakening at night

Reduced frequency of exacerbations

Reduced frequency of p.r.n. inhaled beta$_2$-agonist

Reduced need for corticosteroid burst

Reduced need for Emergency Department treatment

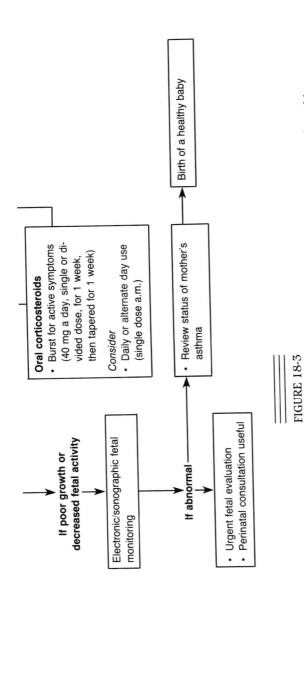

FIGURE 18-3

Management of asthma during pregnancy: chronic severe asthma. Note: Individuals with severe asthma should be evaluated by an asthma specialist. *All therapy must include patient education about prevention (including environmental control where appropriate) as well as control of symptoms. † PEFR percent baseline refers to the norm for the individual, established by the clinician. This may be percent predicted based on standardized norms or percent of patient's personal best. ‡‡ If exceed 3–4 doses a day, consider additional therapy other than inhaled beta$_2$-agonist.

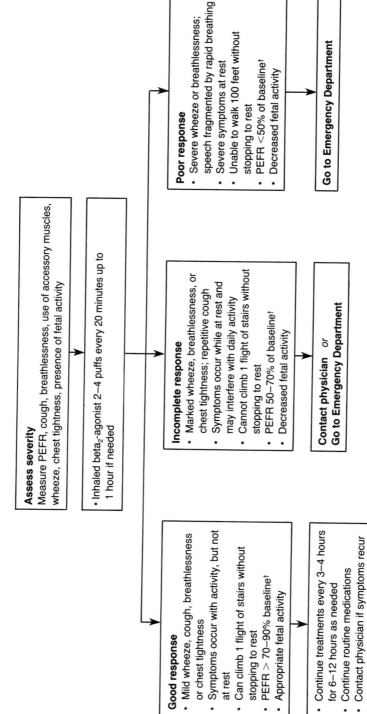

Assess severity
Measure PEFR, cough, breathlessness, use of accessory muscles, wheeze, chest tightness, presence of fetal activity

- Inhaled beta$_2$-agonist 2–4 puffs every 20 minutes up to 1 hour if needed

Good response
- Mild wheeze, cough, breathlessness or chest tightness
- Symptoms occur with activity, but not at rest
- Can climb 1 flight of stairs without stopping to rest
- PEFR > 70–90% baseline†
- Appropriate fetal activity

- Continue treatments every 3–4 hours for 6–12 hours as needed
- Continue routine medications
- Contact physician if symptoms recur

Incomplete response
- Marked wheeze, breathlessness, or chest tightness; repetitive cough
- Symptoms occur while at rest and may interfere with daily activity
- Cannot climb 1 flight of stairs without stopping to rest
- PEFR 50–70% of baseline†
- Decreased fetal activity

Contact physician *or*
Go to Emergency Department

Poor response
- Severe wheeze or breathlessness; speech fragmented by rapid breathing
- Severe symptoms at rest
- Unable to walk 100 feet without stopping to rest
- PEFR <50% of baseline†
- Decreased fetal activity

Go to Emergency Department

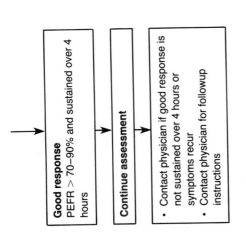

Good response
PEFR > 70–90% and sustained over 4 hours

Continue assessment

- Contact physician if good response is not sustained over 4 hours or symptoms recur
- Contact physician for followup instructions

FIGURE 18-4

Acute exacerbations of asthma during pregnancy: home management. ˡPEFR percent baseline refers to the norm for the individual, established by the clinician. This may be percent predicted based on standardized norms or percent of patient's personal best.

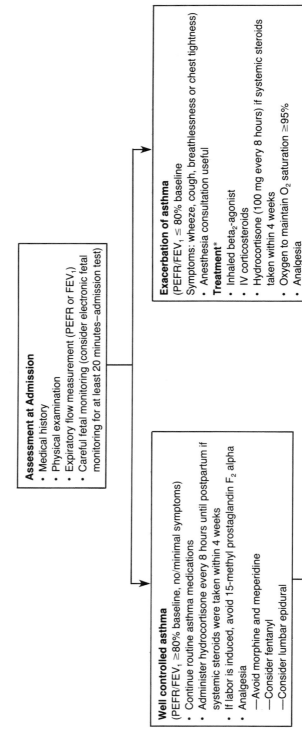

Assessment at Admission
- Medical history
- Physical examination
- Expiratory flow measurement (PEFR or FEV$_1$)
- Careful fetal monitoring (consider electronic fetal monitoring for at least 20 minutes–admission test)

Well controlled asthma
(PEFR/FEV$_1$ ≥80% baseline, no/minimal symptoms)
- Continue routine asthma medications
- Administer hydrocortisone every 8 hours until postpartum if systemic steroids were taken within 4 weeks
- If labor is induced, avoid 15-methyl prostaglandin F$_2$ alpha
- Analgesia
  —Avoid morphine and meperidine
  —Consider fentanyl
  —Consider lumbar epidural

Exacerbation of asthma
(PEFR/FEV$_1$ ≤ 80% baseline
Symptoms: wheeze, cough, breathlessness or chest tightness)
- Anesthesia consultation useful
Treatment*
- Inhaled beta$_2$-agonist
- IV corticosteroids
- Hydrocortisone (100 mg every 8 hours) if systemic steroids taken within 4 weeks
- Oxygen to maintain O$_2$ saturation ≥95%
- Analgesia
  —Avoid narcotic analgesics
  —Consider epidural analgesia

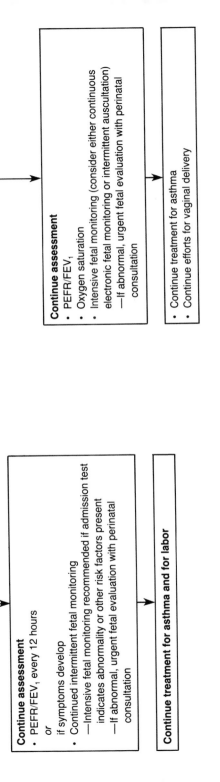

Continue assessment
- PEFR/FEV$_1$ every 12 hours
  or
  if symptoms develop
- Continued intermittent fetal monitoring
  —Intensive fetal monitoring recommended if admission test indicates abnormality or other risk factors present
  —If abnormal, urgent fetal evaluation with perinatal consultation

Continue treatment for asthma and for labor

Continue assessment
- PEFR/FEV$_1$
- Oxygen saturation
- Intensive fetal monitoring (consider either continuous electronic fetal monitoring or intermittent auscultation)
  —If abnormal, urgent fetal evaluation with perinatal consultation

- Continue treatment for asthma
- Continue efforts for vaginal delivery

FIGURE 18-5

Management of asthma during labor. *See chart and discussion "Acute Exacerbations of Asthma: Emergency Department Management" in the full report: Management of Asthma During Pregnancy. Bethesda, MD: Department of Health and Human Services, National Heart, Lung, and Blood Institute, 1992.

Assessment at Admission

- Medical history
- Physical examination
- Expiratory flow measurement (PEFR or FEV_1)
- Oxygen saturation (oximeter or arterial blood gas)
- Careful fetal monitoring

Well controlled mild, moderate, or severe asthma

(PEFR/FEV_1 ≥ 80% baseline, no/minimal symptoms)

- Continue routine inhaled asthma medications
- Transfer routine oral asthma medications to IV route
- Administer hydrocortisone (100 mg every 8 hours until postpartum) if systemic steroids were taken within 4 weeks
- Analgesia
  —Avoid morphine and merperidine
  —Consider fentanyl
  —Consider lumbar epidural with diluted concentrations of local anesthetic and narcotics
- Anesthesia, if necessary
  —Pre-anesthetic atropine and glycopyrrolate
  —Low concentrations of halogenated anesthetics

Exacerbation of asthma

(PEFR/FEV_1 ≤ 80% baseline
Symptoms: wheeze, cough, breathlessness or chest tightness)

Treat exacerbation*

- Inhaled $beta_2$-agonist
- IV corticosteroids
- Hydrocortisone (100 mg every 8 hours until postpartum) if systemic steroids were taken within 4 weeks
- Oxygen to maintain O_2 saturation ≥95%

Continue efforts for vaginal delivery

- Notify anesthesia consultant and pediatrician
- Analgesia
  —Avoid narcotic analgesics
  —Consider epidural analgesia
- Anesthetic, if necessary
  —Pre-anesthetic atropine and glycopyrrolate
  —Low concentrations of halogenated anesthetic

Respiratory failure

(PEFR/FEV_1 ≤25% and CO_2 ≥ 35 mm Hg)
Symptoms: extreme distress, confusion

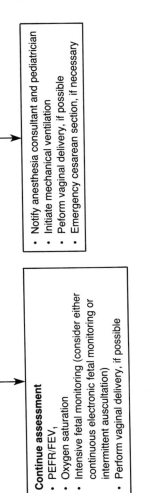

Continue assessment
- PEFR/FEV$_1$
- Oxygen saturation
- Intensive fetal monitoring (consider either continuous electronic fetal monitoring or intermittent auscultation)
- Perform vaginal delivery, if possible

- Notify anesthesia consultant and pediatrician
- Initiate mechanical ventilation
- Peform vaginal delivery, if possible
- Emergency cesarean section, if necessary

FIGURE 18-6

Management of asthma during delivery. *See chart and discussion "Acute Exacerbations of Asthma: Emergency Department Management" in the full report: Management of Asthma During Pregnancy. Bethesda, MD: Department of Health and Human Services. National Heart, Lung, and Blood Institute. 1992.

Intravenous access should be achieved, both for administration of medications and for hydration, which may help prevent inspissation of mucus plugs and may aid in expectoration.

The first-line pharmacologic therapy of acute severe asthma in pregnancy consists of adrenergic agonists, either epinephrine or terbutaline. Tables 18-2, 18-3, and 18-4 list the more common agents, their dosages, and their routes of administration.

Corticosteroids should be used early in the course of acute severe asthma. Pharmacologic effects thought to play a role in acute asthma include:

1. Direct bronchial smooth-muscle relaxation.
2. Constriction of the bronchial microvasculature, with reduced capillary permeability and reduced edema formation.
3. Decreased activity and number of circulating inflammatory cells.
4. Increased production of lipomodulin, resulting in decreased availability of substrate for prostaglandin formation.
5. Perhaps most importantly, increased responsiveness to beta-adrenergic stimulation.

This last method of action is a result of increased down-regulation after repeated use. This potentiation of beta-adrenergic therapy is seen within one to two hours of steroid administration. Finally, corticosteroids have been noted to improve V/Q mismatching in status asthmaticus, possibly as a result of altered prostaglandin metabolism and pulmonary perfusion.

REFRACTORY STATUS ASTHMATICUS AND RESPIRATORY FAILURE

When maternal respiratory status continues to decline despite aggressive pharmacologic therapy, consideration should be given to intubation. Specific indications for intubation of the gravida with status asthmaticus include 1) inability to maintain a Pa_{O_2} of >60 mm Hg with 90% hemoglobin saturation despite supplemental oxygen, 2) inability to maintain a P_{CO_2} of <40 mm Hg, or 3) evidence of maternal exhaustion. Guidelines to

TABLE 18-2

Drugs and dosages for asthma and associated conditions preferred for use during pregnancy*

Drug Class	Specific Drug	Dosage
Anti-inflammatory	Cromolyn sodium	2 puffs q.i.d. (inhalation) 2 sprays in each nostril b.i.d.-q.i.d. (intranasal for nasal symptoms).
	Beclomethasone	2–5 puffs b.i.d.-q.i.d. (inhalation) 2 sprays in each nostril b.i.d. (intranasal for allergic rhinitis).
	Prednisone	Burst for active symptoms: 40 mg a day, single or divided dose for 1 week, then taper for 1 week. If prolonged course is required, single A.M. dose on alternate days may minimize adverse effects.
Bronchodilator	Inhaled beta₂-agonist	2 puffs every 4 hours as needed.
	Theophylline	Oral: dose to reach serum concentration level of 8–12 μg/mL.
Antihistamine	Chlorpheniramine	4 mg by mouth up to q.i.d. 8–12 mg sustained-release b.i.d.
	Tripelennamine	25–50 mg by mouth up to q.i.d. 100 mg sustained-release b.i.d.
Decongestant	Pseudoephedrine Oxymetazoline	60 mg by mouth up to q.i.d. 120 mg sustained-release b.i.d. Intranasal spray or drops up to 5 days for rhinosinusitis.
Cough	Guaifenesin Dextromethorphan	2 tsp by mouth q.i.d. —
Antibiotics	Amoxicillin	3 weeks therapy for sinusitis.

*This table presents drugs and suggested dosages for the home management of asthma and associated conditions. Drugs and dosages for the treatment of exacerbations in the emergency department or hospital are presented in the full report of the working group.

TABLE 18-3

Sympathomimetics used in the treatment of asthma

Drug	Predominant Receptor Effect	Route of Administration	Recommended Dosages
Epinephrine	Alpha, beta-1, beta-2	Subcutaneous	0.3–0.5 mL of a 1:1000 solution
		Inhaled	0.2–0.3 mg/puff
			1 to 2 puffs every 4 h
Terbutaline	Beta-2	Subcutaneous	0.25 mg every 15 min × 3
		Per oral	2.5 mg every 4–6 h
Isoproterenol	Beta-1, beta-2	Inhaled	1:1000, 1:200 solutions 3–7, 5–11 inhalations respectively, every 4–6 h
		Intravenous	0.5–5 μg/min infusion
Metaproterenol	Beta-2	Inhaled:	
		Metered dose	0.65 mg puff, 2–3 puffs every 3–4 h
		Nebulizer	0.3 mL of 5% solution every 4 h

TABLE 18-4

Corticosteroid regimens used in acute severe asthma

Drug	Relative Anti-Inflammatory Potency	Route of Administration	Recommended Dosages
Hydrocortisone	1.0	Intravenous	1–2 mg/kg loading dose followed by 0.5 mg/kg/h infusion
Methylprednisolone	5.0	Intravenous	125 mg every 6–8 h
Prednisone	3.5	Per oral	10–40 mg/day
Dexamethasone	30.0	Intravenous	4–20 mg every 8–12 h

avoid complications from mechanical ventilation in status asthmaticus include:

1. Use of the largest possible diameter of endotracheal tube to reduce expiratory resistance.
2. Use of a volume-cycled ventilator.
3. Increased humidity, to facilitate clearance of mucus.
4. Allowance of adequate expiratory time.
5. Sedation and possibly paralysis to minimize barotrauma.

Continuous positive airway pressure (CPAP) not only improves ventilation, but also dramatically reduces the work of breathing by unloading the inspiratory muscles during severe bronchial asthma.

CONSIDERATIONS FOR LABOR AND DELIVERY

Attention to the gravida with a recent history of severe asthma will avoid several pitfalls during labor, delivery, and the puerperium. Stress-dose steroids should be given to any parturient exposed to steroids within the preceding 9 months. When choosing a sedative for labor, one of the non-histamine-releasing narcotics, such as fentanyl, may be preferable to others, such as morphine.

As endotracheal intubation has been associated with severe bronchospasm, consideration should be given to the early placement of epidural anesthesia. Finally, in the event of postpartum hemorrhage, PGE_2 and other uterotonics should be used in lieu of PGF_2, which has been associated with clinically diminished pulmonary function.

SUGGESTED READING

Greenberger PA, Patterson R. The outcome of pregnancy complicated by severe asthma. Allergy ProC 1988;9:539–543.

Greenberger PA, Patterson R. Management of asthma during pregnancy: current concepts. New Engl J Med 1985;312:897–902.

Hankins GDV, Berryman GK, Scott RT Jr, Hood D. Maternal arterial desaturation with 15-methyl prostaglandin F2 alpha for uterine atony. Obstet Gynecol 1988;72:367–370.

Masey KL, Gotz VP. Iptratropium bromide. Drug Intell Clin Pharm 1985;19:5–12.

Schatz M, Harden K, Forsythe A, et al. The course of asthma during pregnancy, postpartum, and with successive pregnancies: a prospective analysis. J Allergy Clin Immunol 1988;81:509–517.

Schatz M, Zeiger RS, Harden KM, et al. The safety of inhaled beta-agonist bronchodilators during pregnancy. J Allergy Clin Immunol 1988;82:686–695.

Siegel D, Sheppard D, Gelb A, et al. Aminophylline increases the toxicity but not the efficacy of inhaled beta-adrenergic agonists in the treatment of acute exacerbations of asthma. Am Rev Resp Dis 1985;75:1–12.

CHAPTER NINETEEN

Amniotic Fluid Embolism

Amniotic fluid embolism (AFE) is perhaps the most devastating condition known in obstetrics, with a mortality rate as high as 80%. It results from an uncommon maternal reaction to fetal tissue and amniotic fluid exposure. Although it is uncommon in an absolute sense, this condition, along with pulmonary thromboembolism, are the leading causes of maternal mortality in the United States.

A biphasic pattern of hemodynamic disturbance has been postulated (Figure 19-1). The initial response of the pulmonary vasculature to the presence of amniotic fluid is vasospasm, producing transient pulmonary hypertension, ventilation-perfusion mismatch, and profound hypoxia. The initial period of intense hypoxia may account for the roughly 50% of patients who succumb to AFE within the first hour after the onset of clinical symptoms. It would also account for cases of survival with severe neurologic impairment or brain death secondary to profound initial hypoxia. The transient nature of this initial hemodynamic response, completely resolved in the animal model within 15–30 minutes, may account for its infrequent documentation in humans.

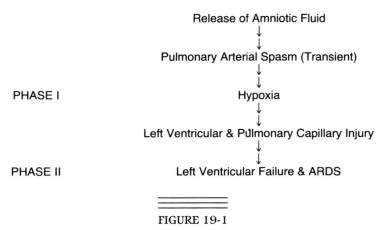

FIGURE 19-1

Hemodynamic alterations in human AFE. Phase I is generally resolved within 30 minutes of the acute event, whereas Phase II has been documented an hour or more following presumed embolization.

Those patients who survive the initial phase experience a secondary phase of hemodynamic compromise that involves left heart failure, with a variable secondary elevation of pulmonary artery pressure (PAP) and return of normal right-heart function. This is the hemodynamic picture most commonly documented in humans. The origin of the documented left ventricular dysfunction in humans remains obscure. Animal data would suggest that hypoxic injury to the left ventricle may be involved; recent studies in rats have demonstrated a decrease in coronary artery blood flow in experimental AFE. The in vitro observation of decreased myometrial contractility in the presence of amniotic fluid suggests the possibility of a direct depressant effect of amniotic fluid or an endogenously released mediator on the myocardium as well.

In addition to hemodynamic collapse and pulmonary injury, patients surviving the initial hemodynamic insult often manifest a coagulopathy, ranging from decompensated disseminated intravascular coagulation to minor disturbances in platelet count.

In both animal and human studies, the amount of particulate

matter found in the pulmonary vasculature has not been consistently related to clinical findings. In addition, pathologic effects have been noted in some animal species following intra-arterial injection of amniotic fluid. Observations have been made that some fetal debris may routinely enter the venous circulation of pregnant women and that clinical AFE is not a function of either an abnormal volume of amniotic fluid entering the maternal circulation or physical plugging of pulmonary capillaries with fetal debris, but rather is related to an abnormal substance within the amniotic fluid of susceptible women or to endogenously released mediators.

CLINICAL PRESENTATION

The classic presentation is that of sudden dyspnea and hypotension, often followed within minutes by cardiorespiratory arrest. In many cases, these initial events may be heralded by seizure activity. DIC often follows. If the patient survives the initial hemodynamic collapse, a secondary noncardiogenic pulmonary edema (adult respiratory distress syndrome [ARDS]) or acute tubular necrosis may occur as well. Patients surviving to receive invasive hemodynamic monitoring generally demonstrate left ventricular dysfunction or failure. Systemic vascular resistance (SVR) may be decreased. In patients who develop a significant coagulopathy, the clinical hemorrhage is often compounded by the simultaneous occurrence of uterine atony. In some cases, a transient rise in fibrin split products or fall in platelet count may be the only manifestation of a subclinical coagulopathy. In other patients, DIC and fatal hemorrhage may be the only clinical manifestations.

Most reported cases of AFE occur in association with labor. A pattern of vigorous labor or hypertonic uterine contractions have in the past been implicated in the pathogenesis of this condition. This association, however, is probably related to catecholamine release associated with the initial hemodynamic insult and cannot be viewed as causal.

DIAGNOSIS

Diagnosis of AFE in the past has classically been made at autopsy, with the demonstration of squamous cells or other fetal debris in the pulmonary artery vasculature. More recently, it has been demonstrated that squamous cells and other debris of presumed fetal origin may be demonstrated in blood aspirated from the central venous or pulmonary artery circulation of living patients with AFE syndrome. Recent studies of pregnant women undergoing pulmonary artery catheterization for a variety of medical indications have suggested that the detection of squamous cells or other fetal elements in the maternal pulmonary artery circulation is a common finding. Such findings are corroborated by early investigations that detected squamous cells in the uterine venous blood of normal patients undergoing cesarean hysterectomy.

Thus, there is no single clinical or laboratory finding that, in itself, can either diagnose or exclude AFE syndrome. The diagnosis must be made on the basis of clinical presentation and supportive laboratory studies. The differential diagnosis of AFE includes local anesthetic toxicity, septic shock, aspiration pneumonia, acute myocardial infarction, pulmonary thromboembolism, and, when coagulopathy is a dominant feature, placental abruption.

TREATMENT

Treatment is directed toward three goals: 1) oxygenation, 2) maintenance of both cardiac output and blood pressure, and 3) combating coagulopathy.

Fetal distress is almost universal during the cardiovascular collapse associated with AFE. The decision regarding operative intervention in an unstable mother is extremely difficult and must be individualized, based upon maternal and fetal condition and fetal age.

Amniotic fluid embolism

Goals of Therapy

1. To maintain systolic blood pressure >90 mm Hg, urine output >25 mL/h, and arterial Po_2 >60 mm Hg, or SaO_2 >90.
2. To correct coagulation abnormalities.

Management Protocol

1. Initiate cardiopulmonary resuscitation if indicated.
2. Administer oxygen at high concentrations. If the patient is unconscious, she should be intubated and ventilated with 100% FIO_2.
3. AFE is often associated with and, in fact, may be heralded by fetal distress. Therefore, the fetal heart rate should be carefully monitored if gestational age is sufficient to warrant intervention for fetal distress.
4. Hypotension is usually secondary to cardiogenic shock. Treatment involves optimization of cardiac preload by rapid volume infusion. Subsequent dopamine infusion would be appropriate if the patient remains hypotensive.
5. Pulmonary artery catheterization may be helpful in guiding hemodynamic management.
6. After correction of hypotension, fluid therapy should be restricted to maintenance levels to minimize pulmonary edema due to developing ARDS.
7. Administer fresh whole blood or packed red blood cells and fresh-frozen plasma to treat bleeding secondary to disseminated intravascular coagulation.

Critical Laboratory Tests

Arterial blood gas, complete blood count (CBC), platelet count, fibrinogen, fibrin split products, prothrombin time (PT), partial thromboplastin time (PTT).

Consultation

Pulmonary medicine, hematology.

SUGGESTED READING

Adamsons K, Mueller-Heubach E, Myer RE. The innocuousness of amniotic fluid infusion in the pregnant rhesus monkey. Am J Obstet Gynecol 1971;109:977.

Azegami M, Mori N. Amniotic fluid embolism and leukotrienes. Am J Obstet Gynecol 1986;155:1119.

Clark SL, Cotton DB, Gonik B, et al. Central hemodynamic alterations in amniotic fluid embolism. Am J Obstet Gynecol 1988; 158:1124.

Clark SL. Amniotic fluid embolism: a review. Obstet Gynecol Surv 1990;45:360.

Hankins GDV, Synder RR, Clark SL, et al. Acute hemodynamic and respiratory effects of amniotic fluid embolism in the pregnant goat model. Am J Obstet Gynecol 1993;168:1113.

CHAPTER TWENTY

Systemic Lupus Erythematosus in Pregnancy

DIAGNOSIS

Antibodies to double-stranded (native) DNA (dsDNA) are the most specific for systemic lupus erythematosus (SLE) and are found in 80%–90% of untreated patients. The presence and titer of anti-dsDNA may be related to the disease activity. SLE patients may also have antibodies to nucleic acids or nucleic acid–protein conjugates, including single-stranded DNA, the Sm antigen, ribonucleoprotein (nRNP), the Ro/SSA antigen, and the La/SSB antigen. Anti-Ro/SS-A and La/SS-B, found in the sera of SLE patients and patients with Sjögren's syndrome, are of particular importance to obstetricians since they are associated with neonatal lupus.

The 1982 American Rheumatism Association (ARA) criteria for SLE are outlined in Table 20-1. To be classified as having SLE, an individual must have at least 4 of the 11 criteria (at one time or serially).

TABLE 20-1

Revised ARA Classification Criteria for SLE (1982). To be classified as having SLE, one must have at least 4 of the 11 criteria at one time or serially.

Malar rash

Discoid rash

Photosensitivity

Oral ulcers

Arthritis (nondeforming polyarthritis)

Serositis (pleuritis and/or pericarditis)

Renal disorder (proteinuria >0.5 g/day or cellular casts)

Neurological disorder (psychosis and/or seizures)

Hematological disorder (leukopenia or lymphopenia/hemolytic anemia/thrombocytopenia)

Immunological disorder (anti-DNA/anti-Sm/LE cell/false-positive STS)

Antinuclear antibody

THE INFLUENCE OF PREGNANCY ON SLE

Several recent studies have shown no increase in exacerbations in pregnant patients compared with nonpregnant controls. Table 20-2 summarizes the results of several controlled trials that examined the influence of pregnancy on SLE.

Recent studies have also shown a low risk of flare in the postpartum period. There is no evidence that termination of pregnancy improves maternal outcome or alters the risk of exacerbation. Therefore, termination should not be performed with the expectation of improving the symptoms of SLE.

Active disease at the time of conception may also increase the risk of exacerbation during pregnancy in patients with SLE. In addition, the rate of exacerbation may be even greater in patients with active renal disease at conception, with some studies suggesting flares in 50% or more. Recent series suggest that the course of renal disease in pregnant women with lupus nephritis (LN) is generally not altered. Deterioration of renal status occurs in about a quarter of the patients undertaking pregnancy. Ten percent of pregnancies are associated with a moderate permanent deterioration in the patient's renal status (Table 20-3).

INFLUENCE OF SLE ON PREGNANCY
PREGNANCY LOSS

Fetal outcome is adversely affected by SLE. Most authors have reported an increased risk of spontaneous abortions, fetal deaths, preterm deliveries, and small-for-gestation fetuses in infants born to mothers with lupus. Table 20-3 lists fetal outcome in several large, recent series. Overall, fetal loss rates range from 10% to 46%. The same risk factors that may slightly increase the chance of SLE flare also appear to worsen the prognosis for the fetus. These include renal disease, active disease at conception, and first presentation during pregnancy or the postpartum period. In patients in remission and without other risk factors (renal disease, hypertension, antiphospholipid syndrome), fetal mortality is at most marginally higher than in the general population.

The 10% to 30% of SLE patients with antiphospholipid antibodies (aPL) are at increased risk for fetal loss, especially second- and third-trimester fetal death. It appears that aPL are the most predictive risk factors for fetal death in lupus pregnancy. In one series, 10 of 11 fetal deaths in 42 lupus pregnancies were predicted by the presence of anticardiolipin (aCL), lupus anticoagulant (LA), or both. Moreover, among patients with aPL, pregnancies proceeding to live birth are often complicated by preeclampsia and growth retardation. The aPL that have most consistently been associated with fetal loss are the lupus anticoagulant and IgG anticardioplipin antibody.

PREGNANCY-INDUCED HYPERTENSION

Overall, 20%–30% of SLE pregnancies are complicated by preeclampsia. In one series, preeclampsia occurred in 8 of 11

TABLE 20-2

Rates of exacerbations of SLE in pregnancy. Only the study by Petri et al. demonstrated a significant difference between pregnant and nonpregnant controls

| Author and Year | Pregnant Patients | | |
	Number of Patients	Number of Pregnancies	Flares
Lockshin, 1984*	28	33	7 (21%)
Mintz, 1986	NA	92	55 (60%) 0.0605†
Meehan, 1987	18	22	10 (45%)
Petri, 1991§	36	39	23 (59%) 1.6337‡ ± 0.30

*Figures in table derived from flares as defined by the requirement for an increase in medication. Flares were also analyzed using a scoring system (see Lockshin et al. for definition), and there was no difference between pregnant patients and nonpregnant controls.

†Flares per month at risk.

‡Flare rate per person years (mean ± SEM). See reference by Petri et al. for definition of flare rate.

§Two control groups used.

(72%) pregnancies in women with SLE and nephropathy, but in only 12 of 53 (22%) pregnant women with SLE alone.

Distinguishing an exacerbation of SLE involving active nephritis from preeclampsia may be difficult. Elevated levels of anti-DNA weigh in favor of active SLE. Normal levels of classical pathway complements weigh against active SLE, but decreased levels are less helpful since they may be seen in preeclampsia or active SLE. Some investigators have found that lupus activity in pregnancy is associated with elevated levels of Ba or Bb, frag-

Controls

Number of Patients	Flares	Nature of Control Patients
33	6 (18%)	Matched nonpregnant
NA	NA 0.0406[†]	"Similar group of young females" using progesterone oral contraceptives
22	12 (54%)	Matched nonpregnant
185	NA 0.6518[‡] ± 0.05	Matched nonpregnant
29	NA 0.6392[‡] ± 0.15	Same patients after delivery

ments of protein B activation in the alternative pathway of complement activation. The terminal attack complex, Sc5b-9, may also be elevated in patients with active SLE. While elevated concentrations of Ba, Bb, and Sc5b-9 may also be found in occasional patients with preeclampsia, the combination of these with a decreased CH50 strongly suggests SLE flare. Other clinical and laboratory features that might be useful in distinguishing SLE flare and preeclampsia are summarized in Table 20–4.

Two tests are particularly helpful in distinguishing between

TABLE 20-3

Deterioration of renal disease during pregnancy in patients with
SLE nephropathy. Only patients with LN diagnosed prior to
pregnancy are included.

Author	Patients	Pregnancies	No Exacerbation
Hayslett			
Remission PTC*	23	31	21/31 (68%)
Active PTC	24	25	13/25 (52%)
Fine	13	14	N/A
Jungers			
Remission PTC	8	11	9/11 (82%)
Active PTC	8	15	4/15 (27%)
Imbasciati	6	18	18/18 (44%)
Devoe	14	17	13/17 (76%)
Bobrie	35	53	35/53 (66%)
Total	131	184	68/117 (61%)
Median			66%

*PTC = prior to conception.

active nephritis and preeclampsia. An active urinary sediment
strongly suggest active lupus nephritis. Cellular casts and hematuria are frequently present in diffuse proliferative glomeru-
lonephrosis, and to a lesser degree in focal proliferative glomeru-
lonephrosis, the two conditions most likely to be confused with
preeclampsia. The second test of immense benefit is the renal
biopsy. In severe and confusing cases, the biopsy results usually
make the correct diagnosis.

PRETERM DELIVERY

Preterm delivery occurs in 30% of women with SLE. Preterm
delivery is most often iatrogenic due to preeclampsia, abnormal
fetal surveillance, or lupus flare. Preterm labor is not more common among women with SLE.

Exacerbation	No Deterioration	Deterioration	Permanent Deterioration
10/31 (32%)	24/31 (77%)	7/31 (23%)	2/31 (6%)
12/25 (48%)	16/25 (64%)	9/25 (36%)	5/25 (20%)
N/A	10/14 (71%)	4/14 (29%)	2/14 (14%)
2/11 (18%)	9/11 (82%)	2/11 (18%)	1/11 (9%)
11/15 (73%)	13/15 (87%)	2/15 (13%)	1/15 (7%)
10/18 (56%)	14/18 (78%)	4/18 (22%)	2/18 (11%)
4/17 (24%)	12/17 (71%)	5/17 (29%)	2/17 (12%)
18/53 (34%)	NA	NA	4/53 (8%)
67/170 (39%)	98/131 (75%)	33/131 (25%)	19/184 (10%)
34%	77%	23%	10%

SMALL-FOR-GESTATIONAL AGE (SGA) INFANTS

SGA infants are probably more prevalent among women with SLE than among normal patients; however, supporting data are sparse. In one large prospective series, 23% of infants were SGA. Other smaller series also suggest a high rate of SGA infants. One important risk factor for SGA infants may be aPL.

NEONATAL LUPUS (NLE)

NLE is an uncommon syndrome of the fetus/neonate characterized by dermatologic, cardiac, or hematologic abnormalities. Typical skin lesions are similar to those of adult subacute cutaneous lupus and usually appear after birth. The hallmark cardiac lesion is congenital complete heart block (CCHB), but wide-

TABLE 20-4

Pregnancy loss in patients with SLE. Only pregnancies occurring after the diagnosis of SLE are included. Elective pregnancy terminations are excluded.

Author	Number of Patients	Number of Pregnancies
Fraga	20	42
Zurier	13	25
Zulman	23	24
Varner	31	34
Gimovsky	39	65
Lockshin	28	32
McHugh	NA	47
Mintz	75	92
Wong	17	19
Medians		

*Losses before 13 completed weeks' gestation are considered spontaneous abortions.

†Losses ≥14 weeks' gestation are considered fetal deaths.

‡Included all losses <21 weeks' gestation.

§Included all stillbirths ≥21 weeks' gestation.

spread endomyocardial involvement may also occur. Hematologic lesions include hemolytic anemia and thrombocytopenia. NLE is attributed to immune damage mediated by maternal autoantibodies which cross the placenta. The most strongly associated is antibody to SSA (Ro), a cytoplasmic ribonucleoprotein. Anti-SSA (Ro) has been found in 83%–100% of mothers of affected infants and in the serum of most infants with NLE. Fifty to 70% of these mothers also have anti-SSB (La). CCHB is thought to be mediated by inflammation and fibrosis of the conduction system, although this process occurs throughout the myocardium.

The risk to a patient with SLE for delivering an infant with NLE is unclear. Most mothers with anti-Ro/SSA or anti-La/SSB

Spontaneous Abortions*	Fetal Death†	Total Losses
NA	NA	17 (40%)
7 (28%)	2 (8%)	9 (36%)
0	3 (12%)	3 (12%)
3 (9%)	2 (6%)	5 (15%)
23 (35%)	7 (11%)	30 (46%)
3 (9%)	7 (22%)	10 (31%)
NA	NA	16 (34%)
16(17%)‡	4 (4%)§	20 (22%)
2 (10%)	0	2 (10%)
10%	8%	31%

have normal fetuses and neonates. Among all mothers with SLE, the risk of NLE is low, probably less than 5%. Among mothers with SLE and anti-Ro/SSA, the risk of skin lesions indicative of definite NLE is about 15%. Fortunately, the risk of CCHB, the only seriously morbid or mortal aspect of NLE, is quite low among women with SLE, even if they have anti-SSA. However, the risk may be higher in women who have previously delivered an infant with CCHB; 25%–60% of these mothers may have another fetus with CCHB. Some investigators suggest prophylactic treatment in such cases with corticosteroids and plasmapheresis or corticosteroids and intravenous immune globulin; however, the reports are anecdotal.

Cutaneous and hematologic manifestations do not pose

long-term risks to the infant because they resolve by six months without treatment. However, CCHB usually appears in utero and can be fatal. There is no proven therapy for in utero treatment, although steroids and plasmapheresis have been used. Most infants who survive the neonatal period do well, although many require permanent pacemakers.

MANAGEMENT OF SLE PREGNANCY

A preconceptional or first-trimester evaluation for renal disease (24-hour urine for CrCl and total protein), aPL, and anti-Ro/La is prudent. Serial testing for serum anti-nuclear anti-body (ANA) titers and complement levels is generally not useful. Increased maternal surveillance for the development of flares and preeclampsia, as well as fetal surveillance for growth and well-being, are recommended. One approach is to see patients at least every 2 weeks and obtain fetal scans every 4 weeks starting at 20 weeks' gestation. Fetal surveillance (non-stress tests [NSTs] and amniotic fluid volumes [AFVs]) is started at 30–32 weeks, or sooner if the clinical situation demands. Patients with aPL should undergo fetal heart rate monitoring starting as early as 24–26 weeks' gestation if there is any suspicion of uteroplacental insufficiency.

Glucocorticoids are the mainstay of the treatment of SLE in pregnancy. Prednisone or hydrocortisone are preferred corticosteroids because the placenta oxidizes these steroids to a relatively inactive 11-keto form. A large body of evidence suggests that these glucocorticoids are not associated with a clinically important risk for fetal malformations in the human. It is important to screen for glucose intolerance in patients receiving corticosteroids. Stress doses of steroids may be used at the time of delivery in patients on chronically administered steroids to avoid adrenal insufficiency.

There is less information available about other drugs commonly used to treat SLE. Antimalarials have been reported to cause loss of vision and ototoxicity and are avoided by most authors, although some feel that the benefits outweigh the risks. Cyclophosphamide and chlorambucil are contraindicated in the first trimester and should be used only in extreme circumstances thereafter. Azathioprine has been associated with SGA infants and neonatal immune suppression and should be used with caution. Nonsteroidal anti-inflammatory drugs (NSAIDs) are best avoided due to concerns about premature closure of the ductus and fetal renal effects. Aspirin taken late in pregnancy may cause neonatal bleeding.

Several well-designed studies indicate that prophylactically administered low-dose aspirin (LDA) may prevent or ameliorate preeclampsia in patients at risk for this disease. In addition, LDA is thought to be safe in pregnancy. Since patients with SLE are at substantial risk for preeclampsia, LDA should be considered, especially in patients with underlying renal disease.

SUGGESTED READING

Bobrie G, Liote F, Houillier P, Grunfeld JP, Jungers P. Pregnancy in lupus nephritis and related disorders. Am J Kidney Dis 1987; 339.

Buyon J, Roubey R, Swersky S, et al. Complete congenital heart block: risk of occurrence and therapeutic approach to prevention. J Rheum 1988;15:1104.

Buyon JP, Swersky SH, Fox HE, et al. Intrauterine therapy for presumptive fetal myocarditis with acquired heart block due to systemic lupus erythematosus. Arthritis Rheum 1987;30:44.

Hayslett JP, Lynn RI. Effect of pregnancy in patients with lupus nephropathy. Kidney Int 1980;18:207.

Jungers P, Dougados M, Pelissier C, Kuttenn F, Tron F, Lesavre P, Bach JF. Lupus nephropathy and pregnancy. Arch Intern Med 1982;142:771.

Lockshin MD, Bonfa E, Elkon D, Druzin, ML. Neonatal lupus risk to newborns of mothers with systemic lupus erythematosus. Arthritis Rheum 1988;31:6,697.

Lockshin MD. Pregnancy does not cause system lupus erythematosus to worsen. Arthritis Rheum 1989;32:6,665.

Lockshin MD, Reinits E, Druzin ML, Murrman M, Estes D. Case-control prospective study demonstrating absence of lupus exacerbation during or after pregnancy. Am J Med 1984;77:893.

Meehan RT, Dorsey JK. Pregnancy among patients with systemic lupus erythematosus receiving immunosuppressive therapy. J Rheumatol 1987;14:252–258.

Mintz R, Niz J, Gutierrez G, Garcia-Alonso A, Karchmer S. Prospective study of pregnancy in systemic lupus erythematosus. Results of a multidisciplinary approach. J Rheum 1986; 13:4,732.

Petri M, Howard D, Repke J. Frequency of lupus flare in pregnancy: The Hopkins Lupus Pregnancy Center experience. Arthritis Rheum 1991;34:12,1538.

Taylor PV, Scott JS, Gerlis LM, et al. Maternal antibodies against fetal cardiac antigens in congenital complete heart block. N Engl J Med 1986;315:667.

Varner MW, Meehan RT, Syrop CH, Strottman MP, Goplerud CP. Pregnancy in patients with systemic lupus erythematosus. Am J Obstet Gynecol 1983;145:8,1025.

CHAPTER TWENTY-ONE

Acute and Chronic Renal Failure in Pregnancy

Acute renal failure (ARF) remains an unusual but life-threatening complication of pregnancy. ARF requiring dialysis occurs in less than one in 10,000–15,000 pregnancies. The most common pregnancy-related causes of acute renal failure are septic abortion (especially *Clostridium perfringes*), renal obstruction due to stones, carcinoma, or uterine compression, preeclampsia with severe oliguria, hemolytic uremic syndrome, acute fatty liver, lupus nephritis, and severe hemorrhage.

DIFFERENTIAL DIAGNOSIS OF ARF

ARF is diagnosed on the basis of a decrease in glomerular filtration rate (GFR), as evidenced by an increase in blood urea nitrogen (BUN) and serum creatinine or a decline in creatinine clearance. Oliguria alone does not signify ARF. Diagnostic features of obstetric ARF are outlined in Table 21-1 and 21-2. Urine sodium and specific gravity may be used to distinguish acute tubular necrosis (ATN) from prerenal azotemia (Table 21-3).

TABLE 21-1

Clinical features of obstetric ARF

	Blood Pressure	Urinalysis Volume	Urine Sodium
Preeclampsia	↑	1+ to 4+ protein may be oliguric	Low
Acute tubular necrosis (ATN)	May be normal, ↑ or ↓	Muddy brown casts may be oliguric	>40 mEq/L
Renal cortical necrosis (RCN)	May be normal, ↑ or ↓	2 to 3+ protein oligo/anuria	
Acute fatty liver	Normal to mild ↑	Benign sediment	<10 mEq/L
Hemolytic uremic syndrome	Normal to great ↑	2+ to 3+ protein RBCs	

PT = prothrombin time; PTT = partial thromboplastin time; Hct = hematocrit; DIC = disseminated intravascular coagulopathy; H/o = history of; GI = gastrointestinal; LDH = lactic dehydrogenase; RBCs = red blood cells.

Liver Function Tests	Clotting Studies	Hemtaologic Changes	Other Findings
Transaminases may be mildly to markedly increased (>1000 possible)	PT, PTT may ↑; platelets may ↓	Hct normal or ↑ microangiopathic changes on smear	Peripheral edema; may have pulmonary edema
Normal	May have DIC	Hct normal or ↓ 2° to bleeding	H/o sepsis hemorrhage
Normal	May have DIC	Hct normal or ↓ 2° to bleeding	H/o abruptio placentae, retained dead fetus, absent cortical blood flow on angiogram
Transaminases mildly to moderately elevated (<1000) jaundice	PT ↑, PTT ↑ platelets ↓	Hct ↓; smear may have microangiopathic changes	GI bleeding hepatic encephalopathy, hypoglycemia; fatty infiltration on liver biopsy
LDH transaminases normal to mildly elevated jaundice	PT, PTT normal platelets ↓	Hct ↓; microangiopathic changes on smear	Neurologic symptoms

TABLE 21-2

Urinary sediment findings in patients with different causes for acute renal failure (ARF)

Urinary Sediment	Possible Cause ARF
Hematuria	Adult hemolytic uremic syndrome
Casts	
Muddy brown	Acute tubular necrosis
Red cell	Acute glomerulonephritis
White cell	Interstitial disease
	Pyelonephritis
Benign sediment	Obstruction
	Preeclampsia
	Acute fatty liver

MANAGEMENT OF ARF: ASSESSMENT AND CORRECTION OF VOLUME STATUS

Whether faced with prerenal azotemia or ARF, the initial goal is to return the intravascular volume to normal (Figure 21-1). Prerenal azotemia will generally improve and, in ARF, the additional insult of volume contraction can be avoided. It is extremely difficult to assess intravascular volume in a pregnant or postpartum woman by physical examination alone.

In a woman who does not have pulmonary congestion or hypertension, a single fluid challenge of 200–300 mL of normal saline can usually be undertaken safely. However, for more precise volume manipulation, a pulmonary artery catheter is often necessary during the first few days of renal failure. Insensible loss less metabolic water production is about 8 mL/kg, and slightly lower values (6–8 mL/kg) can be used to offset the total body salt and water excess that is always present if the patient is postpartum. Therefore, in a patient who stabilizes quickly and is able to eat, fluid balance can be maintained by allowing a total fluid intake of 6–8 mL/kg plus urine output. Estimates of insensible loss should be increased for fever. Often, the medication and nutritional needs of the patient make conservative management difficult, and fluid balance must be controlled by dialysis.

Although there is no consensus that diuretics improve the prognosis in patients with ARF, these agents may make fluid management easier if a few pitfalls are avoided. Care should be taken to establish that the patient is volume repleted before using diuretics, especially in patients with PIH. Within the first 48 hours of oliguria, furosemide can be given in doses up to 500 mg I.V. Repeated high doses may cause hearing loss.

HYPERKALEMIA

A serum potassium greater than 6.8 mEq/L should be treated promptly without waiting for dialysis. Electrocardiogram (EKG) changes of hyperkalemia include peaked T waves, flattening of the P wave, prolongation of the PR interval, widened QRS interval. When EKG changes other than peaked T waves are present, 10–30 mL of a 10% solution of calcium gluconate should be given I.V. Although the administration of calcium does not change the serum potassium level, such therapy serves to protect the heart from the pathologic effects of hyperkalemia. Two additional treatments can be used to shift potassium into cells, thereby temporar-

TABLE 21-3

Distinguishing acute tubular necrosis from prerenal azotemia (U/Pcr = urine-to-plasma creatinine ratio

	Acute Tubular Necrosis	Prerenal Azotemia
Urine sodium (mEq/L)	>30	<10
Specific gravity	1.010–1.012	>1.012
U/PCr	Decreased	Increased
Renal failure index	>1	<1

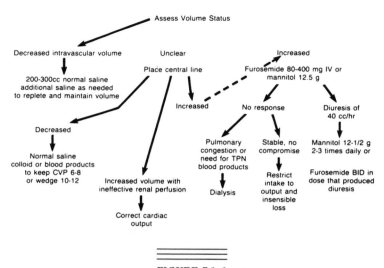

FIGURE 21-1

Volume control in oliguric patients.

ily relieving hyperkalemia. Fifty milliliters of a 50% solution of glucose with 10 units of regular insulin should be given I.V. The sodium–potassium exchange resin Kayexalate actually removes potassium from the body when given orally or by rectal enema. Fifty grams is given in 50 mL of 70% sorbitol every 2–4 hours. Measurement of serum potassium should be done hourly to make sure that treatment has been effective, and the patient should undergo continuous cardiac monitoring until the serum potassium is below 7 mEq/L. Large doses of sorbitol cause an osmotic diarrhea with greater losses of water than sodium; thus the patient should also be monitored for the development of hypernatremia.

ACIDOSIS

In a patient with chronic failure, serum bicarbonate drops by about 2 mEq/L per day. In the catabolic patient early in the course of ARF, the serum bicarbonate can drop by 15–20 mEq/L per day. Bicarbonate should be administered to keep the serum bicarbonate in the 18–22 range, appropriate for the respiratory alkalosis of pregnancy. In the patient with severe ongoing acid production, this can be accomplished only by dialysis. The space of distribution of bicarbonate is 60% of body weight. The dose of bicarbonate needed to bring the serum bicarbonate up to 15 can be calculated by the following formula:

$$15 - \text{serum bicarbonate} \times 0.6 \times \text{body weight}.$$

DRUG DOSES

Drugs that are renally excreted have a changed half-life in renal failure. There are additional changes with peritoneal dialysis and hemodialysis, and appropriate doses should be checked. Drug formulas that use the serum creatinine for calculation are not useful when the serum creatinine is rising, in which case the GFR should be assumed to be zero.

HYPONATREMIA

In the patient with ARF, salt and water losses are unregulated. A common problem is hyponatremia resulting from excessive administration of hypotonic fluids. Fluid replacement should be designed to replace the composition as well as quantity of losses. Insensible loss, including respiratory loss, is free water, while sweat is approximately half normal saline. Gastrointestinal losses are usually isotonic, but the hydrogen ion concentration varies with the origin of such losses and whether histamine receptor blockers are used. When the patient is not oliguric, urine sodium may be measured to assess urinary sodium losses.

NUTRITION

Optimal nutrition is of critical importance in the treatment of patients with ARF. Proper dietary management aimed at minimizing protein catabolism not only limits the accumulation of nitrogenous wastes, nonvolatile acids, and potassium in the extracellular fluid compartment, but also prevents malnutrition, which may lead to delayed wound healing and decreased resistance to infection. Various nutritional regimens have been credited with improving survival, decreasing the interdialytic rise in BUN, shortening the period of oliguria, and hastening the healing process within the kidney.

In the stable patient who does not appear to be catabolic, at least 100 g of glucose and at least 0.6 g/kg/day of high-biologic-value protein should be given to reduce endogenous protein breakdown. Protein intake should be increased if the patient is receiving dialysis because 10–13 g of amino acids are lost with every hemodialysis treatment, and as much as 10–20 g per day may be lost in peritoneal dialysis. Protein intake should be increased to 1.5 g/kg/day if this can be done without raising the BUN above 100 mg/dL. Caloric requirements should be calculated using requirements for ideal body weight plus a stress factor for extrarenal illnesses. In the patient who is still pregnant, the basal needs for pregnancy should be used. When the gastrointestinal tract functions, but the patient cannot eat because of anorexia, a feeding tube should be used.

The most widely used parenteral nutrition solutions contain hypertonic glucose plus essential amino acids. In the catabolic patient, about 70% of calories are provided by carbohydrate and 20%–30% by amino acids and fat emulsion. Water-soluble vitamins are lost in dialysis and should be supplemented. Potassium and phosphorus are added as dictated by serum chemistries.

DIALYSIS

Indications for dialysis in patients with ARF include hyperkalemia, fluid overload, hyponatremia, severe acidosis, and uremic complications such as bleeding, central nervous system (CNS) symptoms, pericarditis, and severe nausea and vomiting. Dialysis should be instituted early in the course of ARF, preferably before these complications appear. There is evidence that the mortality associated with ARF may be reduced modestly by prophylactic dialysis.

Acute renal failure (ARF) in pregnancy

Goals of Therapy

1. Maintain euvolemia.
2. Avoid hyperkalemia, acidosis, hyponatremia, hypocalcemia.
3. Maintain adequate nutrition.
4. Avoid severe hypertension.
5. Institute dialysis early, if necessary.
6. Assess fetal well-being.
7. Identify and eliminate or treat cause of ARF.

Management Protocol

1. Volume status.
   A. Consider pulmonary artery catheterization for closer assessment of volume status.
   B. Fluid intake: 6–8 mL/kg + urine output.
   C. Lasix 40–500 mg I.V., to assist in fluid balance.
   D. Dialysis if volume overload occurs.
2. Hyperkalemia:
   A. K+ > 8.0 mEq/L or EKG changes (other than peaked T waves).
      1. Calcium gluconate 10–20 mL of 10% solution.
      2. 10 units of regular insulin and 50 mL of 50% glucose.
      3. Sodium bicarbonate 50–150 mEq (if patient is not volume overloaded).
      4. Dialysis.
      5. Cardiac monitor.
   B. K+ 6.8–7.9 mEq/L
      1. 10 units of regular insulin and 50 mL of 50% glucose.
      2. Sodium bicarbonate 50–150 mEq/L (if the patient is not volume overloaded).
      3. Kayexalate 20–30 g every 2–4 hours orally, 50–100 g rectally.
      4. Dialysis.
      5. Cardiac monitor.
   C. K+ 5.6–6.8 mEq/L.
      1. Kayexalate as in step B.
         and/or
      2. Dialysis.
3. Acidosis: Maintain bicarbonate above 15 mEq/L and pH above 7.2.
   A. Euvolemic patient: sodium bicarbonate dose to achieve desired increase in bicarbonate × 0.6 body weight.

   B. Volume overloaded, hypernatremic, or severely catabolic patient: dialysis with high bicarbonate dialysate.

4. Hyponatremia:
   A. Serum sodium >125 mEq/L: restrict free water.
   B. Serum sodium 120–125 mEq/L: dialysis.
   C. Serum sodium <120: dialysis with high sodium dialysate; administration of hypertonic saline during dialysis.

5. Hypocalcemia: administer calcium intravenously only if positive Chvostek's sign or carpal pedal spasm is present. Oral supplements to maintain serum calcium above 7.5 mg% and to keep phosphorus below 5.5 mg%.

6. Nutrition:
   A. Management without dialysis: at least 100 g of glucose, 25–50 kcal/day, 0.6 g of protein/kg ideal body weight, up to 1.5 g/kg if BUN can be kept less than 100 mg% or if the patient is still pregnant.
   B. Management with dialysis:
      1. Oral intake: 1–5 g of protein/kg; 25–50 kcal to prevent catabolism, potassium 50 mEq, sodium 2 g in the form of food or enteral-elemental diet preparation; supplemental multivitamins.
      2. Total parenteral nutrition (TPN): total parenteral nutrition, 25–50 kcal day, 70% as glucose with 1–1.5 g protein as essential amino acids; maximum lipid is 500 mL of a 10% intralipid solution, supplemental multivitamins; electrolytes added indicated by lab values.

7. Adjust drug doses for renal failure.

8. Indications for dialysis:
   A. Uremia: BUN >100 mg% or uremic symptoms.
   B. Volume overload.
   C. Hyperkalemia.
   D. Acidosis with volume overload or hypernatremia.
   E. Pericarditis.
   F. Need for TPN, blood products, or other fluid in excess of what can be tolerated with conservative therapy.

Critical Laboratory Tests

Serum electrolytes (including HCO_3; bicarbonate), BUN, creatinine, total serum protein and albumin, calcium, phosphorus, creatinine clearance, arterial blood gases, serum osmolality, urine sodium-osmolality, chest x-ray.

Consultation

Nephrology.

SUGGESTED READING

Bobrie G, Liote F, Houillier P, et al. Pregnancy in lupus nephritis and related disorders. Am J Kid Dis 1987;9:339–343.

Feinstein EI, Blumencrantz MJ, Healy M, et al. Clinical and metabolic responses to parenteral nutrition in acute renal failure. Medicine 1981;60:124–137.

Grunfeld JP, Ganeval D, Bournerias F. Acute renal failure in pregnancy. Kidney Int 1980;18:179–191.

Hayslett JP. Postpartum renal failure. N Engl J Med 1985;312:1556–1559.

Loughlin KR, Bailey RB. Internal ureteral stents for conservative management of ureteral calculi during pregnancy. N Engl J Med 1986;315:1647–1649.

Maikranz P, Coe FL, Parks J, Lindheimer MD. Nephrolithiasis in pregnancy. Am J Kid Dis 1987;9:354–358.

Vintzileos AM, Turner GW, Campbell WA, et al. Polyhydramnios and obstructive renal failure: a case report and review of literature. Am J Obstet Gynecol 1985;152:883–885.

CHAPTER TWENTY-TWO

Dialysis and Renal Transplant in Pregnancy

METHOD OF DIALYSIS

Both hemodialysis and peritoneal dialysis have been used in the treatment of ARF in pregnancy. Relative contraindications to peritoneal dialysis include the presence of prosthetic material in the peritoneal cavity, a colostomy, severe respiratory distress, severe catabolism, severe hyperkalemia, and extensive recent abdominal surgery. Peritoneal dialysis may be performed following cesarean section. Two absolute contraindications to peritoneal dialysis are connection between the peritoneal and pleural space and the presence of a ventriculoperitoneal shunt.

In patients with a very high blood urea nitrogen (BUN), peritoneal dialysis minimizes the risk of circulatory instability and disequilibrium syndrome because it provides a more gradual decrease in BUN. However, if urea production is high, peritoneal dialysis may not be efficient enough to provide adequate removal of nitrogenous wastes. The use of continuous peritoneal dialysis, now commonly used in patients with chronic renal failure, has been applied to patients with ARF, with some improvement in nitrogenous waste removal. Infection, hyperglycemia, and peritoneal access problems are the most frequent complications of acute peritoneal dialysis. In severely catabolic patients, hemodialysis is more effective than peritoneal dialysis for removal of potassium and nitrogenous wastes. Blood pressure can be supported with albumin. In pregnant patients, bicarbonate rather than acetate should be used as the source of base, to minimize hemodynamic instability associated with acetate. Fluid removal is best controlled by a volumetric machine allowing most patients to tolerate the use of dialyzer with a high urea and creatinine clearance. Vasopressor agents may serve as temporary expedients for maintaining blood pressure and blood flow through the dialysis machine.

When blood pressure cannot be maintained due to rapid fluid removal and there is a contraindication to peritoneal dialysis, fluid can be removed more gradually by cannulating the femoral artery and vein and attaching a filter containing a semipermeable membrane made of polysulfone or polyacrylonitrile. In this setup, ultrafiltration is driven by the patient's own blood pressure, and an excessive rate of fluid removal is avoided. Continuous systemic heparinization is indicated in such patients.

When intravenous catheters are used for temporary vascular access, a double-lumen catheter is preferable because it minimizes the amount of recirculation. Use of femoral and subclavian vessels for catheter access devices carries the risk of infection and the troubling complications of both clotting within the catheter and subclavian vein stenosis.

PREGNANCY IN WOMEN ON CHRONIC DIALYSIS

Fertility is uncommon in chronic dialysis patients. Successful pregnancy is even more unusual, with only 19%–23% of all pregnancies ending in live births.

Maternal risks during pregnancy include severe hypertension, bleeding complications and anemia, clotting of vascular access, and infection. Fetal risks include intrauterine fetal death, prematurity, intrauterine growth retardation (IUGR), and exposure to viral illnesses.

HYPERTENSION

Hypertension remains the most common life-threatening complication of pregnancy in these women. Every home-dialysis patient should be instructed to take her blood pressure several times daily, and every center-dialyzed patient should be instructed to take her blood pressure at home on nondialysis days. An attempt should be made to keep the blood pressure below 140–150/90–100 during pregnancy. As in other dialysis patients, the first line of treatment for hypertension is correction of volume overload by dialysis. If this approach is unsuccessful, pharmacologic therapy may be indicated.

MODIFICATIONS OF HEMODIALYSIS PRESCRIPTION FOR PREGNANCY

Approximately 800 mg of calcium are absorbed during each 4-hour dialysis with a dialysate calcium of 3.5 mEq/L. The combination of oral calcium as a phosphate binder and increased absorption of calcium as a result of increased dialysis appears to provide enough calcium for fetal skeletal development. Hypercalcemia may occur, and serum calcium levels should be monitored before and after dialysis weekly and the dialysate calcium reduced if hypercalcemia is noted. Phosphorus removal during dialysis in patients with a predialysis phosphorus of 5–6 mg/dL averages 1 g. With more frequent dialysis, it may be possible to lower the dose of phosphate binders. Aluminum should be avoided because it is toxic to the mother and its effects on the fetus are unknown.

Avoidance of hypotension on dialysis is extremely important for the pregnant patient as it may be associated with fetal distress. Continuous electronic fetal heart-rate monitoring should be considered in the late second- or third-trimester fetus. Daily dialysis minimizes the amount of fluid that must be removed with each dialysis, and this may minimize the risk of hypotension.

PREGNANCY IN RENAL
TRANSPLANT RECIPIENTS

Fertility is often restored in women with renal transplants. Transplant patients are generally advised to avoid pregnancy until $1\frac{1}{2}$–2 years after transplant and to undertake it only if renal function is stable, with a creatinine below 2 mg/dL. When this advice is followed, the perinatal outcome is generally favorable.

Most patients with renal transplant go through pregnancy without incurring permanent loss of graft function. In women whose graft function is impaired at the time of conception, there is a substantial risk of worsening graft function. However, there are occasional instances where irreversible loss of graft function has occurred during pregnancy in women with good, stable graft function prior to pregnancy and normal blood pressure throughout gestation.

A 30% decline in renal function in the third trimester is normal in allograft recipients and generally does not need to be evaluated aggressively. When a decline in renal function occurs during the first two trimesters or more than a 30% decline in renal function occurs in the third trimester, the patient should be evaluated for changes in volume status and the history reviewed for exposure to nephrotoxins. Obstruction by the enlarging uterus is unusual but may occur. Obtaining a baseline renal sonogram at 20 weeks' gestation may assist in the evaluation of possible hydronephrosis later in pregnancy.

A difficult diagnostic dilemma that often occurs in the pregnant transplant patient is the need to distinguish between acute rejection, cyclosporin toxicity, preeclampsia, and pregnancy-associated progression of the underlying disease or a combination of these factors. Cytomegalovirus (CMV) infection may also be associated with reduced graft function, most commonly in the immediate posttransplant period. Hypertension may be present in any of the processes that cause ARF in the pregnant transplant patient. Only in their most severe forms may preeclampsia and severe acute graft rejection have distinguishing clinical features. In the early posttransplant period, acute rejection may be accompanied by high fevers and a swollen tender graft, but an isolated rise in serum creatinine is not unusual. In its most severe form, preeclampsia may be accompanied by abnormal liver function tests, pulmonary edema, and evidence of disseminated intravascular coagulation (DIC). However, interpretation of even these late signs of preeclampsia may be confusing, as azathioprine can cause both abnormal liver function tests and thrombocytopenia, and CMV infection may be associated with abnormal liver function tests and pulmonary picture indistinguishable from preeclampsia-induced pulmonary edema.

The initial approach to this diagnostic dilemma includes hospitalizing the patient because both acute rejection and preeclampsia can progress rapidly. If hypertension is easily controlled and renal function is not changing rapidly, attempts may be made to reduce the cyclosporin dose, particularly if the dose or blood level is high. If renal function is deteriorating rapidly or does not improve after 3 days, biopsy should be done. Acute rejection should be treated with high-dose steroids. Monoclonal antibodies should be used only if the rejection episode does not respond to steroids. If the biopsy suggests preeclampsia and the fetus is mature, delivery is indicated. It is occasionally justifiable to temporize if the fetus is premature, if blood pressure elevations are moderate and signs of severe preeclampsia are absent, and if the decline in renal function is mild and not rapidly progressive. The pregnancy need not be terminated for acute rejection or cyclosporin toxicity, but the fetus should be monitored carefully, as delivery may be indicated for fetal distress. If renal function declines as a result of progression of the underlying disease, termination of the pregnancy generally fails to bring about a lasting improvement in renal function; thus, terminating the pregnancy in cases of prematurity may not be justified.

SUGGESTED READING

Cattran DC, Benzie RJ. Pregnancy in a continuous ambulatory dialysis patient. Perit Dial Bull 1983;3:13–14.

Hou S. Peritoneal and haemodialysis in pregnancy. Clin Obstet Gynaecol (Balliere's) 1987;1:1009–1025.

Hou SH, Grossman SD, Madias NE. Pregnancy in women with renal disease and moderate renal insufficiency. Am J Med
1985;78:185–194.

Katz AI, Davison JM, Hayslett JP, et al. Pregnancy in women with
kidney disease. Kidney Int 1980;18:192–206.

Penn I, Makowski EL, Harris P. Parenthood after renal transplanta-
tion. Kidney Int 1980;18:221–233.

Redrow M, Cherem L, Elliot J, et al. Dialysis in the management of
pregnant patients with renal insufficiency. Medicine 1988;67:199–
208.

Schiff E, Peleg E, Goldenberg M, et al. The use of aspirin to prevent
pregnancy induced hypertension and to lower the ratio of thromboxane A_2 to prostacyclin in relatively high risk pregnancies. N
Engl J Med 1989;321:351–356.

Surian M, Imbasciati E, Cosci P, et al. Glomerular disease and pregnancy. Nephron 1984;36:101–105.

Whetham JCG, Cardella C, Harding M. Effect of pregnancy on graft
function and graft survival in renal cadaver transplant patients.
Am J Obstet Gynecol 1983;145:193–197.

CHAPTER
TWENTY-THREE

Peripartal Adult Thrombotic Thrombocytopenic Purpura and Hemolytic-Uremic Syndrome

THROMBOTIC THROMBOCYTOPENIC PURPURA

Thrombotic thrombocytopenic purpura (TTP) is a clinical diagnosis. The majority of patients express their disease in the postpartum period, although illness may occur during the late second and early third trimester of pregnancy. To make the diagnosis accurately requires that all three major criteria and two of the minor criteria be present (Table 23-1). It must be emphasized, however, that the clinical pentad of TTP is variable and often incomplete at initial presentation. Pregnant patients usually present with a variety of clinical features (Table 23-2). Nonspecific constitutional symptoms such as musculoskeletal discomfort can also be present. Often, the fever in these multisystem diseases is at or near 102°F, the platelet count is usually less than 50,000/mm, and neurologic manifestations may be highly variable and evanescent.

The most striking histopathologic feature of TTP is the presence of widespread subendothelial and intraluminal hyaline consisting of platelets and fibrin. The former are unique to TTP-hemolytic-uremic syndrome (HUS) patients and absent in

---

TABLE 23-1

Adult thrombotic thrombocytopenic purpura (TTP) syndrome description and definition

Major Criteria

---

1. Severe thrombocytopenic purpura.
2. Coombs' test negative for microangiopathic hemolytic anemia.
3. Fluctuating neurologic abnormality or complaint.

Minor Criteria

---

4. Fever.
5. Renal abnormalities (BUN ≤40 mg/dL, creatinine ≤3 mg/dL), hematuria, proteinuria, hypertension.
6. Microthrombi on tissue biopsy.
7. No evidence of DIC.
8. Normal antithrombin III activity.

BUN = blood urea nitrogen; DIC = disseminated intravascular coagulopathy.

---

preeclampsia–eclampsia syndrome. These thrombi occlude capillaries and small arterioles in the absence of a surrounding inflammatory reaction or tissue necrosis. A spectrum of abnormalities is seen under the electron microscope, including simple endothelial cell swelling, subendothelial deposits of hyaline material in nonoccluded larger arterioles, vessels with lumen occluded by loose platelet aggregates, and occlusive thrombi. Although detectable throughout the vascular system, hyaline thrombi predominantly involve the brain, heart, kidneys, pancreas, and adrenal gland.

During life, changes in the maternal red cell facilitate diagnosis. Microangiopathic hemolytic anemia is characterized by severe anemia, reticulocytosis, and red-cell fragmentation on a peripheral blood smear. Burr cells, schistocytes, microspherocytes, and other varieties of abnormally shaped cells are invariably present in advanced TTP. Intravascular hemolysis is reflected by a high serum lactic dehydrogenase (LDH), elevated indirect bilirubin, reduced haptoglobin, hemoglobinemia, and occasional hemoglobinuria. Direct Coombs' testing should be negative.

Thrombocytopenia, which precedes the development of hemolysis, usually becomes severe, with less than 50,000 platelets/mm. However, in contrast to preeclampsia, there is no evidence for primary endothelial damage. Coagulation studies—including prothrombin time (PT), partial thromboplastin time (PTT), antithrombin III (AT III), fibronectin, fibrinogen, protein C, and ratio of factor VIII antigen to activity—are usually normal. The presence of moderate amounts of fibrin split prod-

---

TABLE 23-2

The spectrum of clinical features in adult TTP-HUS syndromes

Presenting Symptoms	Presenting Signs

Neurologic (often intermittent)
    Confusion
    Mental status changes
    Dizziness
    Headache
    Focal/central losses
	Fever
	Neurologic
	    Tremor
	    Hemiparesis
	    Seizures
	    Coma

Bleeding (usually mild traumatic)
    Easy bruisability
	Hemorrhage
	    Petechiae
	    Ecchymoses

Gastrointestinal
    Abdominal pain
    Diarrhea
    Nausea
    Vomiting
	Blood pressure
	    Normotension (TTP)
	    Hypertension (HUS)

Nonspecific
    Weakness
    Fatigue
    Agitation
	Nonspecific
	    Pallor
	    Agitation

Occasional prodromal illness	

ucts (FSP), however, is a nonspecific finding and does not detract from the diagnosis of TTP.

Peripheral thrombocytopenia is accompanied by marked marrow megakaryocytic hyperplasia. Histological confirmation by bone marrow core biopsy or skin biopsy of a petechial spot can sometimes substantiate the diagnosis in confusing cases when the characteristic thrombotic vascular lesion of platelet-capillary microthrombotic occlusion is observed. Ordinarily, patients with TTP have minimal elevations of BUN and creatinine. They are not oliguric, although they have some sediment findings, proteinuria, and microscopic hematuria (Table 23-3).

TABLE 23-3
Laboratory features of TTP

---

1. Microangiopathic hemolytic anemia (MHA)
   Anemia, often severe
   Reticulocytosis
   Red cell fragmentation
   Nucleated red cells, spherocytes, myelocytes, schistocytes, helmet cells
   High lactate dehydrogenase (LDH)
   Negative direct Coombs' test
   Indirect hyperbilirubinemia
   Hemoglobinemia (occasional)
   Leukocytosis
   Absent serum haptoglobin

2. Thrombocytopenia: usually severe

3. Azotemia: usually mild–moderate

4. Normal coagulation parameters: PT, PTT, thrombin time (TT), fibrinogen, FSP, AT III, fibronectin

5. Abnormal urinary sediment
   Microscopic hematuria
   Proteinuria
   Hemoglobinuria

6. Bone marrow aspirate: marked megakaryocytic hyperplasia

7. Gingival/skin biopsy of petechial spot: platelet microthrombi

---

HEMOLYTIC-UREMIC SYNDROME

In both adult TTP and adult HUS, in vivo platelet aggregation is considered to be the primary problem, although both the pathogenesis of and the basic pathophysiologic mechanism leading to these clinical syndromes are unknown. In adult HUS, the kidney is the major organ affected. Adult HUS, like adult TTP, is characterized by the finding of platelet aggregates, platelet fibrin thrombi, or subendothelial deposition of mucinous material in the small blood vessels of many organs but especially in the afferent arterioles and glomeruli of the kidneys.

At the ultrastructural level, there is swelling of endothelial cells. The formation and localization of the platelet thrombi and the differences in their characteristic organ distribution account for the neurologic symptoms and signs in adult TTP and for impaired renal function in adult HUS. In adult HUS, the glomeruli show varying degrees of damage, ranging from focal necrosis to total infarction. In contrast to the severe renal damage and acute renal failure of adult HUS patients, in adult TTP, there is usually only mild impairment of kidney function. Glomerulosclerosis secondary to adult HUS with associated tubal atrophy can be present with irreversible renal impairment.

Hypertension secondary to renal impairment is a universal feature of adult HUS, whereas it is less commonly present in adult TTP. Because of the renal changes and associated secondary hypertension, DIC is occasionally encountered in patients with adult HUS. Although the kidney is the primary target organ in HUS, almost all patients with this disorder also have gastrointestinal complaints, whereas only 30% of patients with TTP have nausea and vomiting or abdominal pain. Neurologic symptoms are always present in TTP, but they are uncommon in HUS, unless they occur secondary to metabolic problems. In HUS patients, there appears to be a good correlation between the pathological findings on renal biopsy and the eventual clinical outcome. Persistent renal insufficiency seems to be related to the severity and duration of disease as well as the number of sclerotic glomeruli. The various forms of HUS are outlined in Table 23-4. TTP and HUS are regarded by most authors as two

---

TABLE 23-4
The adult HUS syndromes: clinical classification

Classic form: infants

Microepidemic

Postinfectious forms
  Shigella dysenteriae
  Streptococcus pneumoniae
  Salmonella typhi
  Certain viruses

Hereditary forms
  Autosomal dominant
  Autosomal recessive

Immunologic form
  Complement activation

Secondary forms
  Connective tissue disorders
  Hypertension
  Renal irradiation
  Immunosuppressive drugs

Pregnancy/oral contraceptive form
  Postpartum renal failure

---

expressions of a more general syndrome of thrombotic microangiopathy.

The pathogenesis and pathophysiology of the microangiopathic TTP and HUS disorders continue to be elusive and controversial. Disorders that may mimic TTP-HUS are outlined in Table 23-5.

For the obstetrician encountering a pregnant patient with thrombotic microangiopathy syndrome, the most important disease to rule out in the differential diagnosis is any form of severe preeclampsia. When adult TTP or HUS are present prior to or during the first trimester of gestation, the diagnosis is relatively easy to make, and some successful pregnancies after therapy have been reported. Later in gestation, the differential diagnostic problem is more difficult because of the strik-

TABLE 23-5
Differential diagnosis of the adult TTP-HUS syndromes

DIC

Evans's syndrome (immune mediated thrombocytopenic purpura + immune mediated hemolytic anemia)

Vasculitis
- Systemic lupus erythematosus (SLE)
- Severe glomerulonephritis
- Other

Other causes of MHA
- Vascular malformation
- Prosthetic valves
- Metastatic adenocarcinoma
- Malignant hypertension

Adult TTP-HUS-like syndromes
- Acute fatty liver of pregnancy
- Postpartum acute renal failure
- Severe preeclampsia–eclampsia–HELLP

ing similarities between the HELLP syndrome form of severe preeclampsia–eclampsia and adult TTP. It is important to differentiate between adult TTP-HUS syndromes and severe preeclampsia–eclampsia–HELLP syndromes because patients with the latter disorder usually respond dramatically to delivery while the former situation requires other therapy. Because severe preeclampsia–eclampsia is a more common condition, it should generally be assumed to be present if clinical and pathological data are not helpful in differentiating these disorders. Because AT III activity is usually normal in patients with adult TTP and diminished in patients with preeclampsia, measurement of AT III activity may be helpful, especially in critical preterm circumstances, so that unnecessary early delivery of a TTP gestation is not undertaken.

TREATMENT

The small number of pregnant patients studied retrospectively with thrombotic microangiopathy and the lack of prospective investigations render it impossible to make dependable, well-tried, and proven recommendations for treatment. A large number of therapies have been proposed, and most have been empiric (Table 23-6). Some form of plasma manipulation is the cornerstone of therapy for these disorders, although the exact type of plasma manipulation to recommend remains controversial. There seems to be general agreement that patients who demonstrate mild renal and neurologic involvement need only supportive care because their prognosis is benign, especially with adult

---

TABLE 23-6

Therapeutic approaches to adult TPP-HUS syndromes

Primary therapy
    Fresh-frozen plasma infusion
    Plasma exchange
    Hemodialysis (HUS)
Secondary therapy
    Glucocorticoids
    Antiplatelet agents
        Aspirin
        Dipyridamole
        Dextran 70
        Splenectomy (TTP)
Experimental therapy
    Prostacyclin infusion
    Vincristine sulfate (TTP)
    Vitamin E infusion
    Hyperimmune gamma globulin
Defunct therapy
    Heparin
    Bilateral nephrectomy

HUS. However, parturients who have severe clinical manifestations and are therefore more likely to suffer serious consequences of their disease are considered to be candidates for more aggressive therapy.

Infusion of fresh-frozen plasma, presumably intended to replace a deficient plasma factor, is recommended therapy immediately after the diagnosis of mild to moderate adult TTP-HUS is confirmed and/or as a measure to prevent relapse and protect a remission. The volume to be administered and the intervals of treatment are individualized, given both the hazard of volume overload and the length of time required to infuse a large volume. Recommended volumes are 30 mL/kg over the first 24 hours, followed by 15 mL/kg per day (or enough to maintain the LDH concentration below 500 units/mL, achieve a spontaneous increase in platelet count to near-normal values, and achieve a disappearance of both neurologic manifestations and renal compromise). Infusion of more than 6 units per day of plasma is often poorly tolerated, with overhydration of the patient. Alternatively, one plasma volume over the first 24 hours can be administered by plasma exchange with donor plasma. As many as 60%–70% of patients overall respond to fresh-frozen plasma infusions with clinically evident improvement, followed by a spontaneous increase in the platelet count and a progressive decrease in serum LDH levels. Individual variation is to be expected, with little correlation having been observed between disease severity and response rate. Relapse occurs in some patients when therapy is discontinued, and repeated induction or maintenance plasma infusions may be required at variable intervals.

Plasma exchange on a cell separator, usually with fresh-frozen plasma as the only replacement fluid, should be instituted: 1) on all patients with adult TTP unresponsive to plasma infusions alone; 2) after 48 hours, or earlier if the facilities are readily available; or 3) if the disease is severe and becoming rapidly progressive. Some investigators feel that intensive plasma exchange should routinely be the initial management of TTP. Optimal guidelines for volume and duration of therapy are difficult to establish. One approach is to exchange two to four liters of plasma with each exchange on a daily basis until a platelet count of 150,000/mm or higher is observed and then to convert to an alternate-day or every-third-day cycle. Reported overall response rates are slightly better than simple plasma infusion and range from 60% to 86% using an intensive plasma exchange and replacement regimen.

In gravidas with adult HUS syndrome, it is critically important to initiate comprehensive supportive therapy first, with correction of fluid and electrolyte imbalance, and to use dialysis in the control of renal failure (BUN >100 mg%) second. Meticulous attention to salt and water management with prevention of hyperkalemia is imperative. Thereafter, or in concert, plasma infusions are administered and/or plasma exchange begun in a protocol similar to that for adult TTP. The aggressive use of plasma exchange with fresh-frozen plasma fluid replacement may be the superior therapy in adults with this microangiopathy. Use of plasma exchange with a hollow fiber plasma separator has been suggested for patients with adult HUS because this equipment permits the patient to receive dialysis and plasmapheresis sequentially with great convenience and safety.

Antiplatelet agents may also be used in the treatment of TTP and HUS. The combination of aspirin and dipyridamole as secondary therapeutic agents for maintenance therapy may reduce systemic embolization and correct altered platelet turnover. Use of aspirin in daily dosages not exceeding 100 mg may be efficacious and devoid of adverse effects. When a remission is achieved, maintenance therapy with oral antiplatelet agents is usually initiated and continued for a few months. The ideal nonpregnant treatment regime for these drugs is also undetermined, but aspirin 300 mg twice daily and dipyridamole 400–600 mg daily in divided doses every 6 hours is a widely recommended combination.

The infusion of platelet concentrates should be restricted to circumstances of life-threatening hemorrhage or to preparation of patients who have platelet counts <50,000/mm immediately prior to surgery or invasive procedures. Administration of platelet concentrates has been associated with worsening of intravascular thrombus formation. The use of heparin is not indicated.

Prostacyclin or vincristine infusion, the administration of high-dose gamma globulin, or splenectomy may be considered in refractory cases.

Adult TTP-HUS syndrome

Goals of Therapy

1. To improve neurologic and renal status (serum creatinine, creatinine clearance).
2. To control hypertension.
3. To reverse thrombotic microangiopathy (stable hematocrit, platelet count >100,000/mL, LDH <500 IU/mL).

Management Protocol

1. Transfer to tertiary care facility.
2. Mild aTTP-aHUS: infuse 30 mL/kg fresh-frozen plasma over 24 hours (6–8 units in divided administrations) and follow with 15 mL/kg daily.
3. Moderate to severe aTTP-aHUS: initiate plasma exchange therapy, 40 mL/kg in exchange daily, days 1 through 5, and follow with 30 mL/kg in exchange, days 7 and 9. Use a continuous automated erythrocytapheresis procedure if equipment is available.
4. Perform concurrent dialysis if necessary to control renal failure.
5. Initiate antihypertensive therapy for diastolic BP >110 mm Hg.
6. Transfuse as necessary to maintain the hemoglobin above 10 g%.
7. Following clinical response, administer dipyridamole 50 mg P.O. t.i.d., aspirin 325 mg P.O. b.i.d., prednisone 100 mg P.O. q.d., multivitamin, and folate.
8. If above modalities fail, consider splenectomy, prostacyclin infusions, and vincristine sulfate.
9. Careful fetal monitoring is crucial, with intervention for standard obstetric criteria only.

Critical Laboratory Tests

CBC with platelet count and red cell morphology, LDH, bilirubin, BUN, creatinine, electrolytes, PT and PTT, thrombin clotting time, fibrinogen, fibrin split products, direct and indirect Coombs' test, uric acid, urinalysis, antiplatelet antibody testing. LE prep/antinuclear antibody and serum complement levels. Bone marrow, gingival, or petechial skin biopsy in suspected aTTP.

Consultation

Nephrology, hematology, neurology.

SUGGESTED READING

Ambrose A, Welham RT, Cefalo RC. Thrombotic thrombocytopenic purpura in early pregnancy. Obstet Gynecol 1985;66:267.

Aster RH. Plasma therapy for thrombotic thrombocytopenic purpura: sometimes it works, but why? N Engl J Med 1985;312:985.

Atlas M, Barkai G, Menczer J, et al. Thrombotic thrombocytopenic purpura in pregnancy. Br J Obstet Gynaecol 1982;89:476.

Bukowski RM, King JW, Hewlett JS. Plasmapheresis in the treatment of thrombotic thrombocytopenic purpura. Blood 1977;50:413.

Caggiano V, Fernando LP, Schneider JM, et al. Thrombotic thrombocytopenic purpura: report of fourteen cases—occurrence during pregnancy and response to plasma exchange. J Clin Apheresis 1983;1:71.

Cochetto DM, Cook L, Cato AF, et al. Rationale and proposal for use of prostacyclin in thrombotic thrombocytopenic purpura therapy. Semin Thromb Haemost 1981;7:43.

Cutner J. Thrombotic thrombocytopenic purpura: a ten year experience. Blood 1980;56:302.

Drummond KN. Hemolytic uremic syndrome—then and now. N Engl J Med 1985;312:116.

Finn NG, Wang JC, Kong KJ. High-dose intravenous Y-immunoglobulin infusion in the treatment of thrombotic thrombocytopenic purpura. Arch Intern Med 1987;147:2165.

Kwaan HC. The pathogenesis of thrombotic thrombocytopenic purpura. Semin Thromb Hemost 1979;5:181.

Lazebnik N, Jaffa AJ, Peyeser MR. Hemolytic-uremic syndrome in pregnancy: review of the literature and report of a case. Obstet Gynecol Surv 1985;40:618.

Lichtin AE, Schreiber AD, Hurwitz S, et al. Efficacy of intensive plasmapheresis in thrombotic thrombocytopenic purpura. Arch Intern Med 1987;147:2122.

May HV Jr, Harbert GM Jr, Thornton WN Jr. Thrombotic thrombocytopenic purpura associated with pregnancy. Am J Obstet Gynecol 1976;126:452.

Obrig TG, Del Vecchio PJ, Karmali MA, et al. Pathogenesis of haemolytic uraemic syndrome. Lancet 1987;2:687.

Petitt RM. Thrombotic thrombocytopenic purpura: a 30-year review. Semin Thromb Hemost 1981;7:1.

Rossi EC, del Greco F, Kwaan HC, et al. Hemodialysis-exchange transfusion for treatment of thrombotic thrombocytopenic purpura. JAMA 1980;244:1466.

Spencer CD, Crane KM, Kumar J, et al. Treatment of postpartum hemolytic uremic syndrome with plasma exchange. JAMA 1982;247:2808.

Walker BK, Ballis SK, Martinez J. Plasma infusion for thrombotic thrombocytopenic purpura during pregnancy. Arch Intern Med 1980;140:981.

Weiner CP. Thrombotic microangiopathy in pregnancy and the postpartum period. Sem Hematol 1987;24:119.

CHAPTER TWENTY-FOUR

Acute Fatty Liver of Pregnancy

Acute fatty liver (AFL) is a rare condition with an estimated incidence of 1 in 15,000 pregnancies. Its cause is unknown.

AFL usually occurs in primigravid women beyond 30 weeks into gestation, or in the immediate puerperium. In women affected by acute fatty liver, there is an increased frequency of twin gestations and male fetuses. There is no firm association of acute fatty liver with increasing maternal age or ethnic background.

Prodromal symptoms and signs include malaise, anorexia, lethargy, tachycardia, and nausea and vomiting. Fever is not typically present in the early stage of the disease but may develop later. After one to three weeks, jaundice develops, usually in association with right-upper-quadrant pain, hepatic tenderness, and ascites. The liver typically is small and nonpalpable. Preeclampsia is present in approximately 40% of affected patients. Generalized edema, gastrointestinal hemorrhage, disseminated intravascular coagulation, pleural effusion, and renal insufficiency also are common clinical manifestations. Eighty percent of patients experience prominent central nervous system aberrations, including restlessness, confusion, disorientation, asterixis, seizures, psychosis, and ultimately, coma.

LABORATORY ABNORMALITIES

The white blood cell count usually is elevated to the range of 20,000–30,000/mm^3. Toxic granulations may be present in leukocytes. Platelets usually are decreased in number. Anemia may be present either as a consequence of pregnancy itself or as the result of gastrointestinal bleeding. Normoblasts typically are evident in the peripheral blood smear.

Serum transaminase concentrations are increased but much less so than would be expected in the face of profound hepatic failure. The serum alkaline phosphatase level and bilirubin concentration also are elevated moderately. Serum concentration of bilirubin usually is less than 10 mg/dL; however, values as high as 25 mg/dL have been recorded. Serum ammonia levels typically are elevated. In women who survive the acute phase of their illness, liver function tests usually return to normal within four to eight weeks after delivery.

In the presence of acute hepatic failure, synthesis of coagulation factors is impaired severely. Accordingly, coagulation tests such as the prothrombin time and partial thromboplastin time usually are prolonged. Frank disseminated intravascular coagulation also may occur during the course of acute fatty liver. Renal dysfunction frequently is associated with hepatic failure. Urine volume and creatinine clearance are decreased. Serum concentration of uric acid and blood urea nitrogen are increased. With the onset of jaundice, urobilinogen usually is present in the urine.

PATHOLOGY

The liver typically is smaller than normal and weighs approximately 1000–1500 grams. It is a uniform pale yellow color. The capsule is thin, transparent, and wrinkled. Subcapsular hemorrhages may be apparent on gross examination, although the lobular structure usually is well preserved.

Characteristic histologic changes are evident in both permanent and frozen sections of the liver. On microscopic examination, individual parenchymal cells are swollen. There is a diffuse fatty infiltration within the hepatocytes; this infiltration is best demonstrated by special stains such as oil-red-O. Fatty infiltration takes the form of fine cytoplasmic vacuoles that give the cells a distinct foamy appearance. These microvesicular deposits may not be evident if only hematoxylin and eosin stains are used. The fat deposits primarily are free fatty acids rather than triglycerides. The myriad of tiny vacuoles are separated from each other by thin eosinophilic cytoplasmic strands. The vacuoles typically do not coalesce to form a single large vacuole. The cell nucleus is located centrally and is normal in size and appearance.

With rare exceptions, necrosis and inflammation are conspicuously absent. Serial liver biopsies in affected patients have confirmed that, even over time, the characteristic lesions do not progress to a stage of necrosis. Characteristic histologic changes may be present up to 3 weeks after the onset of jaundice.

Histologic changes usually are most prominent in the central portion of the lobule. Frequently, there is a thin rim of normal hepatocytes at the periphery of each affected lobule. Bile thrombi may be present, but the gallbladder and extrahepatic biliary system are normal.

DIFFERENTIAL DIAGNOSIS

Three principal disorders should be considered in the differential diagnosis of acute fatty liver of pregnancy: acute viral hepatitis, cholestasis of pregnancy, and preeclampsia. Table 24-1 summarizes the similarities and differences among these four diseases.

The clinical manifestations of fulminant viral hepatitis and acute fatty liver may be quite similar. Histologic changes of fulminant viral hepatitis are characterized by extensive necrosis and inflammation, features not typically observed in acute fatty liver. This distinction, however, may not always be absolute; in one recent review, histologic findings from biopsy specimens were initially misinterpreted as acute hepatitis in four of seven cases.

The distinction between acute fatty liver of pregnancy and preeclampsia may not be possible on the basis of clinical presenta-

TABLE 24-1

Differential diagnosis of acute fatty liver of pregnancy

	Fatty Liver of Pregnancy	Acute Viral Hepatitis
Trimester	Third	Variable
Parity	Nullipara	No association
Clinical manifestations	Malaise, nausea, jaundice, altered sensorium	Malaise, nausea, jaundice, anorexia, altered sensorium
Bilirubin	Increased	Increased
Transaminases	Minimal increase	Marked increase
Alkaline phosphatase	Normal for pregnancy	Minimal increase
Histology	Fatty infiltration, no inflammation or necrosis	Marked inflammation and necrosis
Perinatal mortality	Marked increase	Minimal increase
Maternal mortality	Marked increase	Minimal increase
Recurrence in subsequent pregnancy	No	No

tion and laboratory evaluation alone, especially in view of the fact that preeclampsia may be a superimposed illness for at least 40% of women with primary acute fatty liver. Elevation in serum transaminase, bilirubin, and uric acid may occur in both diseases. In preeclampsia, blood urea nitrogen usually is not increased to as high a level as that noted in acute fatty liver. Further, while thrombocytopenia is not uncommon in preeclampsia, DIC is rarely seen in this condition in the absence of placental abruption.

In many situations, liver biopsy may be the only diagnostic test that can distinguish between the two conditions. Unfortunately, the presence of coagulation defects may make liver biopsy impossible during the acute phase of the patient's illness.

Cholestasis	Severe Preeclampsia
Third	Third
No association	Nullipara
Pruritus, jaundice	Hypertension, edema, proteinuria, oliguria, CNS hyperexcitability, coagulopathy
Increased	Normal or increased
Minimal increase	Normal or minimal to moderate increase
Moderate increase	Normal for pregnancy
Biliary stasis, no inflammation	Inflammation, necrosis, fibrin deposition
Minimal increase	Moderate increase
No increase	Moderate increase
Yes	Yes

Several recent reports have examined the utility of computerized tomography in the diagnosis of acute fatty liver. All investigators have described diffuse decreased attenuation over the liver, consistent with fatty infiltration.

TREATMENT

Patients with acute fatty liver of pregnancy should be hospitalized in an intensive care setting. The first objective is to ensure that there is a patent airway and that effective ventilation and oxygenation are maintained. The second objective is to provide optimal nutrition and to reduce the endogenous production of nitrogenous wastes. The patient should receive approximately 2000–2500 calories per day, primarily in the form of glucose. Twenty to 25% glucose solutions should be administered by nasogastric tube or by intravenous infusion. During the acute phase of the illness, protein intake should be excluded. Protein should be restored gradually to the diet when the patient begins to show clinical improvement.

Magnesium citrate should be given orally in a dose of 30–50 mL to promote colonic emptying. Fleet enemas also may be used for this purpose. Neomycin, 6–12 grams orally per day, is of value in decreasing production of ammonia by intestinal bacteria. With rare exceptions, any drug that requires hepatic metabolism should be withheld from the patient.

The third objective of therapy is to correct electrolyte abnormalities and metabolic disturbances such as hypoglycemia. A fourth objective is to identify and correct promptly any coagulation abnormalities that develop. This objective is accomplished most effectively by administration of vitamin K, platelets, and fresh-frozen plasma.

The final objective is to minimize the risk of gastrointestinal hemorrhage. The most important preventative measure is correction of coagulation abnormalities. In selected patients, administration of antacid solutions may be indicated.

Finally, after the diagnosis is established, preparations should be made for delivery. Prompt delivery appears to result in improved maternal and neonatal survival. There are no reported cases in which patients have recovered from acute fatty liver prior to delivery.

There is no prospective controlled study, however, that demonstrates that immediate cesarean section offers an advantage over vaginal delivery, provided that supportive care is optimal and progress in labor is rapid. The decision about method of delivery should be based on assessment of maternal and fetal condition and the favorability of the cervix for induction of labor. Fetal distress, possibly on the basis of uteroplacental insufficiency, appears to be more common in these patients. If cesarean delivery is performed, regional anesthesia should be used, provided that coagulation abnormalities can be corrected. If general anesthesia is necessary, agents with potential hepatotoxicity (e.g., halothane) should be avoided.

In patients who continue to deteriorate despite supportive care, several experimental modalities may be considered. Such forms of therapy include exchange transfusion, hemodialysis, plasmapheresis, extracorporal perfusion, and liver transplant. Unfortunately, there is virtually no published information concerning the efficacy of these measures in the treatment of acute fatty liver of pregnancy.

PROGNOSIS

Before 1980, investigations of acute fatty liver reported perinatal mortality rates in excess of 75%. Most of the fetal deaths occurred as the direct result of death of the mother. The majority of neonatal deaths resulted from complications of prematurity. More recent data indicate a fetal mortality of 14%. This more favorable prognosis presumably reflects earlier diagnosis and improved supportive care for the infant.

Similarly, in reports published from 1940 to 1980, the maternal mortality associated with acute fatty liver has been in the range of 75%–80%. Recently, however, there have been reports in which maternal mortality was reduced to the range of 8%–10%. In these latter investigations, the improved survival was attributed to early diagnosis and prompt delivery.

In women who survive the acute phase of their illness, recovery of hepatic, renal, and neurologic function usually is complete. The disorder does not appear to recur in subsequent pregnancies.

Acute fatty liver of pregnancy

Goals of Therapy

1. To normalize liver function tests, electrolytes, clotting profile, and serum ammonia.
2. To prevent renal failure.
3. To maintain serum glucose >60 mg%.
4. To return patient to normal mental status.
5. To deliver the fetus.

Management Protocol

1. Hospitalize in intensive care unit.

2. If the patient is comatose, provide a secure airway and maintain effective ventilation and oxygenation.

3. Provide optimal nutrition. Administer 2000–2500 calories per 24 hours. Administer most of the calories in the form of concentrated glucose solutions.

4. Decrease endogenous ammonia production. Restrict protein intake during acute phase of illness. Evacuate colonic contents by administering magnesium citrate orally or by instilling Fleet enema solutions via rectum. Administer oral neomycin, 6–12 g/24 h, to decrease production of ammonia by intestinal bacteria.

5. Avoid use of medications that require hepatic metabolism.

6. Correct electrolyte and metabolic derangements.

7. Identify and correct coagulation abnormalities. Administer vitamin K, fresh-frozen plasma, or platelets as indicated.

8. Maintain surveillance for nosocomial infection, especially pneumonia, urosepsis, bacteremia.

9. Prevent gastrointestinal hemorrhage.

10. Deliver the patient promptly after the diagnosis is established.

Critical Laboratory Tests

Complete blood count (CBC), platelet count, partial thromboplastin time (PTT), prothrombin time (PT), fibrinogen, fibrin split products, serum glutamic pyruvic transaminase (SGPT), serum glutamic oxaloacetic transaminase (SGOT), alkaline phosphatase, total and direct bilirubin, blood urea nitrogen (BUN), creatinine, serum electrolytes, serum ammonia, liver biopsy (if coagulopathy is not present).

Consultation

Internal medicine, gastroenterology.

SUGGESTED READING

Kaplan MM. Acute fatty liver of pregnancy. N Engl J Med
  1985;313:367.

Mabie WC, Dacus JV, Sibai BM, et al. Computed tomography in
  acute fatty liver of pregnancy. Am J Obstet Gynecol
  1988;158:142.

Moise KJ, Shah DM. Acute fatty liver of pregnancy: etiology of fetal
  distress and fetal wastage. Obstet Gynecol 1987;69:482.

Riely CA, Latham PS, Romero R, et al. Acute fatty liver of pregnancy. A reassessment based on observations in nine patients.
  Ann Int Med 1987;106:703.

Rolfes DB, Ishak KG. Acute fatty liver in pregnancy: a
  clinicopathologic study of 35 cases. Hepatology 1985;5:1149.

CHAPTER TWENTY-FIVE

Trauma in Pregnancy

The most frequent cause of death in women 35 years of age or less is trauma. Trauma is also the leading nonobstetric cause of maternal mortality, accounting for 20% of such deaths. The risks of trauma increase as pregnancy progresses; the incidence of all trauma is 8.8% in the first trimester, 40% in the second, and 52% in the third. This chapter will be limited to considerations unique to the pregnant patient.

GENERAL CONSIDERATIONS

During the first trimester of pregnancy, the uterus and urinary bladder are confined to the bony pelvis and are thereby at reduced risk in cases of abdominal trauma. As pregnancy progresses to about the thirteenth to fourteenth week, the uterus becomes an abdominal organ and thereby is more disposed to injury. It does, however, shield other intra-abdominal organs from penetrating injury. The bladder, when distended, passively becomes an abdominal organ in the second and third trimester. Penetrating injury to the bladder becomes more frequent as pregnancy advances.

The smooth-muscle-relaxant property of the elevated levels of progesterone has a profound and clinically important effect on the gastrointestinal (GI) tract. Gastric motility is decreased, and gastric emptying time is increased. As a result, the pregnant woman is predisposed to regurgitation and aspiration. Airway management, particularly in the obtunded patient, is of critical importance.

Distension of the abdomen can obscure clinical findings suggestive of intraperitoneal injury. Evidence of guarding or peritoneal irritation may be absent even after documented bowel injury. These findings have led some to conclude that indications for peritoneal lavage and abdominal exploration should be liberalized during pregnancy.

The pancreas and spleen are not significantly affected by pregnancy. Serum amylase levels, sometimes elevated with blunt trauma, are otherwise normal in pregnancy. However, lipase levels may be decreased in pregnancy, and normal values do not exclude the possibility of pancreatic injury.

Of major clinical significance in the care of a traumatized pregnant patient is her markedly diminished tolerance for apnea because of her reduced functional residual capacity (FRC).

When measured with the patient in the supine position, cardiac output declines dramatically in the third trimester secondary to aortocaval compression by the enlarged uterus. One crucial factor in the management of a traumatized gravida is avoidance of the supine position. Even in patients with cervical spine injury, lateral uterine displacement may be accomplished without movement of the head.

Blood volume is also increased by 50% in pregnancy. In a pregnant trauma patient with bleeding, hemodynamic instability, indicating the need for transfusion, may not occur until blood loss approaches 1500–2000 mL. Alterations in pulse and blood pressure may be found later than usual in hypovolemic gravidas. Although heart rate increases by 10%–15% during pregnancy, tachycardia (above 100 beats per minute) still should be considered abnormal in pregnancy.

The "ABCs" of basic cardiac life support apply equally well

to the traumatized gravida. The absence of spontaneous and effective cardiac function mandates initiation of cardiopulmonary resuscitation (CPR) with mechanical chest compression and ventilation with appropriate pharmacologic therapy. When prompt maternal response to CPR is not evident, perimortem cesarean delivery should be considered if the fetus is potentially viable.

Concern is frequently expressed over the use of ionizing radiation during pregnancy. However, even in the first trimester, radiation doses below 5–10 rads are not associated with adverse outcome. In many cases, proper shielding can minimize fetal exposure. However, important diagnostic tests should never be omitted out of fetal concerns in the critically ill mother. (See Table 25-1.)

SPECIFIC INJURY PATTERNS

BLUNT ABDOMINAL TRAUMA

Automobile accidents are the most common cause of serious abdominal trauma in pregnancy. Uterine rupture, unlikely in the first trimester, has been reported with blunt trauma to the gravid abdomen. The incidence of this catastrophic event is less than 1%. In studying subhuman primates subjected to acute deceleration injuries, Crosby and coworkers reported marked increases in intrauterine pressure. They speculated that such an increase is etiologic in uterine rupture. However, because the forces generated lasted only a short time, fetal effects were unlikely to be clinically significant unless uterine rupture or placental abruption occurred.

Lower abdominal trauma may predispose the gravida to pelvic fractures. Unstable pelvic fractures can potentially cause injury to the uterus, urethra, or urinary bladder. Even if preterm labor ensues, a pelvic fracture is not an absolute contraindication to vaginal delivery. X-ray or CT pelvimetry may be helpful in such cases.

Fetal injury following abdominal trauma is rare. The fetus is cushioned by the amniotic fluid, the anterior abdominal wall,

TABLE 25-1

Physiologic adaptations to pregnancy that affect maternal response to trauma

System	Alteration	Clinical Effect
Genitourinary	Uterine enlargement	Protects bowel
	Bladder becomes intra-abdominal	Predisposes to injury
	Ureteral dilation	Abnormal intravenous pyelogram (IVP)
Gastrointestinal	Decreased motility	Prolonged gastric emptying; regurgitation-aspiration
	Distended abdomen	Reduces peritoneal signs
Pulmonary	Increased minute ventilation; increased oxygen consumption; reduced functional residual capacity (FRC)	Predisposes to hypoxemia with apnea
Cardiovascular	Increased cardiac output	
	Aortocaval compression	Supine hypotension
	Increased blood volume	Protects in case of hemorrhage
	Decreased peripheral resistance	Increased skin temperature
Hematologic	Larger relative increase in plasma volume	Physiologic anemia leukocytosis

and the distensible gravid uterus; therefore, forces are distributed more uniformly when blunt trauma is applied to the gravid uterus. Varying injuries have been reported, and no consistent relationship exists between type of trauma and type of injury. Nonetheless, both skull and long-bone fractures have been documented.

The use of seat belts has generated some measure of controversy, particularly during pregnancy. Isolated reports of fetal and maternal injury presumably caused by seat belts have appeared in the literature. The fetal skull can be fractured by being crushed between the seat belt and the sacral promontory. In spite of the isolated reports, the preponderance of evidence supports the safety of seat belt use during pregnancy. The most frequent cause of fetal death remains death of the mother, which occurs more frequently when she is ejected from a motor vehicle or strikes the steering column. Proper positioning of a three-point restraint system (lap and shoulder belts) is recommended for gravidas during automobile travel. These restraints reduce the risk of fetal and maternal death and play an insignificant role in fetal injury.

The greatest clinical concern is generated by placental abruption. This adverse perinatal event has been reported in 5.9% of patients involved in severe automobile collisions; abruption is the leading cause of fetal death when mothers survived automobile accidents. Abruption following significant abdominal trauma also may be delayed. Twenty-four to 48 hours of continuous fetal heart rate monitoring is recommended in such patients.

Kleihauer–Betke determinations should be considered in patients suffering blunt abdominal or multiple trauma. A positive test should be an indication for prolonged fetal heart rate monitoring. Additionally, in the Rh-negative mother, hyperimmune anti-D globulin should be administered in the hopes of preventing sensitization. A single 300-μg dose protects against 15 mL of fetal red blood cells. The Kleihauer–Betke test also may be helpful in determining the number of vials of anti-D globulin necessary.

The final diagnostic consideration in the hemodynamically stable gravida sustaining blunt abdominal trauma is peritoneal lavage (Table 25-2). This technique may be invaluable in the early diagnosis of intraperitoneal injury or hemorrhage. An open technique is recommended. In brief, a vertical infraumbilical incision is made under local anesthesia. The peritoneum is incised; under

TABLE 25-2

Criteria for interpretation of peritoneal lavage

Positive

1. Free-flowing blood on aspiration.
2. Grossly bloody lavage fluid.
3. Appearance of lavage fluid in Foley catheter.
4. Red cell count >100,000/mm^3.
5. White cell count >500/mm^3.
6. Amylase >175 international units per deciliter (IU/dL).

Indeterminate

1. Red cell count between 50,000 and 100,000/mm^3.
2. White cell count between 100 and 500/mm^3.
3. Amylase 75 to 175 IU/dL.

Negative

1. Red cell count <50,000/mm^3.
2. White cell count <100/mm^3.
3. Amylase <75 IU/dL.

(Reproduced with permission from Rothenberger DA, Quattlebaum FW, Zabel J, et al. Diagnostic peritoneal lavage for blunt trauma in pregnant women. Am J Obstet Gynecol 1977;129:479.)

direct visualization, a peritoneal dialysis catheter is placed and directed caudad. If aspiration yields free-flowing blood, the test is considered positive and laparotomy is performed. In the absence of blood, 1 L of warmed Ringer's lactate is infused and allowed to drain by gravity. The returning fluid then is analyzed for cell count (white and red blood cells) and amylase. Table 25-2 lists criteria for interpretation of the test. Positive tests generally mandate laparotomy, and indeterminate tests are repeated. An intermediate step is the use of ultrasound for the diagnosis of hemoperitoneum or as a guide to the performance of paracentesis.

GUNSHOT WOUNDS

After a gunshot victim is stabilized, she should undergo exploratory laparotomy via a midline abdominal incision. Careful exploration of the abdomen, including the entire length of the large and small bowel, stomach, diaphragm, and retroperitoneal surfaces, should be made. With appropriate general and urologic surgical consultation, definitive repair of injuries should be accomplished. Repair of minor uterine injuries also should be considered. The high incidence of fetal injury (59%–89%) should be weighed carefully against the risks of premature delivery in patients sustaining uterine injury. If no significant uterine injury is observed, little is to be gained by incidental cesarean delivery. However, with significant uterine injury in a viable fetus, cesarean delivery is often indicated.

STAB WOUNDS

Stab wounds are the second most frequent type of penetrating injury. Mortality is generally lower than with gunshot wounds. Generally, the extent of intra-abdominal injury is also less, because bowel may slide away from the knife blade. Stab wounds to the upper abdomen are more likely to injure the bowel because the enlarged uterus has crowded the intestines together and shifted their position cephalad.

Controversy exists as to whether all knife wounds need exploration. Use of peritoneal lavage, laparoscopy, or even a fistulogram may reduce the incidence of laparotomy. However, exploration is often indicated when the extent of injury is in question. Intraoperative management and decisions regarding cesarean delivery are similar to those discussed in the section dealing with gunshot wounds.

ELECTRICAL INJURY

The fetus may be at risk with common household electrical injuries that permit current to travel from the hand to the foot, through the uterus and its contents. The frequency of these in-

juries is probably underreported. In one series of six patients
who sustained a household electrical injury, three incurred intrauterine fetal death. In two, an immediate decrease in fetal movement was felt, and fetal death was probably immediate. In two
others, oligohydramnios was noted at delivery. These findings
led the authors to recommend frequent fetal surveillance with
assessment of amniotic fluid and nonstress testing.

THERMAL INJURY

The frequency of burns among pregnant patients is unknown.
Fetal wastage may be as high as 36% with serious first-trimester
burns. Second- and third-trimester burn patients may experience
preterm labor. In view of the metabolic complications associated
with thermal injury, tocolysis should be approached with caution.

Multiple trauma in pregnancy

Goals of Therapy

1. To stabilize maternal condition.
2. To undertake thorough diagnostic evaluation.
3. To evaluate fetal condition.
4. To administer definitive therapy.

Management Protocol

1. Determine cardiopulmonary status.
2. Initiate resuscitation if necessary.
3. Control hemorrhage.
4. Place the patient in a lateral decubitus position.
5. Maintain maternal Po_2 >60 mm Hg to achieve adequate fetal oxygenation.
6. Start one or two large-bore intravenous lines.
7. Implement volume replacement; stabilize vital signs.

8. Initiate fetal monitoring.
9. Insert Foley catheter.
10. Use nasogastric or orogastric tube if warranted.
11. Administer tetanus prophylaxis with or without tetanus-immune globulin.
12. Apply antibiotic coverage as appropriate.
13. Use definitive therapy.

Critical Laboratory Tests

CBC, type and cross-match, arterial blood gas, serum electrolytes, serum amylase, urinalysis; peritoneal lavage and radiographic studies, as appropriate.

Consultation

General surgery, urology, neurosurgery.

SUGGESTED READING

Buchsbaum HJ. Accidental injury during pregnancy. Contemp OB/GYN 1982;20:27.

Chan YF, Sivassambo R. Lightning accidents in pregnancy. J Obstet Gynecol Br Common 1972;79:761.

Crosby WM, Costiloe JD. Safety of lap-belt restraint for pregnant victims of automobile collisions. N Engl J Med 1971;284:362.

Davison JS, Davison MC, Hay DM. Gastric emptying time in late pregnancy and labour. J Obstet Gynecol Br Cwlth 1970;77:37.

Deitch EA, Rightmire DA, Clothier J. Management of burns in pregnant women. Surg Gynecol Obstet 1985;161:1.

Hankins GDV. Trauma during pregnancy, ACOG Technical Bulletin 161. American College of Obstetrics and Gynecologists, 1991.

Higgins SD, Garite TJ. Late abruptio placenta in trauma patients: implications for monitoring. Obstet Gynecol 1984;63:105.

Iliya FA, Hajj SN, Buchsbaum HJ. Gunshot wounds of the pregnant uterus: report of two cases. J Trauma 1980;20:90.

Lavin JP, Polsky SS. Abdominal trauma during pregnancy. Clin Perinatol 1983;10:423.

Lieberman JR, Mazo RM, Molchio J, et al. Electrical accidents during pregnancy. Obstet Gynecol 1986;67:861.

Lowe R. Should laparotomy be mandatory or selective in gunshot wounds of the abdomen? J Trauma 1977;17:903.

Rothenberger DA, Quattlebaum FW, Zabel J, et al. Diagnostic peritoneal lavage for blunt trauma in pregnant women. Am J Obstet Gynecol 1977;149:479.

Schmitz JT. Pregnancy patients with burn. Am J Obstet Gynecol 1971;110:57.

CHAPTER TWENTY-SIX

Intracranial Hemorrhage in Pregnancy

Intracranial hemorrhage (ICH) is a life-threatening complication that may occur in the gravid population. The major cause of ICH in pregnancy is subarachnoid hemorrhage (SAH) from cerebral aneurysm or arteriovenous malformation (AVM) rupture. The incidence of SAH in the pregnant population is 1 in 10,000, with an immediate mortality of 43%. Pregnancy-induced hypertension (PIH) is also associated with intracerebral pathology including ICH, which may account for up to 60% of the deaths associated with eclampsia (Table 26-1). The pathophysiology and management of ICH associated with these SAH, AVM, and eclampsia are discussed in this chapter. Less common etiologies include moyamoya disease, dural venous sinus thrombosis, mycotic aneurysm, choriocarcinoma, vasculitides, and coagulopathies. Recently, cocaine and phenylpropanolamine have also been associated with ICH in pregnant patients.

TABLE 26-1

Causes of death in toxemic patients

	Donnelly et al.	Hibbard	Lopez–Llera	Evans et al.
Cerebral				
Hemorrhage	180	21	62	14
Edema	—	13	—	6
Pulmonary				
Edema	133	3	—	3
Insufficiency	29	4	10	—
Hepatic				
Rupture	30	—	1	3
Necrosis	—	10	—	2
Renal				
Failure	—	2	—	7
Necrosis	—	5	1	—
Coagulopathy	39	6	7	6
Anesthesia	12	—	—	—
Sepsis	18	—	—	—
Drug overdose	—	2	—	—
Undetermined	92	1	3	8
Total	533	67	86	49

(Modified with permission from Evans S, Frigoletto FD, Jewett JF. Mortality of eclampsia: a case report and the experience of the Massachusetts Maternal Mortality Study. N Engl J Med 1983;309:1644.)

SUBARACHNOID HEMORRHAGE

PATHOPHYSIOLOGY

Aneurysms and AVMs are believed to develop secondary to congenital defects in cerebral vasculature formation. Aneurysms generally are located at an angle of bifurcation of vessels in or near the circle of Willis. AVMs, on the other hand, can be located anywhere between the frontal region and the brain stem, but they occur with a slightly higher frequency in frontoparietal and temporal regions. Hemodynamic factors and hormonal changes exist that theoretically may predispose these cerebrovascular abnormalities to bleed during pregnancy. These factors include increases in blood volume, stroke volume, and cardiac output, along with hormonal factors such as increased estrogens, which may result in vasodilation of already abnormal vessels. However, there are no clear clinical data indicating that the incidence of SAH is increased during pregnancy. Parity seems to have little effect on the incidence of SAH, and SAH-associated mortality is not increased by pregnancy. When SAH does occur in association with pregnancy, it most often is identified in the latter half of gestation.

There are three major complications that may occur in a patient suffering from SAH who survives transport to the hospital: 1) hydrocephalus, 2) vasospasm, and 3) rebleed. Hydrocephalus may occur any time in the first 2 weeks following SAH. It appears to be due to blood obstructing the reabsorption of cerebrospinal fluid (CSF) in the subarachnoid villi. The chief danger of hydrocephalus is compression of the brain stem, leading to deterioration in the level of consciousness and, eventually, death. Thus, serial computerized tomography (CT) scans are performed to diagnose this process before it is manifested by a deterioration in the physical exam. The immediate treatment of hydrocephalus is drainage of CSF through a ventriculostomy. Hydrocephalus usually resolves when blood is cleared from the CSF, but some patients require a permanent shunt.

Cerebral ischemia due to vasospasm represents a major threat to survival of patients following SAH, especially those with aneurysm rupture. The mechanism of vasospasm is not clear, but its severity correlates with the amount of blood found in the basilar cisterns. Radiologically, vasospasm appears as cerebral arterial narrowing, sometimes with a beaded pattern. Vasospasm is associated with decreased cerebral blood flow as measured by radioactive tracers such as ^{133}Xenon and by transcranial Doppler. Clinically, the patient may exhibit a relentless progression of hemiparesis, somnolence, and death.

Recurrent bleeds are associated with a much higher mortality than that seen with first bleeds. Aneurysms tend to rebleed at 7–10 days, whereas AVMs are associated with infrequent and late rebleeding. Aneurysms are associated with a 64% and an 80% mortality with the first and second rebleeds, respectively.

CLINICAL PRESENTATION

The clinical presentation of SAH is similar whether resulting from aneurysm or from AVM and may not be distinguishable from intracerebral bleeding associated with severe preeclampsia. Patients with SAH generally present with the sudden onset of a "bursting" headache. The headache generally is accompanied by other symptoms, such as nausea and vomiting, dizziness, and diplopia, and there may be an abrupt decrease in level of consciousness. The symptoms depend on the size, location, and rapidity of the bleed. If the patient is conscious, signs of meningeal irritation (such as nuchal rigidity), as well as cranial nerve palsies or hemiplegia, may be present on physical exam. In other patients, the SAH will have been so massive that the patient presents as moribund.

The condition of the patient at presentation is the most important prognostic indicator of outcome. Clinical grading scales have been developed to categorize the severity of the patient's condition in order to determine management and prognosis. The Hunt and Botterell scales combine the level of consciousness and the presence of neurologic deficit to describe the patient as follows:

Grade I: Alert with or without nuchal rigidity
Grade II: Drowsy or severe headache with no neurologic deficits other than those of the cranial nerves
Grade III: Focal neurologic deficit such as mild hemiparesis
Grade IV: Stupor with severe neurologic deficits
Grade V: Moribund

DIAGNOSIS

It is of primary importance that all suspicious neurologic signs and symptoms in the gravida be evaluated thoroughly. CT of the brain, lumbar puncture (if necessary), and cerebral angiography is the common sequence of testing. The CT scan can predict, with a high degree of accuracy, the type of hemorrhage and its site of origin. In addition, cerebral CT can be useful in determining the presence of life-threatening hematomas requiring surgical evacuation, as well as in following the development of hydrocephalus. If the CT scan is normal, the CSF should be examined for blood or xanthochromia. Nonclearing bloody CSF found at lumbar puncture supports the diagnosis of SAH, but it may also be seen with preeclampsia. Cerebral angiography remains the best diagnostic tool for identifying any vascular abnormality. In addition, important anatomic (and therefore prognostic) information usually is obtained by using this invasive technique. If no lesion is identified, a repeat angiogram may be necessary to rule out false-negative results secondary to vasospasm or clot filling of the aneurysm. Abdominal shielding should always be considered during any radiologic examination of the gravid patient.

MANAGEMENT

Pregnancy alters the standard management of SAH only slightly, as the clinical goals remain the prevention and treatment of neurologic complications. In all patients thought to be viable, immediate management includes evacuation of life-threatening hematomas and treatment of hydrocephalus. A number of considerations have led neurosurgeons to perform aneurysm clipping in the early (<4 days) post-SAH period for patients with Grades I–III. These considerations include the disastrous consequences of rebleeding, the decreased severity of vasospasm with early removal of cisternal blood, and newer developments in neurosurgery and neuroanesthesia. Patients with significant neurologic deficits (Grades IV and V) are not usually subjected to aneurysm clipping due to an extremely high operative mortality. Rather, such patients receive medical therapy until their condition improves. The proper timing for resection of AVMs is more controversial due to the smaller number of available cases. Some surgeons advocate operative intervention in AVMs only to remove clinically significant hematomas. One alternative is embolization of the AVM under angiographic control prior to surgical excision.

Medical therapy is directed toward reducing the risks of

rebleeding and alleviating cerebral ischemia due to vasospasm. Patients are generally confined to bed rest in a dark, quiet room, and they are administered stool softeners, sedatives, and analgesics. Because of the presumed benefits of volume expansion, colloid solutions are frequently administered. Calcium-entry blockers such as nimodipine are begun after angiography in nonpregnant patients.

In surviving patients, most aneurysm ruptures have initially bled only a few milliliters before a platelet plug sealed the leak. This tenuous hemostasis is strengthened over several days by a process of fibrosis. Interference of early physiologic fibrinolysis therefore theoretically improves the patient's chances of avoiding rebleed. Epsilon-aminocaproic acid (EACA) and tranexamic acid block the activation of plasminogen, a precursor of plasmin, a major fibrinolytic protein. Clinical trials initially found a reduction in the incidence of rebleeding with these agents; however, later work failed to demonstrate significant improvement in outcome. Opposition to the use of EACA in pregnancy has been raised by Beller, who suggests that interference with fetal fibrinolysis may be linked to the development of hyaline membrane disease. In this setting, however, practicality must take precedence over theory.

There are two intraoperative therapies of aneurysm clipping—hypotension and hypothermia—that are commonly instituted to reduce complications, which raise special concerns in the pregnant patient. Hypotension is sometimes instituted to reduce the risk of rupture of the aneurysm during dissection. Although maternal hypotension may pose a threat to fetal well-being, it has been successfully induced with sodium nitroprusside or isoflurane in a number of cases. Based on experimental evidence, administration of sodium nitroprusside in pregnant patients has raised concerns regarding potential fetal cyanide toxicity. Thus, it is recommended that infusion rates not exceed 10 μg/kg/min. The fetal effects of maternal hypotension should be evaluated throughout the perianesthetic period with electronic fetal heart rate monitoring. Adverse changes in fetal cardiac activity suggest the need for elevation in maternal blood pressure if safe and feasible from the maternal standpoint. Excessive hyperventilation has been shown to further decrease uterine blood flow during sodium nitroprusside administration and should be avoided. Because the fetus may not tolerate maternal hypotension, some authors recommend cesarean delivery prior to surgery if acceptable fetal maturity is present.

Hypothermia is instituted during cerebral aneurysm clipping as a means of cerebral protection from potential ischemia due to aneurysm rupture, retractor injury, or hypotension. Strange and Haldin have suggested that hypothermia is well tolerated by the mother and fetus, provided that other confounding variables (such as respiratory exchange, acidosis, and electrolyte balance) are controlled. Regardless of the neurosurgical technique employed, maternal outcome remains the most important predictor of fetal outcome.

After a successful repair of an aneurysm or AVM, the most frequent obstetrical concern relates to mode of delivery. Although earlier authors routinely recommended elective cesarean section for these patients, more recent data suggest that labor and vaginal delivery pose no additional risk to mother or fetus. These recommendations probably also hold true for the patient who begins labor before surgical correction is attempted or in the case where the intracranial lesion is inaccessible to surgical intervention. Young and associates have suggested that the physiologic blood pressure increases known to occur with labor are counterbalanced with a parallel increase in CSF pressure. This would result in no overall change in transluminal vascular pressure and represents one explanation for the foregoing clinical observations. However, most authorities still advocate minimizing the hemodynamic stresses of labor by using epidural anesthesia and by shortening the second stage of labor with outlet forceps. In contrast to the foregoing recommendations, Robinson et al. recommend elective cesarean section with concomitant fertility sterilization in patients with AVMs because of a presumed increased risk of subsequent rebleed with vaginal delivery.

PREECLAMPSIA-ASSOCIATED INTRACEREBRAL HEMORRHAGE

Intracerebral hemorrhage is the most common cause of death in the eclamptic patient (Table 26-1). Intracerebral hemorrhage is more likely to occur in the older parturient and is correlated better with advancing maternal age and hypertension than with seizure activity. When hemorrhage does occur, it often does not coincide with the onset of seizures but rather is usually manifested at least six hours after the onset of convulsions.

The clinical report of flashes of light and other fluctuating neurologic signs and symptoms in these patients supports the concept of intermittent ischemia, although the definitive pathologic events involved still remain to be elucidated.

CLINICAL PRESENTATION

A detailed presentation of the clinical aspects of eclampsia has been presented elsewhere in this text. In brief, the eclamptic patient traditionally presents with hypertension and tonic-clonic convulsions. The occurrence of seizure activity, however, does not necessarily result in the subsequent development of intracerebral hemorrhage even if a transient neurologic deficit is identified in the postictal period. When small intracerebral hemorrhages do occur, the patient may present initially with only drowsiness or complaints of flashes of light. If the disease progresses, stupor and focal neurologic deficits worsen. Hemiplegia or rapidly progressive coma and cerebral death may result when a more massive cerebral bleed occurs.

DIAGNOSIS

The diagnosis of preeclampsia is well ingrained in the practicing obstetrician's mind; however, the clinician may not always be alert to the fact that a variety of subtle neurologic abnormalities such as lethargy, visual disturbances, and even acute psychosis can herald the onset of an intracerebral hemorrhage. It is interesting to note the infrequency with which most obstetricians recommend a further workup of these neurologic abnormalities. Few advocate CT scanning to rule out other pathology or to evaluate the significance of a potential bleed. In truth, the clinical approach to the patient will only rarely be altered by this relatively expensive diagnostic evaluation. In addition, most preeclamptic patients are in the process of labor and delivery when they suffer seizures, which makes the logistics of obtaining a CT scan difficult. However, given the increasing availability of CT scanning, more information regarding its utility in the eclamptic patient should be forthcoming. Other diagnostic techniques such as magnetic resonance imaging (MRI) have also been utilized recently in this patient population to better define intracranial pathology. Certainly, any preeclamptic gravida with residual neurologic findings after both acute events and/or delivery deserves the benefit of a complete neurologic evaluation.

MANAGEMENT

Acute surgical intervention, even for the removal of a large intracerebral hematoma, is rarely of benefit. Control of seizure activity and severe hypertension, however, is always indicated. DIC is not an uncommon complication of preeclampsia and aggravates the intracerebral bleeding process. Appropriate management requires monitoring of coagulation indices and replacement therapy as indicated. If the patient's outcome appears to be grave, consideration of perimortem cesarean delivery should be made.

ADJUNCTIVE APPROACHES TO THE PATIENT WITH INTRACRANIAL HEMORRHAGE

Potent glucocorticoids such as dexamethasone have been used widely for the treatment of cerebral edema and ischemia. Support for this use comes not only from laboratory evidence of steroid-induced membrane stabilization but also from the often dramatic clinical improvement of patients with brain tumors. However, little clinical evidence exists for the efficacy of steroids, in any dose, in altering the progress and outcome of patients with cerebral hypoxia or ischemia. There is evidence that the administration of steroids may worsen neurologic outcome in the presence of increased intracranial pressure (ICP).

Cerebral edema can result in elevated ICP. The neurosurgeon may wish to monitor this variable in some patients to avoid severe intracranial hypertension. In patients with SAH, monitoring usually is done with a ventriculostomy so that CSF can be drained if hydrocephalus is present. The ventriculostomy may be connected to a transducer for continuous monitoring. ICP elevations resulting from cerebral edema may be treated with mannitol, an osmotic diuretic. The mechanism of action for mannitol is felt to be primarily desiccation of normal brain tissue. Mannitol is a nonmetabolized sugar that is available in 20% and 25% solutions. Typically, 12.5–50 g is administered intravenously, as needed, to keep the ICP below 20 mm Hg. The development of hyperosmolality is a potential hazard of mannitol therapy and can be monitored by serum osmolality determinations. Normal values are 280–300 mosm/L; the drug should be withheld when a level of 315–320 mosm/L is reached. Care must be taken to prevent hypovolemia resulting from the accompanying diuresis, which could aggravate placental and cerebral hypoperfusion.

In the presence of either ICH or cerebral edema, rapid initiation of diagnostic procedures and therapy is essential. Although pregnancy may complicate the diagnosis, once the life-threatening conditions are recognized, pregnancy should not in any way slow or alter the mode of therapy.

Intracranial hemorrhage in pregnancy

Goals of Therapy

---

1. To prevent cerebral ischemia.
2. To reduce intracranial pressure (ICP).
3. To minimize cerebral edema.
4. To surgically correct lesions when and where appropriate.

Management Protocol

---

1. Ruptured aneurysm: Grades I, II, and III—early surgical intervention. Grades IV and V—stabilization and conservative management.
    A. Bed rest, quiet environment.
    B. Sedative, analgesic support, supplemented by a stool softener.
    C. Surgery after stabilization.

2. Arteriovenous malformation (AVM): Early surgical intervention versus embolization labor and delivery after repair.
   A. Cesarean for obstetric indications only.
   B. Labor with epidural anesthesia.
   C. Outlet forceps to shorten second stage of labor.
3. Cerebral edema: Mannitol 12.5–50 g I.V. (serum osmolality not to exceed 315 mosm/L).

Critical Laboratory Tests

MRI or CT scan of head, lumbar puncture, cerebral angiography, prothrombin time, partial thromboplastin time, fibrinogen, platelets.

Consultation

Neurosurgery, neurology, intensivist.

SUGGESTED READING

Dearden NM, Gibson JS, McDowall DG, et al. Effect of high-dose dexamethasone on outcome from severe head injury. J Neurosurg 1986;64:81–88.

Giannotta SL, Daniels J, Golde SH, et al. Ruptured intracranial aneurysms during pregnancy: a report of four cases. J Reprod Med 1986;31:139.

Hunt HB, Schifrin BS, Suzuki K. Ruptured berry aneurysms and pregnancy. Obstet Gynecol 1974;43:827.

Kassell NF, Boarini DJ, Adams HP, et al. Overall management of ruptured aneurysm: comparison of early and later operation. Neurosurg 1981;9:120.

Ljunggren B, Brandt L, Saveland H, et al. Outcome in 60 consecutive patients treated with early aneurysm operation and intravenous nimodipine. J Neurosurg 1984;61:864.

Minielly R, Yuzpe AA, Drake CG. Subarachnoid hemorrhage secondary to ruptured cerebral aneurysm in pregnancy. Obstet Gynecol 1979;53:64.

Newman B, Lam AM. Induced hypotension for clipping of a cerebral aneurysm during pregnancy: a case report and brief review. Anesth Analg 1986;65:675.

Robinson JL, Hall CS, Sedzimir CB. AV malformations, aneurysms, and pregnancy. J Neurosurg 1974;41:63.

Tuttelman RM, Gleicher N. Central nervous system hemorrhage complicating pregnancy. Obstet Gynecol 1981;58:651.

CHAPTER
TWENTY-SEVEN

Nonneoplastic Complications of Molar Gestation

Today, mortality attributable to hydatidiform mole is rare, largely because of early recognition and treatment. Still, hydatidiform mole remains a high-risk pregnancy because of the threat of trophoblastic malignancy and numerous medical complications related to the molar gestation itself. In this chapter, we discuss preevacuation and perioperative and immediate postoperative problems and their management.

CARDIORESPIRATORY INSUFFICIENCY

Acute respiratory embarrassment, defined as either sudden hypoxemia or tachypnea with associated tachycardia occurs in 2%–11% of molar gestations. The incidence increases to 27% in patients with uteruses exceeding 16 weeks' size. Although in most instances spontaneous resolution occurs, maternal deaths have been reported. Initially felt to be secondary to trophoblastic embolization, the etiology of this condition is most likely multifactorial. Even though all factors may be potentially contributory in any given case, each of these factors is best discussed individually.

TROPHOBLASTIC EMBOLIZATION

There are many reports of presumed or documented pulmonary trophoblastic deportation. However, among those reports, the combined overall occurrence of clinical embolism, well documented or not, is only around 3%. Thus, it is doubtful that this is the main cause of cardiorespiratory insufficiency. Data from autopsy and central catheterization series reveal that the magnitude of trophoblastic deportation varies markedly. The term "embolism" should be reserved for clinically significant deportation. The incidence of trophoblastic embolization appears to be greatest in those patients with uteruses large for dates, particularly if the uterine size exceeds 16–20 weeks, in an earlier gestation.

Trophoblastic deportation has been associated temporally with uterine manipulation. However, because all methods of evacuation increase uterine activity, this factor is not entirely controllable. Suction dilatation and curettage, first reported in 1966, has become a standard for molar evacuation. It increases uterine activity only indirectly. Use of uterine stimulants (oxytocin, prostaglandin) as the primary evacuation method is less desirable because of a potential for increased deportation and sudden uncontrolled hemorrhage. However, it is speculated that the perioperative addition of oxytocin at the initiation of suction curettage will initially cause clamping down of the myometrium around venous sinusoids as the uterus is emptied. This would tend to decrease both the degree of deportation and blood loss. Hysterectomy in those patients without complications from the molar gestation who are stable and who do not desire further fertility remains a reasonable option for treatment.

Recent data from invasive monitoring of patients undergoing molar evacuation support the idea that trophoblastic embolization as a cause of acute cardiorespiratory insufficiency is rare. Despite the findings of transient cardiorespiratory dysfunction and pulmonary edema in several patients, these small series failed to identify unequivocally the presence of circulating trophoblastic cells in patients with pulmonary complications. It appears that most cases of pulmonary insufficiency associated with hydatidiform mole are due to factors other than trophoblastic deportation. These are discussed in the following section.

PULMONARY EDEMA

A high index of suspicion for molar gestation should be maintained when a woman of childbearing age presents with pulmonary edema, as occasionally a patient may be unaware that she is pregnant. In one report, a patient with infiltrates due to pulmonary edema was mistakenly treated for presumed pneumonia for a week prior to the discovery of an existing molar gestation.

The genesis of pulmonary edema in patients with molar pregnancy is probably multifactorial. Contributory factors may include cardiac depression by anesthetic agents, preexisting dilutional anemia, and overestimated blood loss with iatrogenic fluid overload, thyrotoxicosis, and heart failure due to either trophoblastic embolization or preexisting cardiopulmonary disease. The coexistence of preeclampsia may further compound the problem.

General anesthesia with nitrous oxide, fentanyl, or other narcotics can transiently depress ventricular performance. Limited available data on patients with molar gestations greater than 16-week size monitored perioperatively with pulmonary artery catheters confirm this effect. A low ratio of colloid osmotic pressure (COP) to pulmonary capillary wedge pressure (PCWP) gradient, combined with aggressive volume resuscitation in the presence of a depressed myocardial function, may further contribute to the development of pulmonary edema.

A state of relative or dilutional anemia may exist in molar gestation just as in normal pregnancy, becoming more pronounced with gestations in the second trimester. This anemia is, in normal pregnancy, a physiologic response, which acts to provide a reserve for hemorrhage, among other protective effects. Pritchard documented that a large patient can lose up to 2 L of blood at delivery without serious sequelae. This reflects the fact that the anemia is due to a relative decrease in hemoglobin or red blood cell concentration and that a hypervolemic state actually exists. One notable exception is seen in patients with coexisting preeclampsia in which a hypovolemic state may be present. These patients are hemoconcentrated and have a falsely normal hematocrit determination.

So-called blood loss at evacuation of a molar pregnancy largely represents sanguinous molar tissue and should not be included in the estimate of circulating blood volume loss. Preexisting severe anemia may be corrected with packed red blood cells (PRBC). Any attempt to replace losses with whole blood or other large volumes of fluid in an already hypervolemic state will increase the likelihood of developing pulmonary edema. Patients with preeclampsia or hypertension, in whom there may be an increase in systemic vascular resistance (SVR) and a contracted blood volume, tolerate acute volume loads even less well. An inverse relationship between the intrinsic work capability of the left heart, measured by left ventricular stroke work index (LVSWI) and SVR, has been documented in eclamptic patients. Therefore, if uncertainty exists as to the patient's volume status, especially in those already symptomatic of or coexisting with severe preeclampsia, use of a pulmonary artery catheter is recommended.

Thyrotoxicosis, although rarely encountered in these patients, could certainly contribute to pulmonary edema because it is a known cause of high–output cardiac failure. Those reported cases in which cardiac failure or acute dyspnea complicated hyperthyroidism have resolved spontaneously after evacuation. Several of these patients were being treated medically for hyperthyroidism with a known molar gestation in situ. Their adverse outcome emphasizes the need to evacuate a molar gestation as soon as possible rather than attempt protracted medical treatment.

Several small series have reported molar pregnancy complicated by adult respiratory distress syndrome (ARDS), with its attendant high morbidity and mortality. ARDS may coexist with or be complicated by sepsis, disseminated intravascular coagulation (DIC), preeclampsia, and/or pneumothorax. Molar gestation should be suspected in women of reproductive age with any of these clinical syndromes and, if present, evacuated as soon as possible.

Risk factors for the development of pulmonary edema in molar pregnancy have been summarized by Morrow. They are advancing age of the patient, advanced molar gestation, thecal lutein cysts, large uterine size, hypertension, extensive uterine hemorrhage, and anemia.

Evaluation of pulmonary edema in these patients should begin with the recognition of these risk factors and the maintenance of a high index of suspicion. Especially for patients with large uterine size, laboratory determinations and preoperative preparation should be expeditious. The evaluation should include a complete blood count (CBC), serum electrolytes, and a urinalysis, including a test for protein as part of screening for preeclampsia. Thyroid function tests may be sent, but evacuation should not be delayed pending results. A chest x-ray should be obtained for all patients. Findings may include pulmonary infiltrates or effusions with variable appearance. Those in the high-risk group for pulmonary complications or with symptoms of respiratory insufficiency should have arterial blood gas determination. Finally, a central venous pressure (CVP) or pulmonary artery catheter should be considered in especially high-risk or symptomatic patients. Although a CVP line may be sufficient in some patients, the added information available from a flow-directed catheter makes its use preferable in most instances.

ANEMIA

The development of anemia is due to an increase in plasma volume out of proportion to red blood cell production. This results in development of a hypervolemic state as the gestation progresses into the second trimester. In most patients, a bone marrow evaluation reveals normoblastic cells. However, dietary deficiencies in iron or folate may compound the problem and result in mixed pictures. Also the development of morning sickness or hyperemesis gravidarum may affect adequate nutrition. Acute and chronic blood loss can also contribute or even be a major factor if excessive. Except in rare instances of DIC, hemolysis is not a significant factor in the genesis of the anemia of molar pregnancy.

If correction of the anemia is warranted, replacement should generally be with packed red cells to avoid fluid overload. The decision to transfuse should be based on symptoms and findings and not on any absolute minimum hematocrit value.

COAGULOPATHY

There have been reports of deaths due to DIC complicating molar pregnancy. Although not yet isolated, factors released by hydatidiform moles are known to have thromboplastic and fibrinolytic activity. In vitro studies have shown procoagulant activity in molar vesicle fluid at the level of factor X. This activity is similar to that described for amniotic fluid. Spillage of these factors into uterine maternal blood spaces may account for focal necrosis and uterine bleeding. Honn proposed a systemic effect of prostanoids produced by various tumors, causing platelet aggregation and activation of coagulation cascades. However, even though vesicular fluid contains thromboxane and prostacyclin in high concentrations, plasma levels of these substances remain low. Therefore, a systemic effect is unlikely. The coexistence of ARDS and DIC has been documented, and deposition of platelets on damaged pulmonary epithelium has been seen, but a cause and effect relationship has not been established.

The evaluation of high-risk patients for a coagulopathy should include a coagulation screen. Those affected may show a decreased platelet count, prolonged clotting time, prolonged partial thromboplastin time (PTT), and prolonged prothrombin time (PT). Sepsis as an etiologic factor should also be considered. Appropriate cultures are taken and antibiotics started if indicated. Kohorn has suggested that cervical dilatation and use of oxytocin immediately before suction evacuation may decrease the release of thromboplastins and reduce the risk of coagulopathy.

PREECLAMPSIA/ECLAMPSIA

Although preeclampsia occurs in 12%–50% of molar pregnancies, only 57 cases of eclampsia have been reported. Among these, seven were fatal. In most cases, multiple seizures were noted, 70% of which occurred before evacuation. Prolonged delay in evacuation of the molar gestation was common. All three components of the classic preeclampsia triad-elevated blood pressure, proteinuria, and edema were present in most patients. When specifically assessed, these patients usually qualified for "severe preeclampsia" by virtue of blood pressure or proteinuria. Decreased platelets were documented in only one patient. However, there are also many reports that detail atypical presentation, with hypertension as the only finding. Acosta-Sison noted that 100% of the hypertensive patients in their series had uteruses at or above the umbilicus. They emphasized the importance of tumor volume and uterine size rather than weeks of amenorrhea as a risk factor. Somewhat atypical for preeclampsia is the finding that its incidence in patients with hydatidiform moles is higher in multiparous women.

Any pregnant patient presenting in the second trimester with evidence of preeclampsia should be promptly evaluated with ultrasound for the presence of a molar gestation. Appropriate prophylactic measures with magnesium sulfate should be initiated. Any delay in evacuation will contribute to increased morbidity and mortality.

HYPERTHYROIDISM

Since first noted by Tisne in 1955, there have been numerous reports of hyperthyroidism in patients with molar gestation. However, clinical hyperthyroidism is rare, and the etiology of thyroid hyperfunction remains unclear. The level of thyroid-stimulating hormone (TSH) is low or normal in these patients, and a search to isolate a secondary thyroid-stimulating factor has not been conclusive. Initially, beta human chorionic gonadotropin (hCG) was reported as being the causative factor. This has, however, not been substantiated in larger clinical studies. Some in vitro evidence supports the fact that beta-hCG binds to TSH receptors in the human thyroid gland. However, the methodology has been questioned, and others have reported contradicting data. Because the thyroid-stimulating activity of beta-hCG has been estimated at 1/4000 that of TSH, it may have an effect in very high concentration. These higher beta-hCG levels are seen with large molar gestations, and it is in these cases that hyperthyroidism has been most pronounced. Upon evacuation, clinical and laboratory evidence of hyperthyroidism quickly resolves. It is also evident that there is a decreasing incidence of hyperthyroidism reported in these patients because the diagnosis of molar gestation is being made earlier, due to better prenatal care and the widespread use of ultrasound.

Generally, the correlation between laboratory evidence of increased thyroid function and clinical hyperthyroidism has been poor. However, if clinically suspected, evacuation should not be delayed in awaiting confirmatory thyroid function tests or in an attempt to medically control thyroid hyperfunction. Beta blockade with propranolol 10 mg four times/day increasing to 40 mg four times/day if arrhythmias become apparent, may be attempted to counter symptoms of thyrotoxicosis. Additionally, sodium or potassium iodide may be administered intravenously to reduce the circulating levels of triiodothyronine. Prior to evacuation, administration of propylthiouracil and awaiting its effects on thyroid hormone synthesis is unwarranted.

HYPEREMESIS GRAVIDARUM

The presence of hyperemesis in the pregnant patient after the first trimester should arouse suspicion for the presence of hydatidiform mole. This late occurrence of severe nausea and emesis may be related to elevated beta–hCG levels, although this correlation has not been firmly established. The excessive emesis and poor dietary intake secondary to nausea lead to electrolyte imbalance and dehydration, which should be treated as indicated.

SEPSIS

Infection of molar tissue and metritis complicate up to 20% of hydatidiform moles evacuated electively and up to 56% of those requiring suction. The mechanism is probably an ascending bacterial invasion through an open cervical os in the presence of chronic bleeding. Instrumentation for evacuation also increases the risk. Extrapolation from elective and spontaneous abortion data suggests that broad-spectrum antibiotics sufficient to cover both gram–negative and anaerobic bacteria should be administered if infection is suspected. Evacuation should be accomplished as soon as therapeutic levels of antibiotics are established.

Molar gestation

Goals of Therapy

1. To completely evacuate the uterus.
2. To avoid volume overload and cardiorespiratory compromise.
3. To avoid or be prepared to treat massive hemorrhage.

Management Protocol

1. Administer I.V. D_5RL (5% dextrose in lactated Ringer's solution), at 125 mL/h (16- to 18-gauge angiocath).
2. Consider pulmonary artery catheter if clinically unstable.
3. Carefully use suction/curettage.
4. Match intake and output.
5. Observe carefully for evidence of respiratory distress.

Critical Laboratory Tests

CBC, quantitative beta-hCG, type and cross-match 2–4 units PRBC, platelet count, fibrinogen, PT, PTT, chest x-ray, arterial blood gas.

SUGGESTED READING

Amir SM, Osathanonah R, Berkowitz RS, et al. Human chorionic gonadotropin and thyroid function in patients with hydatidiform mole. Am J Obstet Gynecol 1984;150:723.

Hankins GD, Wendell GD, Snyder RR, et al. Trophoblastic embolization during molar evacuation: central hemodynamic observations. Obstet Gynecol 1981;69:368.

Orr JW, Austin JM, Hatch KD, et al. Acute pulmonary edema associated with molar pregnancies: a high risk factor for development of persistent trophoblastic disease. Am J Obstet Gynecol 1980;136:412.

Schlaerth JB, Morrow CP, Montz FJ, d'Ablaing G. Initial management of hydatidiform mole. Am J Obstet Gynecol 1988; 158(6):1299.

Twiggs LB, Morrow CP, Schlaerth JB. Acute pulmonary complications of molar pregnancy. Am J Obstet Gynecol 1979;135:189.

CHAPTER
TWENTY-EIGHT

Life-threatening Complications of Pregnancy Termination

AVOIDING COMPLICATIONS

The most important single factor in preventing complications is adequate training and experience. A number of excellent references outline additional principles of complication prevention. The following are the author's condensation of the most important principles for risk reduction with respect to pregnancy termination.

1. Do only what you have been trained to do and are capable of performing.
2. Evaluate the health status of each patient carefully. Obtain consultation and hospitalize these patients who need close observation.
3. Determine gestational age accurately.
4. Use ultrasound to clarify uterine size or position when in doubt.
5. Use only the most effective instrumentation, such as Pratt dilators, osmotic dilators, Beyer rongeur, or Sopher forceps, and needle extenders.
6. Dilation must be adequate for the requirement of the termination. When in doubt, use Dilapan® or laminaria.

7. Tissue must be examined postoperatively and assessed carefully for completion of the procedure and confirmation of an intrauterine pregnancy.
8. The patient's vital signs must be monitored during and after the procedure, until she has recovered.
9. Possible, potential, or actual complications should be managed as soon as suspected or detected.
10. Complications must be anticipated with protocols, rehearsals, and ready availability of appropriate emergency equipment.
11. Sensitive quantitative pregnancy tests should be readily available.
12. A triage and tracking system must be in place to follow the patients with possible complications.
13. Postabortal medical coverage and adequate hospital backup coverage must always be available and known to the staff and patients.
14. Local anesthesia should be given slowly and in quantities that are not toxic. When used, general anesthesia must be administered carefully by qualified anesthesia personnel operating with adequate equipment under suitable protocols.

MANAGEMENT OF COMPLICATIONS

GENITAL TRACT INJURY

Genital tract injury may occur during the course of suction curettage or dilatation and evacuation. It is important to recognize that a patient can pass slowly or rapidly from injury of the genital tract to hemorrhage, hypotension, shock, cardiac arrest, and/or death. These are a series of linked events, the end result of which is dependent on the extent of injury, the time of recognition, and the vigor and appropriateness of therapy rendered.

In general, any cervical laceration that is bleeding and/or extensive should be repaired, using absorbable suture. Care should be taken to avoid suturing the bladder or ureter, especially during the repair of injured cervical blood vessels. Prior to discharge, a patient with a repaired cervical laceration should be examined to document that further hemorrhage or hematoma formation has not taken place.

Uterine or cervical perforation with a blunt instrument, a suction curet, or ovum forcep may lead to more serious injury. The appearance of any viscera at the cervical os or in one of the instruments, or perforation with a suction cannula are all indications to stop the procedure immediately and prepare the patient for exploratory laparotomy. There are no circumstances under which mere observation would be appropriate after viscera have been identified in this manner. Occasionally, there may be an unavoidable delay during the period of time from recognition of the injury to arrival in the operating room. During this time, the patient should be monitored carefully, with an intravenous line in place. The additional use of oxytocin, ergotrates, or a prostaglandin derivative is frequently beneficial in reducing the amount of blood loss prior to surgical repair.

More controversial is the management of perforation that is recognized by the passage of a sound beyond the uterine confines at the end of the procedure or by the passage of a sound or dilator early in the procedure before any attempt at suction or use of a grasping instrument. There are several reports of patients being observed within an ambulatory facility or overnight in a hospital who require no further surgical intervention. It is certain that, if the patient has come from a considerable distance or is traveling to an area unknown to the operator, with minimal availability for medical care, it would be more prudent to hospitalize the patient overnight.

Another problem is failure to discover a major injury. It is clearly possible to pass a curet, a suction cannula, or other instruments through the uterine wall, particularly into the broad ligament, causing major or minor damage to the uterine blood supply that may not be recognized during the procedure. Injuries of this type may manifest themselves by uterine bleeding during the procedure, which occasionally may be minimized or stopped by the use of intravenous oxytocic agents. Thus, the operator may be led to believe that the bleeding was due to atony and has been controlled. This reduction in hemorrhage will, however, be maintained only as long as the oxytocic agent is given or if sufficient thrombus formation at the site of injury serves to stop the hemorrhage permanently.

It is also possible that a lesser injury to a vessel may be caused by the incomplete fracturing or laceration of the lower uterine segment laterally (either during dilatation or by the withdrawal of a large, sharp fragment of fetal bone through the cervix). These lacerations may also respond temporarily to the vigorous use of oxytocics. Lateral vessel injuries are difficult to manage because the initial bleed may be controlled without recognizing the etiology of the hemorrhage. A number of instances have also been reported in which the subsequent course of the patient was a secondary hemorrhage, again treated successfully with oxytocics. Thus, unless vessel injury can reasonably be excluded in an unstable or bleeding patient, exploratory laparotomy is indicated.

Abdominal ultrasonography or computerized tomography (CT) scanning may assist in identification of broad ligament hematomas, which, at times, may extend superiorly to the kidneys. Management of these large hematomas is difficult, as evacuation may result in the immediate loss of several liters of blood, leading to hypovolemic shock. Further, conservative management may result in absorption of the blood without the necessity of surgery. However, conservative management of large hematomas must be undertaken with caution.

Upon entering the abdominal cavity, one should be aware that, if no blood is seen and no hematoma is found, an incomplete laceration causing bleeding each time the thrombus is dissolved or expelled may be the cause of the vaginal hemorrhage. This type of occult injury may result in multiple surgical explorations prior to definitive therapy. If the uterus is not atonic and no cause for secondary bleeding can be found (such as retained fetal or placental tissue or subinvolution of the placental site), consideration should be given to ligation of the internal iliac and/or ovarian vessels if no obvious external suturable laceration can be identified. A large external laceration may require uterine removal if the vessels of the uterus cannot be clearly identified and ligated separately.

In cases of extensive hemorrhage secondary to injury, an adequate incision must be made to permit access to the iliac vessels and visualization of the ureters so that hemostasis can be obtained without ureteral kinking or obstruction. In the presence of massive injury and hemodynamic instability, stopping to perform hypogastric artery ligation has not met with great success. Further, older literature on hypogastric artery ligation predates the possibility of using intramuscular or cervical prostaglandins to manage postabortal or postpartum hemorrhage. Several reports exist of selective embolization techniques to stop hemorrhage from vessel disruption after injury. However, this technique has not been reported in the management of postabortal lateral uterine vessel injury.

Extensive injury of the uterus mandates adequate exploration of the peritoneal cavity to rule out abrasions, contusions, or lacerations of the small bowel, rectosigmoid, ureters, bladder, and/or omentum. All of these structures have been injured in the course of pregnancy termination. Laparoscopic examination of the viscera is not adequate in the presence of anything more than a minimal puncture that occurred at the onset of the procedure, detected either by a sound or a dilator. The evaluation of injury after a suction curet or ovum forcep has passed through the uterine wall mandates a more careful observation of the internal organs. Though this can be obtained through an adequate Pfannenstiel incision, it is often prudent to make a vertical midline or left paramedian incision to facilitate complete access to the gastrointestinal tract.

Hemorrhage due to atony or placenta accreta is managed in a manner identical to that seen in later pregnancy.

TOXIC OR ALLERGIC REACTIONS

During the course of vaginal termination procedures, a number of respiratory and cardiac arrests have been reported following toxic or allergic reaction to a local anesthetic or due to sulfites commonly mixed with such drugs. The sudden loss of consciousness preceded by bradycardia or cardiac irregularity should immediately alert the surgeon to start resuscitative measures. This is done initially by maintaining ventilation and supporting the circulatory system with intravenous fluids. Additionally, proper resuscitative equipment must be present, including "artificial" airways, a laryngoscope, a portable ventilator, and equipment for defibrillation. At least one person who is currently certified in advanced cardiopulmonary resuscitation must be present in the facility. For all patients undergoing second-trimester dilatation and evacuation (D&E), intravenous access should be established prior to the injection of local anesthesia. Additionally, intravenous access should be obtained during first-trimester procedures in the following patients:

1. Obese women.
2. Intravenous drug users.
3. Women who have no visible veins.
4. Persons who have some other medical condition that might necessitate urgent treatment, such as asthma, epilepsy, or cardiac arrhythmias.

A history of previous allergy to local anesthetic agents, previous untoward experiences with intravenous anesthesia, recent drug ingestion, previous history of marked hypersensitivity reactions (such as bee- or wasp-sting allergies or penicillin hypersensitivity) should alert the physician to an increased likelihood of adverse anesthetic reactions. When intravenous anesthesia is used, oximetry is a relatively inexpensive and extraordinarily valuable way of monitoring early decreases in blood oxygenation, thus allowing early detection of impending cardiovascular compromise.

EMBOLIZATION

Potentially lethal embolization can take place at any time during suction curettage, dilatation, and evacuation, or during induction of abortion with oxytocic agents. In the first trimester, there is little amniotic fluid present, and amniotic fluid embolization (AFE) is extremely rare, although well described. However, the risk of AFE rises with D&E and reaches even higher levels with amino-infusion or labor-induction procedures. One should constantly be on the lookout for early clinical signs of defibrinogenation and intravascular coagulation. Prolonged bleeding around a needle puncture site may appear several hours after injection of hypertonic saline solution or urea, or increased bleeding may follow placental expulsion at the end of the procedure. Because maximum defibrinogenation occurs physiologically approximately two hours after injection of saline, it is possible that these changes may appear early and may slowly increase in severity as the procedure continues.

Embolization can also take place from thrombi dislodged from the lower extremities or pelvic veins in patients who, by virtue of their pregnancy, are hypercoagulable and thus prone to deep vein thrombosis. Patients with marked lower-extremity varicosities, a history of venous thrombosis or pulmonary embolization in the past or a habit of heavy smoking should be observed especially carefully with a minimal amount of lower-extremity hyperflexion and immobilization during the procedure. The use of support stockings is an additional aid in preventing thromboembolism.

Septic embolization may also occur. If a life-threatening medical condition mandating termination accompanies such pelvic infection (a not-uncommon scenario in women with AIDS), then comprehensive antibiotic coverage with second- or third-generation cephalosporins or any other acceptable regimens for the treatment of extensive pelvic inflammatory disease should be instituted at least 4 hours prior to the procedure and continued postoperatively.

COMPLICATIONS OF LATE MIDTRIMESTER ABORTIONS

Labor-induction procedures carry with them the possibility of several additional serious complications, including absorption of toxic quantities of saline into the circulation by direct injection into a maternal vessel or the rapid uptake of saline from the amniotic cavity due to tetanic contractions. Hypersalinity can be life-threatening due to massive hemolysis and damage to the renal, pulmonary, or cerebral circulation. Death may occur acutely, secondary to arrhythmias or pulmonary edema, or slowly, following renal or hepatic failure. It is for this reason that hypertonic saline solutions should be given by gravity drip and not forced into the amniotic cavity by syringe pressure. To further avoid hypersalinity, it is necessary to ensure that the patient is not sedated, as the entrance of hypertonic saline into the circulation is almost instantaneously perceived by the patient as tasting of extreme saltiness. The urea taste may also be perceived if an inadvertent injection of urea attains access to the circulation; however, the consequences of intravenous hypertonic urea are considerably less serious.

As soon as one becomes aware of inadvertent uptake of hypertonic saline, the infusion should be stopped and attempts made to remove as much amniotic fluid as possible. This fluid is replaced with 5% glucose and water. At the same time, the circulation is rapidly expanded with 1–2 L of 5% glucose, in an attempt to reduce serum hypertonicity. If the injection has been discovered early enough, this will suffice. If more saline has been given before detection, a severe headache may occur, warning of even more severe problems to come, including pulmonary edema or cardiac irregularities. The correction of serum sodium must be carried out rapidly, with careful monitoring in an intensive care unit. Prevention and early detection are far better approaches to this problem.

In some reports, hypertonic saline has also been unintentionally injected into the peritoneal cavity (causing peritonitis), into an ovarian cyst (causing necrosis), or into myometrium (causing necrosis).

Reactions to prostaglandin E vaginal suppositories can generally be treated by immediate removal of the suppository and appropriate supportive measures. Intramuscular prostaglandin F can produce severe bronchiolar changes in patients with a predisposition to asthma, as well as other well-known prostaglandin effects such as hyperthermia.

The concurrent administration of multiple oxytocics for the purpose of expediting or shortening abortion time in the midtrimester requires increased care and attention. The simultaneous use of hypertonic saline infusion, amniotic infusion, prostaglandin suppositories, or oxytocin administration is fraught with the possibility of tetanic uterine contractions. These contractions, even in the midtrimester, have been associated with rupture of old cesarean section or myomectomy scars, large annular lacerations of the cervix, or cervical detachment due to excessive force against an effaced, undilated cervix. As with full-term delivery, labor must be managed carefully to avoid hypertonicity and uterine tachysystole.

SUGGESTED READING

Atrash HK, Cheek TG, Hogue CJR. Legal abortion mortality and general anesthesia. Am J Obstet Gynecol 1988;158:420–424.

Darney PD, Atkinson E, Hirabayashi K. Uterne perferation during second trimester abortion by cervical dibitation and instrumental extraction: a review of 15 cases. Obstet Gynecol 1990;75:441.

Grimes DA, Gates W Jr. Complications from legally induced abortion: a review. Obstet Gynecol Survey 1979;34:177–191.

Grimes DA, Gates W Jr, Tyler CW Jr. Comparative risk of death from legally induced abortion in hospitals and nonhospital facilities. Obstet Gynecol 1978;51:323–326.

Guerre EF, O'Keeffe DF, Elliott JP, et al. Uncontrollable intraabdominal hemorrhage treated with packing and use of a MAST suit: a case report. J Rep Med 1987;32:230–232.

Guidotti RJ, Grimes DA, Cates W. Fatal amniotic fluid embolism during legally induced abortion in the United States, 1972–1978. Am J Obstet Gynecol 1981;141:257.

Hakim-Elahi E, Tovell HMM, Burnhill MS. Complications of first trimester abortion: a report of 170,000 cases. Obstet Gynecol, 1990;76:129.

Kafrissen ME, Barke MW, Schulz KF, et al. Coagulopathy and induced abortion methods: rates and relative risks. Am J Obstet Gynecol 1983;147:344–345.

Pais SO, Glickman M, Schwartz P, et al. Embolization of pelvic arteries for control of postpartum hemorrhage. Obstet Gynecol 1980;55:754–758.

Schulman H. Second trimester abortion: techniques and complications. In: Sciarra JJ, Zatuchni GI, LaFerla JJ, eds. Gynecology and obstetrics (vol 6). Philadelphia: JB Lippincott Co, 1989;1–11.

CHAPTER
TWENTY-NINE

Cardiopulmonary Resuscitation in Pregnancy

PHYSIOLOGY AND TECHNIQUES OF CPR

Time is critical in cases of cardiac or pulmonary arrest. If breathing stops first, the heart often continues to pump blood for several minutes. When the heart stops, oxygen in the lungs and bloodstream is not circulated to vital organs. The patient whose heart and breathing have stopped for less than 4 minutes has an excellent chance for recovery if cardiopulmonary resuscitation (CPR) is administered immediately and followed by advanced cardiac life support (ACLS) within 4 minutes. By four to six minutes, brain damage may occur, and after 6 minutes, brain damage almost always occurs. The initial goals of CPR therefore are 1) delivering oxygen to the lungs, 2) providing a means of circulating it to the vital organs (via closed-chest compressions); followed by 3) ACLS, with restoration of the heart as the mechanism of circulation.

Delivery of oxygen is achieved by positioning the patient, opening the airway, and performing rescue breathing. In the absence of muscle tone, the tongue and epiglottis frequently obstruct the airway. The head-tilt with the chin-lift maneuver (Figures 29-1 and 29-2) or the jaw-thrust maneuver (Figure 29-3)

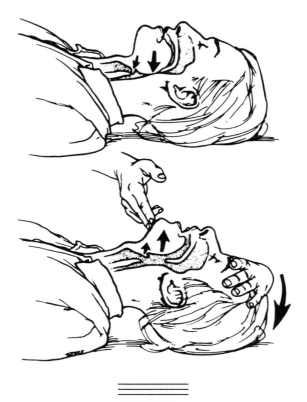

FIGURE 29-1

Opening the airway. Top: Airway obstruction produced by the tongue and the epiglottis. Bottom: Relief via head-tilt and chin-lift maneuvers. (Reproduced with permission. © Instructor's manual for basic life support, American Heart Association, 1987.)

may provide airway access. If foreign material appears in the mouth, it should be removed either manually or with active suction if available. If air does not enter the lungs with rescue breathing, reposition the head and repeat the attempt at rescue breathing. Persistent obstruction requires the sequence of chest thrusts, finger sweeps, and rescue breathing outlined in Table 29-1. Airway obstruction may occur in a choking victim as well as a patient experiencing a cardiopulmonary arrest. With only partial airway obstruction, the conscious woman should be allowed to

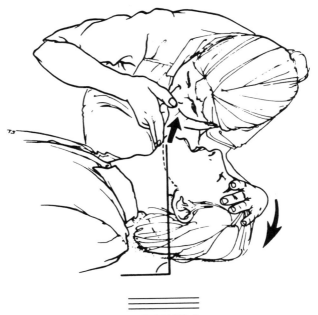

FIGURE 29-2

Head-tilt/chin-lift maneuver. Perpendicular line reflects proper neck extension (i.e., a line along the edge of the jaw bone should be perpendicular to the surface on which the victim is lying). (Reproduced with permission. © Instructor's manual for basic life support, American Heart Association, 1987.)

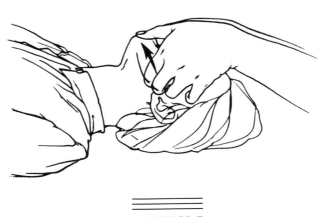

FIGURE 29-3

Jaw-thrust maneuver. (Reproduced with permission. © Instructor's manual for basic life support, American Heart Association, 1987.)

TABLE 29-1

Management of a foreign-body obstruction

Conscious Victim

1. Perform chest thrust.
2. Repeat until obstruction is relieved or victim is unconscious.

Unconscious victim

1. Turn on back.
2. Perform tongue-jaw lift and finger sweep.
3. Open airway with head-tilt and chin-lift maneuvers. Attempt rescue breathing.
4. Perform chest thrusts.
5. Perform tongue-jaw lift and finger sweep.
6. Open airway with head-tilt and chin-lift maneuvers. Attempt rescue breathing.
7. Repeat steps 4–6 until the obstruction is relieved.

attempt to clear the obstruction herself, and finger sweeps by the rescuer are avoided. Finally, failure of nonsurgical procedures to relieve the airway obstruction is an indication for emergency cricothyroidotomy or jet-needle insufflation if appropriate equipment is available.

Chest thrusts in a conscious sitting or standing victim require placing the thumb side of the fist on the middle of the sternum, avoiding the xiphoid and the ribs. The rescuer then grabs his or her own fist with the other hand and performs chest thrusts until either the foreign object dislodges or the patient loses consciousness (Figure 29-4). The unconscious patient requires chest compressions. The rescuer's hand closest to the patient's head is placed two finger-breadths above the xiphoid. The long axis of the heel of the provider's hand rests in the long axis of the sternum (Figure 29-5). The other hand lies over the first, with fingers either extended or interlaced. The elbows are extended and the chest compressed $1\frac{1}{2}$ to 2 inches (Figure 29-6).

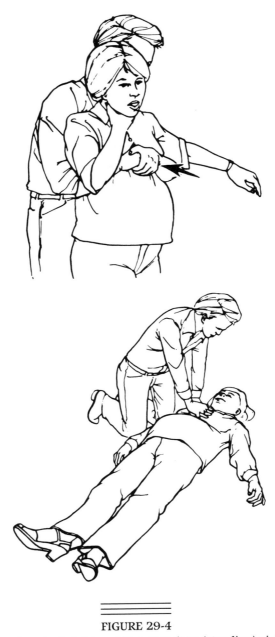

FIGURE 29-4

Top: Chest thrust administered to a conscious (standing) victim of foreign-body airway obstruction. Bottom: Chest thrust administered to an unconscious (lying) victim of foreign body airway obstruction. (Reproduced with permission. © Instructor's manual for basic life support, American Heart Association, 1987.)

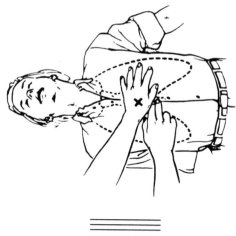

FIGURE 29-5

External chest compressions: locating the correct hand position on the lower half of the sternum. (Reproduced with permission. © Instructor's manual for basic life support, American Heart Association, 1987.)

External chest compressions cause a rise in intrathoracic pressure, which is distributed to all intrathoracic structures. Competent venous valves prevent transmission of this pressure to extrathoracic veins, whereas the arteries transmit the increased pressure to extrathoracic arteries, creating an arterial venous pressure gradient and forward blood flow. The mitral and tricuspid valves remain open during CPR, supporting the concept of the heart as a passive conduit rather than a pump during CPR.

Basic life support (BLS) guidelines call for a ratio of two ventilations to 15 compressions in one-person CPR and a 1:5 ratio in two-rescuer CPR, with a total of 80–100 compressions per minute in both circumstances. ACLS involves the addition of electrical and pharmacologic therapy, invasive monitoring, and therapeutic techniques to correct cardiac arrhythmias, metabolic imbalances, and other causes of cardiac arrest. Standard algorithms recommended by the American Heart Association (AHA) are reviewed in Appendix 2.

THE EFFECT OF PREGNANCY ON CPR

Pregnancy produces physiologic changes that have a potentially dramatic effect on cardiopulmonary resuscitation. Upward displacement of the diaphragm by the enlarging uterus leads to a decrease in the functional residual capacity (FRC) of the lungs. The decrease in FRC combines with the increase in oxygen demand to predispose the pregnant woman to a decrease in arterial and venous oxygen tension during periods of decreased ventilation. The pregnant uterus exerts pressure on the inferior vena cava, iliac vessels, and abdominal aorta. In the supine position, such uterine compression may lead to sequestration of up to 30% of circulating blood volume. For the patient in the latter half of pregnancy, aortocaval compression by the gravid uterus renders resuscitation more difficult than in her nonpregnant counterpart. It does so by decreasing venous return, causing supine hypotension, and decreasing the effectiveness of thoracic compres-

FIGURE 29-6

Proper position of rescuer: shoulders directly over victim's sternum; elbows locked. (Reproduced with permission. © Instructor's manual for basic life support, American Heart Association, 1987.)

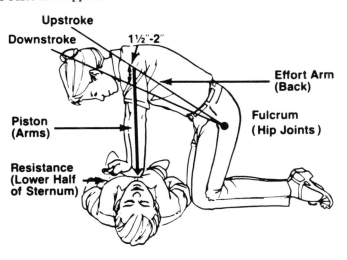

sions. Furthermore, the enlarged uterus poses an obstruction to forward blood flow, particularly when arterial pressure and volume are decreased, as in a cardiac arrest.

Changes in the gravid woman's response to drugs and alterations in the maternal gastrointestinal system also hinder effective resuscitation. Vasopressors used in ACLS, especially alpha-adrenergic or combined alpha and beta agents, are capable of producing uteroplacental vasoconstriction, leading to decreased fetal oxygenation and CO_2 exchange. Decreases in gastrointestinal motility and relaxation of the lower esophageal sphincter lead to an increased risk of aspiration prior to or during endotracheal intubation.

MODIFICATIONS OF BLS AND ACLS IN PREGNANCY

The anatomic and physiologic changes of pregnancy require several modifications in emergency cardiac care (ECC). Most important, to effect an increase in venous return and reduce supine hypotension, the uterus must be displaced to the left. This can be attempted in several ways. Left lateral displacement can be achieved by 1) manual displacement of the uterus by a member of the resuscitation team, 2) positioning the patient on an operating room table that can be tilted laterally, or 3) positioning a wedge under the patient's right hip.

It must also be kept in mind that sodium bicarbonate only very slowly crosses the placenta. Accordingly, with rapid correction of maternal metabolic acidosis, the patient's respiratory compensation will cease with normalization of her partial pressure of carbon dioxide (P_{CO_2}). If the maternal P_{CO_2} increases from 20 to 40 mm Hg as a result of bicarbonate administration, the fetal P_{CO_2} will also increase. However, the fetus will not receive the benefit of the bicarbonate. If the fetal pH was 7.00 before maternal bicarbonate administration, the normalization of maternal pH will be achieved at the expense of increasing the fetal P_{CO_2} by 20 torr, with a resultant fall in fetal pH to approximately 6.84. Accordingly, the merits of such treatment must be questioned, especially in light of the fact that the AHA is deemphasizing the use of sodium bicarbonate in the acute arrest situation.

PERIPARTUM CESAREAN DELIVERY

If a pregnant woman suffers a cardiopulmonary arrest beyond the stage of fetal viability for a given institution, a perimortem cesarean delivery should be considered. A 4–minute limit to initiate delivery, as advocated by several texts, is derived from theoretical physiologic advantages for resuscitating the mother, as well as from extrapolation of data on infant survival. However, a paucity of data, and no standard, exists to address this.

Clearly, the timing of the operation is critical for infant survival, which appears proportional to time between the mother's cardiac arrest and her delivery (Table 29–2). Primate studies confirm brain damage in utero with as little as six minutes of complete asphyxia; severe cellular damage occurs by eight minutes.

TABLE 29-2

Postmortem cesarean delivery with surviving infants with reports of time from death of the mother to delivery

Time from Maternal Death to Delivery (min.)	Surviving Infants	
	Numbers	% (of Births Reported)
0–5	42 normal infants	70
6–10	7 normal infants 1 with mild neurologic sequelae	13
11–15	6 normal infants 1 with severe neurologic sequelae	12
16–20	1 with severe neurologic sequelae	1.7
21+	2 with severe neurologic sequelae 1 normal infant	3.3

Scattered reports describe infant survival at longer intervals following arrest, implying that cesarean delivery should be performed even several minutes postarrest if signs of fetal life are
present.

SUGGESTED READING

Basic Life Support. Dallas: American Heart Association, 1987.

Katz VI, Dotters DJ, Droegemuller W. Perimortem cesarean delivery.
Obstet Gynecol 1986;68:571–576.

Textbook of Advanced Cardiac Life Support (2nd ed.) Dallas: American Heart Association, 1987.

CHAPTER THIRTY

Blood and Component Therapy in Obstetrics

BLOOD AND ITS COMPONENTS

The indications for transfusion are: 1) restoration of circulating volume, 2) improvement in oxygen transport, and 3) correction of coagulation disorders.

To type and screen blood, the ABO group and the RH(D) type of the potential recipient's cells are first determined. Her serum is then mixed with reagent red cells, which contain the antigens with which most of the common clinically significant antibodies will react. The appearance of agglutination indicates the presence in the recipient's serum of an antibody to at least one of the antigens on the reagent red cells.

A type and cross-match follows the same procedure as a type and screen except that the donor erythrocytes are used instead of reagent red cells. Therefore, if blood that had been screened but not cross-matched were to be given, a transfusion reaction might take place only if the recipient's serum contained an antibody to an antigen present on the donor cells but not present on the surface of the reagent red cells. The likelihood of this occurrence is remote. From 0.03% to 0.07% of patients who were determined not to have antibodies on typing and screening were subsequently found to have preexisting antibodies determined by the cross–match.

Significant advantages may be derived from typing and screening rather than cross-matching blood for most obstetrical indications. Not testing for a cross-match decreases blood bank costs. Also, blood that is cross-matched is held exclusively for a single potential recipient, whereas blood that has been screened may be available for more than one potential recipient. Further, by increasing the number of patients for whom a unit of blood may be held, wastage of banked blood may be reduced.

Because of the time and expense required for a cross-match as well as the unpredictable nature of obstetrical hemorrhage, typing and screening of blood for most obstetrical patients seems reasonable. A cross-match may be more appropriate for those patients at greater risk for hemorrhage, as well as those in whom clinically significant antibodies have been discovered by the antibody screen (Table 30-1 and Figure 30-1).

WHOLE BLOOD

A unit of whole blood contains a minimum of 405 mL and an average of 450 mL of blood. To this is added 63 mL of preservative. The average hematocrit of stored whole blood is 36%–

TABLE 30-1
Ordering blood

Type and cross–match
1. Placenta previa
2. Placental abruption
3. Uterine rupture
4. Uterine atony
5. Genital tract lacerations
6. Coagulopathy
7. Several significant antibodies found on screening

Type and screen: all others

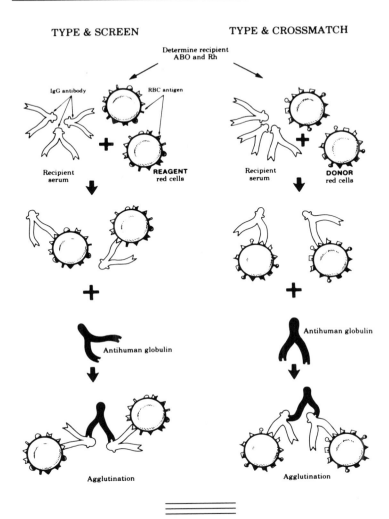

FIGURE 30-1

Type and screen versus type and cross-match. See text for explanation.

40%. A single unit of whole blood will raise the recipient's by about 3%–4%. Whole blood stored longer than 24 hours has few functioning granulocytes or platelets. Stable clotting factors are maintained in adequate concentration for the life of the unit. Levels of the labile clotting factors V and VIII are present in banked blood in reduced but functionally adequate concentrations for one to two weeks.

RED BLOOD CELLS

Red blood cells (RBCs) are prepared by separating the cells from either centrifugation or sedimentation. RBCs stored in citrate-phosphate-dextrose (CPD) or citrate-phosphate-dextrose-adenine (CPDA) have a hematocrit of approximately 70%. A unit of RBCs to which 100 mL of saline-adenine-glucose-mannitol (SAGM) has been added has a hematocrit of 60%. Because a unit of RBCs contains the same number of erythrocytes as a unit of whole blood, it too, will raise the recipient's hematocrit by 3%–4%. RBCs have the advantage of providing oxygen-carrying capacity equivalent to that of a unit of whole blood in only half the volume.

LEUKOCYTE-POOR RED CELLS

Patients who have had several pregnancies and/or multiple transfusions may develop antibodies to leukocyte antigens. Leukocyte antigens are responsible for the majority of nonhemolytic febrile transfusion reactions. Removal of the buffy coat (the layer containing leukocytes and platelets) may be accomplished with leukocyte-depletion filters, inverted centrifugation, or saline washing.

A patient who has had a single febrile reaction is unlikely to have a second. Leukocyte-poor red cells should be reserved only for those patients who have had two or more transfusion reactions. Patients who continue to have nonhemolytic febrile reactions despite receiving leukocyte-depleted filtered red cells may benefit from the use of frozen-thawed-deglycerolized red cells.

RANDOM-DONOR PLATELETS

Random-donor platelets are prepared from individual units of whole blood by centrifugation. The platelets are then suspended in 50–70 mL of plasma. Unlike whole blood and red cells, platelets cannot tolerate storage at 1°–6°C for more than 48 hours. With constant and gentle agitation, they may be stored at 20°–24°C for up to 5 days in containers that are permeable to oxygen.

Because of the risk of hemolysis to the recipient, the donor plasma in platelets ideally should be ABO-compatible with the potential recipient's red blood cells. Because of the potential for transfusion of small amounts of erythrocytes with the platelet transfusion, ideally only platelets from Rh-negative donors should be given to Rh-negative recipients. An Rh-negative recipient receiving platelets from an Rh-positive donor may be given Rh-immune globulin to prevent the formation of anti-D antibodies.

A unit of random donor platelets should contain at least 5.5 $\times$ 10^{10} platelets. The usual dose for a thrombocytopenic patient is 6–10 units. A platelet count above 50,000/mL is unlikely to be associated with bleeding even in a surgical setting, while a high likelihood of spontaneous bleeding exists below 5000/mL (Figure 30-2).

FRESH-FROZEN PLASMA

Plasma is the liquid portion of blood in which cells and solutes are suspended. It consists primarily of water; 7% is proteins and 2% carbohydrates and lipids. Fresh-frozen plasma (FFP) differs from stored whole blood and liquid plasma in that it contains the labile clotting factors V and VIII. It is prepared by separating plasma from whole blood within six hours of phlebotomy and then freezing it at −18°C or lower. The volume of a unit is approximately 200–250 mL. A unit should be transfused within 24 hours of thawing to obtain maximal levels of labile clotting factors.

FFP is indicated for patients with congenital factor deficien-

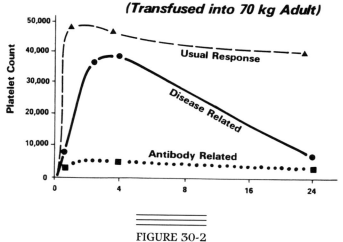

FIGURE 30-2

Results of six units of platelets transfused into a 70-kg adult in three clinical situations. "Usual response" means no increased platelet destruction; "disease related" refers to consumption of platelets; "antibody related" refers to formation of platelet-specific or histocompatibility locus antigen (HLA) antibodies. (Reproduced with permission from Simon, TL: Platelets: uses, abuses and indications. In: Kolins J, McCarthy LJ (eds): Contemporary transfusion practice. Arlington: American Association of Blood Banks, 1987;58.)

cies for which no factor concentrates are available, such as factor V or factor XI deficiencies. It may also be used for treatment of von Willebrand disease (VWD). However, because desmopressin (DDAVP) increases von Willebrand factor (VWF) and factor VIII:c and all but type IIb VWD usually respond to DDAVP, DDAVP is considered primary therapy for most forms of this disease.

CRYOPRECIPITATE

This component is prepared by thawing FFP at 4°C, removing the supernatant liquid plasma, and then refreezing the white precipitate plus 10–15 mL of plasma to −18°C or lower. Cryoprecipitate contains factor VIII:c, factor VIII: VWF, fibrinogen, factor XIII, and fibronectin. Because of the availability of both factor VIII (as concentrates) and DDAVP, the use of cryoprecipitate is currently extremely limited.

ADMINISTRATION OF BLOOD AND BLOOD COMPONENTS: PATIENT IDENTIFICATION

The majority of fatal transfusion reactions result not from technical problems but rather from errors in identification of specimens, components, or recipients. Patients must remain under direct observation for the first 5–10 minutes after the transfusion has begun, and they should be checked periodically throughout the transfusion.

INTRAVENOUS SOLUTIONS AND MEDICATIONS

Only normal saline is acceptable for priming the intravenous line just prior to initiating transfusion. Normal saline may also be used to dilute red blood cells in order to decrease their viscosity and thus increase their rate of flow.

No medication should ever be added to a unit of blood; the high pH of most medications may cause hemolysis.

All blood products must be filtered to avoid transfusion of blood clots and other debris. The standard filter with a 170-μm size should be adequate to trap these debris, as well as cellular macroaggregates.

Blood warming may be useful in massive transfusions. While the slow administration of one to three units of cold blood poses no apparent threat, the administration of three or more litres of cold banked blood at rates in excess of 50 mL/min has been associated with cardiac arrest and ventricular arrhythmias. Blood warming is also indicated for patients having cold autoagglutinins active at 30–37°C. Warming devices must be equipped with a visible thermometer, and they should not warm blood above 37°C, as thermal injury to red cells occurs at temperatures over 40°C.

AUTOLOGOUS TRANSFUSIONS

Among the major forms of autologous transfusions, intraoperative salvage and reinfusion is not currently used in obstetrics because of the potential for contamination from the operative site. Predepositing blood during pregnancy for possible autologous transfusion, however, is possible. The timing and frequency of autologous donations during pregnancy are important considerations. Because of the 42-day shelf life of red cells stored in SAGM, phlebotomy must be performed at a time relatively close to the time of potential transfusion. The risk of iatrogenically lowering the circulating red cell and plasma volume in a patient who may suffer a massive hemorrhage must be carefully weighed against the benefit of autologous blood. A potential solution for this problem is the leapfrog phlebotomy protocol. Following removal of one unit of blood, the oldest previously collected unit is reinfused to the donor just prior to removal of a second unit.

PERFLUOROCARBON EMULSIONS

Perfluorocarbons (PFCs) are cyclic- or straight-chain hydrocarbons in which fluorine has replaced hydrogen atoms. PFCs are immiscible in water. By emulsifying them with surface-active agents, these compounds may be introduced into the vascular system. The tissue retention time of PFCs is approximately seven days. Unlike hemoglobin, which carries oxygen in combination, PFCs carry oxygen in solution. Thus PFCs require that a patient constantly breathe 70%–90% oxygen to maintain oxygen carriage. In animal studies, PFCs have been shown to depress the reticuloendothelial system, possibly resulting in decreased resistance to bacterial endotoxins and viruses. Both animal and human studies have revealed cytotoxic effects of PFCs, particularly on phagocytic cells.

SUGGESTED READING

Braunstein AH, Oberman HA. Transfusion of plasma components. Transfusion 1984;24:281–286.

Committee on Standards. Standards for Blood Banks and Transfusion Services (13th ed.). Arlington: American Association of Blood Banks, 1989.

Kamani AA, McMorland GH, Wadsworth LD. Utilization of red blood cell transfusion in an obstetric setting. Am J Obstet Gynecol 1988;159:1177–1181.

Karn KE, Ogburn PL, Julian T, Cerra FB, Hammerschmidt DE, Vercellotti G. Use of whole blood substitute, Fleuosol-DA 20%, after massive postpartum hemorrhage. Obstet Gynecol 1985;65:127–130.

Kruskall MS, Mintz PD, Bergin JJ, et al. Transfusion therapy in emergency medicine. Ann Emerg Med 1988;17:327–335.

National Institutes of Health Consensus Conference. Perioperative red blood cell transfusion. JAMA 1988;260:2700–2703.

Reisner LS. Type and screen for cesarean section: a prudent alternative. Anesthesiology 1983; 58:476–478.

Toy PTCY, Strauss RG, Stehling LC, et al. Predeposited autologous blood for elective surgery. N Engl J Med 1987;316:517–520.

CHAPTER THIRTY-ONE

Complications of Blood and Component Transfusion

COAGULOPATHY

Clinical and laboratory evidence of platelet and coagulation factor deficiencies are at times found in association with transfusion for massive hemorrhage. In the past, these deficiencies have been attributed to washout of coagulation factors by acellular fluids used to restore intravascular volume. However, clinical evidence suggests that other mechanisms may be operant. Following transfusion of 10 units of packed cells and crystalloid, over one-third of the original blood elements, including platelets and coagulation factors, are still present. Even in the absence of new production of these factors, these levels are usually adequate to maintain hemostasis. The prophylactic administration of fresh-frozen plasma (FFP) and/or platelets does not substantially correct clinical or laboratory coagulation deficiencies in massively transfused subjects.

While the development of coagulopathies has not been correlated with the volume of blood lost or replaced, it has been correlated with the duration of hypotension in massive blood loss. This is consistent with the finding of platelet activation and microthrombus formation in capillaries of animals subjected to acute massive hemorrhage. The postulated sequence of massive bleeding followed by prolonged hypotension and intravascular consumption of platelets and clotting factors thus has both clinical and laboratory support. It therefore seems reasonable to correct hypotension with acellular fluids prior to giving consideration to replacement of platelets and coagulation factors. It also seems reasonable to restrict replacement of these factors to patients exhibiting diffuse or intractable bleeding despite correction of hypotension and establishment of surgical hemostasis.

CITRATE TOXICITY

Citrate is intentionally added to most red-cell storage solutions to bind calcium and thus prevent clotting. In normothermic patients with normal perfusion and normal hepatic function, the citrate is rapidly metabolized in the liver. When transfused at rates in excess of one unit/5 minutes, citrated blood will depress ionic calcium by 50%; despite this, myocardial depression in otherwise healthy transfused adults has not been noted. However, it seems advisable to observe for electrocardiographic (EKG) changes in patients who have profound heart failure, liver disease, or hypothermia. Calcium chloride (0.5–1 mL of 10% solution per 100 mL of transfused blood) may be cautiously infused in patients exhibiting EKG changes.

HYPERKALEMIA

The concentration of extracellular potassium increases with storage time of red cells. Hyperkalemia is unusual, however, unless massive volumes of stored blood are transfused over a very short time interval. It is more common to find hypokalemia, which is due to the metabolic alkalosis resulting from the metabolism of citrate to bicarbonate. Periodic monitoring of potassium levels in massively transfused patients thus seems prudent.

TRANSFUSION REACTIONS

Acute transfusion reactions are seen in 5% of blood recipients and delayed reactions in 7%. Nonhemolytic febrile and allergic reactions accompany 1% of all transfused units and are rarely serious.

HEMOLYTIC TRANSFUSION REACTIONS

Hemolytic transfusion reactions are categorized as acute or delayed. The former are subdivided into intravascular and extravascular, depending on the site of hemolysis. Acute intravascular hemolysis is most often due to transfusion ABO-incompatible blood. ABO-incompatible hemolytic reactions are the most frequent cause of acute fatalities resulting from blood transfusions. Hemolysis due to ABO incompatibility is complement-mediated.

The clinical severity of a hemolytic transfusion reaction is proportional to the volume of incompatible blood transfused and the time interval between the reaction and the initiation of treatment. The conscious patient may complain of heat and pain along the vein into which the blood is being transfused. She may also experience lumbar pain, facial flushing and constricting chest pain. Associated signs include fever, tachycardia, hypotension, disseminated intravascular coagulation (DIC), hemoglobinuria, oliguria, and respiratory distress. In the anesthetized patient undergoing transfusion (e.g., with cesarean section), abnormal bleeding and hypotension disproportionate to blood loss may be the only signs of severe hemolysis.

Intravascular hemolysis may result in renal damage and/or renal failure. Included among the direct causes of renal damage are inadequate perfusion due to systemic hypotension, renal arterial vasoconstriction, and renal intravascular thrombus deposition, alone or in combination. Renal tubular obstruction may result from deposition of hemoglobin and/or acid hematin.

DIC may be found with intravascular hemolysis due to activation of Hageman factor, platelets, and leukocytes by antibody-antigen complexes. Release of thromboplastic lipids from erythrocyte stromata may also initiate DIC.

Laboratory findings consistent with intravascular hemolysis include a decrease in plasma haptoglobin, an increase in serum-free hemoglobin, and the appearance of hemoglobinuria. Hemoglobin does not appear in the urine until the plasma level exceeds 25 mg/dL. Further, gross hemoglobinuria is usually not found below a plasma hemoglobin concentration of 150 mg/dL.

Extravascular hemolysis is mediated by the development of IgG antibodies to such antigens as RH, Kell, Kidd, and Duffy. Clinical findings include fever and anemia. Laboratory findings include increased serum-indirect bilirubin and a positive-direct antiglobulin test. Severe clinical symptoms are less frequent than with ABO incompatibility because extravascular hemolysis is not complement-mediated.

A delayed hemolytic transfusion reaction usually occurs 3–10 days following a transfusion. This is usually mediated by an anamnestic response to an antibody present in undetectable levels at the time of transfusion. Clinical and laboratory findings are similar to those of acute extravascular hemolysis. No specific treatment is usually required. Occasionally, severe delayed reactions, which usually include some degree of intravascular hemolysis, are seen. These patients should be managed as outlined in Table 31-1.

Nonimmune hemolysis may be caused by exposure of erythrocytes to hypotonic or hypertonic solutions, freezing, excessive warming, or bacterial contamination. Because some of the clinical findings cannot be differentiated from those of immune hemolysis, and because mortality from intravascular hemolysis is time-related, laboratory evaluation to rule out immune hemolysis should be undertaken immediately.

FEBRILE NONHEMOLYTIC REACTIONS

Although a fever may be the first sign of intravascular hemolysis or bacterial sepsis, it is more commonly found in patients having antibodies directed against leukocytes and/or platelets. The absence of hemolysis suggests that the fever is due to these antibodies. Management consists both of slowing the rate of transfusion and of administering antipyretics.

TABLE 31-1

Transfusion reactions

Type	Cause	Findings	Management
Acute intravascular hemolysis	ABO incompatibility	1. Fever, chills 2. Shock 3. DIC 4. Hemoglobinuria 5. Oliguria	1. Support BP and respirations 2. Maintain diuresis
Acute and delayed extravascular hemolysis	Non-ABO, anti-RBC antibodies	1. Fever 2. Anemia 3. Hyperbilirubinemia	1. Identify antibody 2. Observation only is usually adequate
Febrile	Antibodies to leukocytes or platelets	1. Fever, chills	1. Antipyretics 2. Leukocyte-poor red cells if recurrent
Allergic	Antibodies to plasma	1. Urticaria 2. Rarely; anaphylaxis	1. Antihistamines 2. Epinephrine and/or steroids if severe 3. Washed red cells if recurrent

ABO = blood groups A,B, and O; DIC = disseminated intravascular coagulopathy; BP = blood pressure; RBC = red blood cell count.

ALLERGIC REACTIONS

Urticarial reactions are usually due to recipient antibodies to donor plasma proteins. Transfusion may be resumed after the urticaria has subsided, following administration of antihistamines. Severe anaphylactic reactions are rare, and they may require treatment with epinephrine and/or steroids. Rarely, a severe allergic reaction may be caused by IgG antibodies to IgA in an IgA-deficient recipient. Therefore, patients with a history of anaphylactic transfusion reactions should be tested for the presence of anti-IgA antibody and/or IgA levels in their plasma. Those in whom the antibody is found should be transfused with only washed red blood cells and IgA-deficient plasma.

Hemolytic transfusion reactions

Goals of Therapy

1. To maintain blood pressure.
2. To avoid respiratory failure.
3. To prevent renal shutdown and maintain urine output >100 mL/ hour.

Management Protocol

1. Stop the transfusion.
2. Maintain an open line with normal saline.
3. Support blood pressure (with dopamine starting dose 2–5 mg/kg/ min, titrated to hemodynamic response) and respiration.
4. Maintain urine output with mannitol, 20–25 mg I.V. over 5 minutes. May be repeated up to 4 times within 24 hours.
5. Check container and patient labels to detect misidentification of patient or blood.
6. Send blood container, transfusion set, I.V. solutions used, and new sample of patient blood to blood bank.
7. Inspect recipient's postreaction plasma for hemolysis; compare with prereaction plasma when available. Pink plasma indicates at least 20 mg/dL of free hemoglobin.

Critical Laboratory Tests

Review labels and records; centrifuge plasma and urine for hemoglobin; direct antiglobulin test on postreaction sample and compare with prereaction sample.

Consultation

Blood bank, hematology, pulmonary medicine.

SUGGESTED READING

Berkman SA. Infectious complications of blood transfusion. Blood Reviews 1988;2:206–210.

Myhre BA. Fatalities from blood transfusion. JAMA 1980;224:1333–1335.

Pindyck J. Transfusion-associated HIV infections: epidemiology, prevention and public policy. AIDS 1988;2:239–248.

Ward JW, Holmbweg SD, Allen JR, Cohn DL, et al. Transmission of human immunodeficiency virus (HIV) by blood transfusions screened as negative for HIV antibody. N Engl J Med 1988; 318:473–478.

Webster BH. Clinical presentation of nonhaemolytic transfusion reactions. Anaesth Intensive Care 1980;8:115–119.

CHAPTER THIRTY-TWO

Fetal Considerations in the Critically Ill Obstetric Patient

ANAPHYLAXIS

Acute maternal allergic reactions pose a threat to the fetus. Treatment directed at the underlying maternal reaction should remedy the accompanying signs of fetal compromise. Prompt reversal usually result from the administration of epinephrine and the infusion of intravenous fluids. To afford the fetus a wider margin of safety, the maternal systolic blood pressure should be maintained above 90 mm Hg. In addition, oxygen should be administered to correct maternal and fetal hypoxia. Maintenance of maternal oxygen tension (Po_2) in excess of 60 mm Hg is essential to assure adequate fetal oxygenation.

SEIZURES

Maternal convulsions usually are associated with a sustained uterine contraction. As a result of the contraction and/or pain, the maternal blood pressure rises suddenly. During the seizure, which generally lasts less than 1.5 minutes, transient maternal hypoxia and uterine artery vasospasm occur and combine to produce a decline in uterine blood flow. In response, spontaneous uterine activity is further increased, resulting in additional compromise of uteroplacental perfusion. Ultimately, fetal hypoxia develops and a fetal heart rate (FHR) deceleration ensues generally within five minutes. Such FHR bradycardia has been reported to last up to 9 minutes. Following the seizure and recovery from the FHR bradycardia, a loss of fetal heart rate variability and a compensatory fetal tachycardia are characteristically seen. The fetal response to the maternal convulsion is quite variable and largely depends both on the condition of the fetus at the time of the seizure and on the severity of the stress.

The cornerstone of patient management during a seizure is to maintain adequate maternal oxygenation and to administer appropriate anticonvulsants. After a convulsion occurs, an adequate airway should be maintained and oxygen administered. To optimize uteroplacental perfusion, the mother is repositioned on her side. Anticonvulsant therapy with intravenous magnesium sulfate to prevent seizure recurrence is recommended in patients with eclampsia. In addition, intrauterine resuscitation with a beta-mimetic or additional magnesium sulfate may occasionally be necessary for eclampsia-induced uterine hypertonus.

CARDIAC SURGERY

With the recent advances in the medical and surgical management of cardiovascular disease, the risk of cardiac surgery to the pregnant woman probably is not increased over that of her nonpregnant counterpart. Paralleling the decline in maternal morbidity and mortality has been a 67% drop in perinatal mortality since 1969. One of the major reasons for the improved fetal outcome has been the use of continuous electronic fetal monitoring during bypass surgery. This approach permits the surgical team to monitor fetal condition continuously throughout the surgery and to identify and treat any evident fetal compromise promptly.

During bypass surgery, fetal bradycardia, followed by a compensatory tachycardia, is the rule. The theoretical basis for the FHR changes has been suggested to be diminished uteroplacental perfusion. This decline in perfusion is thought to be the result of a lack of pulsatile flow, the opening of uterine arteriovenous shunts, uterine artery spasm, or insufficient flow rates. It appears that there is a direct relationship between flow rates and the FHR. Intraoperative correction of fetal bradycardia has been achieved simply by increasing flow rates. In instances where the fetal bradycardia has persisted, repositioning the mother to relieve possible compression of the umbilical cord or the inferior vena cava has been suggested. If these measures fail and the surgery is to be prolonged, cesarean delivery may be required.

Spontaneous uterine activity is increased during and immediately following bypass surgery. Suppression of uterine activity, in the absence of fetal distress, has been suggested during these perioperative periods.

PERIMORTEM CESAREAN DELIVERY

To date, there have been 269 cases of postmortem cesarean delivery reported in the English literature, with 188 (70%) surviving infants.

Since Weber's review of the subject in 1976, the causes of maternal death leading to a postmortem cesarean delivery have not changed substantially. These include hypertension, hemorrhage, and sepsis. With unanticipated or sudden death, such as amniotic fluid embolus syndrome, pulmonary embolus, or acute respiratory failure, the timing of cesarean delivery is a critical issue.

If a pregnant woman does sustain a cardiopulmonary arrest, cardiopulmonary resuscitation (CPR) should be initiated immediately. Optimal performance of CPR results in a cardiac output of 30%–40% of normal in the nonpregnant patient. For best efficiency, the patient should be placed in the supine position. However, in this position, dextrorotation of the uterus may impede venous return and may become severely compromised. Manual uterine displacement may help to remedy this problem.

If maternal and fetal outcomes are to be optimized, the timing of the cesarean delivery is critical. Katz and associates have suggested that "cesarean delivery should be begun within 4 minutes, and the baby delivered within 5 minutes of maternal cardiac arrest" to optimize maternal and fetal outcome. According to these authors, delivery within this time interval permits restoration of maternal cardiac output and the greatest possibility of maternal and fetal survival. Moreover, care must be taken to continue maternal CPR not only until the birth of the fetus but also after the delivery. On occasion, a woman has been resuscitated and has lived postcesarean.

As demonstrated in Table 32-1, fetal survival is linked closely to the interval between maternal arrest and delivery. For optimal fetal results, delivery should be accomplished within 5 minutes of the maternal death, and the fetus should be resuscitated promptly. Although the probability of a surviving, normal infant diminishes the longer the time interval from maternal death, the potential exists for a favorable fetal outcome at more than 20 minutes from maternal cardiac arrest.

While the timing of cesarean delivery is a major determinant of subsequent fetal outcome, the gestational age of the fetus is also an important consideration, the probability of survival being related directly to the neonatal birth weight or gestational age.

Maternal death is not always an unforeseeable event. For instance, patients hospitalized with terminal cancer, class IV car-

TABLE 32-1

Perimortem cesarean delivery with the outcome of surviving infants from the time of maternal death until delivery

Time Interval (min)	Surviving Infants (no.)	Normal (%)
0–5	42	100
6–10	8	88
11–15	7	86
16–20	1	0
21+	3	33

diac disease, pulmonary hypertension, or previous myocardial infarction are at an increased risk of death during pregnancy. Although these cases are infrequent, it seems reasonable to prepare for such an eventuality. One consideration is to have a cesarean delivery pack and neonatal resuscitation equipment immediately available.

In the sudden, unexpected maternal death, consent to deliver the potentially viable fetus does not appear to be required. However, where maternal death is foreseeable, maternal consent for cesarean delivery in the event of death would appear reasonable.

SUGGESTED READING

Bernal JM, Growdon JH. Cardiac surgery with cardiopulmonary bypass during pregnancy. Am J Obstet Gynecol Surv 1986;41:1.

Black PM. Brain death. N Engl J Med 1978;229:338–344, 393–401.

Boehm FH, Growdon JH. The effect of eclamptic convulsions of the fetal heart rate. Am J Obstet Gynecol 1974;120:851.

Clark SL, Paul RH. Intrapartum fetal surveillance: the role of fetal scalp sampling. J Obstet Gynecol 1985;153:717.

Clark SL, Sabey P, Jolley K. Non-stress testing with acoustic stimulation: 5960 tests without a fetal demise. Am J Obstet Gynecol 1989;160:694.

Dillion WP, Lee RV, Tronolone MJ, et al. Life support and maternal brain death during pregnancy. JAMA 1982;248:1089.

Katz VL, Dotters DJ, Droegemueller W. Perimortem cesarean delivery. Obstet Gynecol 1986;68:571.

Koh KD, Friesen RM, Livingstone RA, et al. Fetal monitoring during maternal cardiac surgery with cardiopulmonary bypass. Can Med Assn J 1975;112:1102.

Leveno KJ, Williams ML, DePalma RT, et al. Perinatal outcome in the absence of antepartum fetal heart rate acceleration. Obstet Gynecol 1983;61:347.

Smith CV, Nguyen HM, Phelan JP, et al. Intrapartum assessment of fetal well-being: a comparison of fetal acoustic stimulation with acid–base determination. Am J Obstet Gynecol 1986;155:726.

Stange K, Halldin M. Hypothermia in pregnancy. Anesthesiology 1983;58:460.

Weber CE. Postmortem cesarean section: review of the literature and case reports. Am J Obstet Gynecol 1971;110:158.

CHAPTER
THIRTY-THREE

Anesthesia for the Patient with Pregnancy-induced Hypertension

LABOR AND VAGINAL DELIVERY: EPIDURAL ANESTHESIA

Most obstetric anesthesiologists prefer epidural analgesia for providing pain relief for patients with pregnancy-induced hypertension (PIH). Contraindications to regional analgesia include 1) the presence of a coagulopathy (prolonged prothrombin time [PT] or partial thromboplastin time [PTT], platelet count < 100,000 mL or fibrinogen level <100–150 mg/dL); 2) uncorrected hypovolemia; 3) infection; and 4) patient refusal.

When epidural analgesia is instituted, a sympathetic block occurs and results in vasodilation. If the parturient is hypovolemic, this vasodilation will result in an excessive fall in CO, blood pressure, and subsequently, uteroplacental perfusion. Adequate prehydration and maintenance of left uterine displacement to prevent aortocaval compression will minimize these pressure changes. Such prehydration is especially vital for patients with PIH, in whom intravascular volume contraction is an integral part of the disease process. The optimal fluid for this volume expansion is debated widely, some strongly preferring use of colloid while others prefer crystalloid infusion to avoid hypotension. When hypotension is avoided, epidural analgesia may improve intervillous blood flow by decreasing uterine vascular resistance, at least in part by lessening the catecholamine release that occurs in response to painful contractions.

If hypotension should occur (a drop in the systolic blood pressure >20% below baseline), left uterine displacement should be maintained, and oxygen and fluids should be administered. If the blood pressure does not quickly respond to these maneuvers, a vasopressor, ephedrine, is usually administered (initially 2.5–5 mg I.V.).

In some patients, epinephrine is included in the local anesthetic solution as a test dose for intravascular injection and/or to prolong the local anesthetic's duration of action. When administered epidurally, epinephrine (<50 μg) does not decrease intervillous blood flow. However, the routine use of epinephrine in the local anesthetic solution is not recommended for parturients with PIH because of the possibility of inadvertent intravascular injection, which may result in severe hypertension because of a hyperreactive vascular system in PIH.

In general, the use of subarachnoid block (spinal) in the hypertensive patient is not recommended because of the potential for severe and rapid hypotension. The quick onset of the sympathetic block does not allow sufficient time for hemodynamic compensatory mechanisms to occur as effectively as they may with the slower onset of epidural analgesia.

One complication of the use of conduction anesthesia for severe preeclampsia concerns the risk of pulmonary edema and congestive heart failure secondary to the required volume expansion. Patients with PIH may retain several liters of excess extravascular fluid; rapid mobilization of this fluid in the postpartum period may lead to transiently increased wedge pressures and pulmonary edema even without anesthetic-related volume expansion. This complication is most likely to occur within 96 hours of delivery, and providers should be cognizant of this possibility. Congestive heart failure and pulmonary edema are more likely to occur either in women who are older and have a past history of hypertension *or* alternatively, in women who remain hypertensive and relatively oliguric beyond 24 hours postpartum.

ANETHESIA FOR CESAREAN SECTION: EPIDURAL VERSUS GENERAL ANESTHESIA

Hodgkinson et al. investigated the systemic and pulmonary arterial pressure and PCWP changes that occur during induction of epidural anesthesia and general anesthesia for cesarean section in severe preeclamptic patients. Parturients receiving epidural anesthesia exhibited minimal changes in the monitored parameters. During the induction of general anethesia, tracheal intubation and extubation resulted in an increase in mean arterial pressure of 45 mm Hg, in mean pulmonary artery pressure of 20 mm Hg, and in PCWP of 20 mm Hg. These pressure elevations may place parturients with PIH at risk for cardiac or cerebral complications.

The use of epidural anesthesia minimizes the risk of airway complications. In preeclampsia, edema of both mucosal membranes and the larynx occurs rarely but may result in respiratory distress and possible difficulty in securing the airway. Additionally, epidural anesthesia lowers the risk of pulmonary aspiration of gastric contents, a rare but potentially fatal occurrence in paturients undergoing general anesthesia.

Epidural anesthesia for a cesarean section involves the same previously discussed concerns regarding volume status. With an epidural anesthetic for cesarean section, a more extensive sympathetic block is attained when an adequate dosage is administered (to a sympathetic sensory level of at least T4) than when the epidural is used for labor analgesia (sympathetic sensory level of T8–T10).

GENERAL ANESTHESIA

General anesthesia may be preferred for women with PIH or contraindications to epidural anesthesia or whose fetuses are showing signs of acute distress, particularly in the absence of skilled and trained individuals in high-risk obstetrical anesthesia. Most parturients with PIH will have been treated with magnesium sulfate during labor. Magnesium decreases the amount of acetycholine released, as well as the sensitivity of the end-plate at the neuromuscular junction. Therefore, a defasciculating dose of a nondepolarizing relaxant is not necessary prior to the administration of succinylcholine. In addition, the total muscle relaxant dosage needed to maintain surgical relaxation will be reduced. Neuromuscular monitoring is recommended, to prevent relaxant overdosage and the subsequent need for postoperative mechanical ventilation.

Extremes of blood pressure should be controlled prior to the induction of general anesthesia and tracheal intubation. Failure to do so may result in various cardiovascular or neurologic sequelae. Several drugs may be administered for the purpose of blood pressure control. Hydralazine has historically been the most commonly used vasodilating drug given during pregnancy. Its slow and somewhat unpredictable onset of action limits its usefulness for controlling the brief but severe hypertensive episodes associated with tracheal intubation and extubation.

Intravenous nitroglycerin, primarily a venodilator, produces arterial dilation at higher dosages and has been used effectively to control the hemodynamic changes associated with intubation. Nitroglycerin's effectiveness depends on the volume status of the parturient, and it is less effective in parturients who are volume expanded. Nitroglycerin may diminish cerebral autoregulation and thus allow increases in mean arterial pressure to be reflected in an increase in intracranial pressure. Therefore, nitroglycerin should be used cautiously in parturients with evidence of elevated intracranial pressure.

Sodium nitroprusside, a direct-acting vasodilator, has been used extensively to control severe hypertension in nonpregnant patients. Concerns about placental transfer and potential fetal cyanide intoxication (particularly in an acidotic fetus) have limited the widespread use of this drug. However, the advantages (potent rapid vasodilation) of nitroprusside may outweigh the possible risks during acute hypertensive episodes (i.e., tracheal intubation and extubation).

In nonobstetric patients, intravenous narcotics such as fentanyl have been shown to blunt the hypertensive response to intubation. Concern about neonatal depression and the prolonged length of neonatal effect has limited the use of this concept in obstetrics. Alfentanil 10 μg/kg, an ultrashort-acting synthetic narcotic, has been used in the nonhypertensive parturient effectively to blunt the response to intubation, with no noted impairment of Apgar scores.

Drugs used to induce general anesthesia must be selected carefully. Ketamine, which induces a sympathomimetic response, may worsen the hypertension and tachycardia associated with tracheal intubation and should be avoided in parturients with PIH. Sodium thiopental is the agent most widely used for anesthesia induction. A dose of 4 mg/kg provides maternal anesthesia with minimal fetal effects. Etomidate (0.3 mg/kg), a drug known for its associated cardiovascular stability, may also be used.

After induction and intubation, anethesia is maintained with nitrous oxide and oxygen in equal concentrations until delivery. This combination may be supplemented with an inhalational anesthetic agent. Isoflurane (0.75%) offers several advantages for this purpose because of its lower rate of metabolism, reduced fluoride ion production, and decreased myocardial depressive effects. In addition, isoflurane offers more cerebral protection (by decreasing the cerebral oxygen consumption rate) than the other two inhalational agents, halothane and enflurane. However, there are no human studies supporting isoflurane as the agent of choice in PIH.

Following delivery, narcotics are administered intravenously to supplement the anesthesia. Also, the concentration of nitrous oxide may be increased (to 60% or 70%) after delivery of the infant. Special caution must be exercised immediately postdelivery. A significant and, at times, precipitous drop in blood pressure often occurs after delivery of the infant and the placenta. Usually, the patient has been weaned from any continuous infusions of a vasodilator prior to this time.

Tracheal extubation at the conclusion of surgery is also of concern. Once again, major elevations of blood pressure are common and may require a short, rapid-acting agent to minimize the risk of complications.

SUGGESTED READING

Cotton DB, Lee W, Huhta JC, et al. Hemodynamic profile of severe pregnancy-induced hypertension. Am J Obstet Gynecol 1988;158:523.

Hankins GDV, Cunningham FG. Severe preeclampsia and eclampsia: controversies in management. Williams Obstetrics Suppl 12 Eighteenth Edition. Norwalk, Connecticut: Appleton-Century-Crofts, June/July 1991.

Hodgkinson R, Husain FJ, Hayashi RH. Systemic and pulmonary blood pressure during cesarean section in parturients with gestational hypertension. Can Anaesth Soc J 1980;27:389.

Weinstein L. Preeclampsia/eclampsia with hemolysis, elevated liver enzymes, and low platelet count: a severe consequence of hypertension in pregnancy. Am J Obstet Gynecol 1982;142:159.

CHAPTER THIRTY-FOUR

Anesthesia for the Pregnant Cardiac Patient

MONITORING DURING LABOR AND DELIVERY

Patients with cardiac disease who have remained in New York Heart Association (NYHA) functional class I and II throughout pregnancy usually do not require invasive monitoring. Maternal blood pressure should be monitored carefully. Continuous oxygen saturation monitoring (e.g., pulse oximetry) provides moment-to-moment evidence of adequate maternal oxygen saturation during labor, and (indirectly) of maternal cardiac output stability. Careful fetal heart rate monitoring allows evaluation of the fetus. Strict intake and output records of maternal fluids is important.

Symptomatic NYHA class III and IV patients and parturients with significant pulmonary hypertension, right-to-left shunt, dissecting aortic aneurysm, or severe aortic stenosis may justify additional invasive monitoring in the form of an arterial line and/or a flow-directed pulmonary artery catheter, with or without the use of continuous mixed venous oxygen saturation monitoring.

CARDIOVASCULAR EFFECTS OF DRUGS AND ANESTHETIC TECHNIQUES

Prepared childbirth and psychoprophylaxis during labor and delivery may be appropriate for NYHA class I and II cardiac patients who have demonstrated a normal response to the hemodynamic changes of pregnancy.

Narcotics in moderate doses can produce analgesia and relief of anxiety and fear, but they also may produce peripheral vasodilation and (rarely) hypotension and respiratory depression. Meperidine and ketamine may produce tachycardia and should be avoided in patients with severe mitral stenosis or idiopathic hypertrophic subaortic stenosis (IHSS). While the use of narcotic analgesic agents is not contraindicated in the cardiac patient, these considerations must be kept in mind when contemplating their use.

Inhalational analgesia or the judicious use of subanesthetic concentrations of various inhalational agents during late labor and delivery produces acceptable pain relief in 40%–80% of patients. However, the unpredictability of anesthetic depth and the subsequent increased risk of overdosage and maternal aspiration limit this technique.

The following factors should be considered when contemplating the use of lumbar epidural analgesia using local anesthetics:

1. Such anesthesia produces segmental sympathetic blockade, resulting in vasodilation. The degree of sympathetic block can be minimized by using a two-catheter technique or, alternatively, by supplementing the local anesthetic with an opioid. Such decreases in SVR may lead to worsening of right-to-left shunts but may be helpful in patients who would benefit from afterload reduction.
2. These agents may lead to bradycardia and negative inotropy if the cardiac accelerator fibers are blocked (a sympathetic sensory level of T2–T4).
3. Significant plasma levels of local anesthetic may be obtained secondary to vascular absorption. The choice of local anesthetic may be modified by the presence of cardiac conduc-

tion defects. When faced with conduction defects or low ejection fractions, 2-chloroprocaine may be the drug of choice because other local anesthetics have greater cardiotoxic properties in the intravascular space.

4. Epinephrine test doses and epinephrine-containing solutions may cause beta-receptor stimulation, leading to increased heart rate and decreased peripheral vascular resistance. With valvular stenosis, such tachycardia may be poorly tolerated.

Central nervous system (CNS) opioids have been used successfully intrathecally or epidurally for both labor analgesia and postoperative pain control. Opioids in the CNS do not produce autonomic or motor blockade. Preservative-free morphine, 0.5–1.0 mg in a hyperbaric or isobaric solution, has been used in the subarachnoid space for labor analgesia. Fentanyl, 50–100 μg in 10 mL of preservative-free saline or local anesthetic solution epidurally, is also receiving wide acceptance. Morphine 5 mg, butorphanol 4 mg, meperidine 100 mg, and fentanyl 100 μg are the most popular epidural drugs for postoperative pain control. The disadvantages of CNS-active opioids include pruritus, nausea, vomiting, urinary retention, and the possibility of delayed respiratory depression. All these symptoms are reported more commonly in association with morphine. The combination of epidural narcotics and local anesthetics may be the technique of choice in patients with severe mitral stenosis, primary pulmonary hypertension, or Eisenmenger's syndrome.

Subarachnoid blockade (spinal) is used rarely in severe cardiac disease because the rapid onset of profound sympathetic, sensory, and motor block may lead to profound hypotension and cardiovascular collapse.

General anesthesia, using a balanced technique with at least 50% oxygen, appears to be an appropriate technique for cesarean section for many cardiac lesions. Thiopental or etomidate may be used as induction agents. Alfentanil, 125–250 μg/kg results in stable cardiovascular hemodynamics during endotracheal intubation, although fetal depression may be present initially. Fentanyl or morphine administration to deepen postdelivery maternal analgesia is desirable. Efforts to avoid myocardial depression, hypotension or hypoxia, shunt reversal, and, in patients with mitral stenosis, tachycardia are crucial.

ANESTHESIA CONSIDERATIONS WITH SPECIFIC CARDIAC LESIONS
MITRAL STENOSIS

1. Prevent rapid heart rates, which decrease the time for diastolic filling and thereby decrease cardiac output, by avoiding atropine, meperidine, ketamine, and pancuronium.
2. Pain, hypercarbia, and acidosis should be avoided. A light general anesthesia should be used. Increases in central blood volume can be minimized both by avoiding acute volume loading and placing the patient in the Trendelenburg position. Monitoring of PCWP is necessary.
3. Marked decreases in SVR, which may result in reflex tachycardia, should be avoided. SVR can be maintained with metaraminol infusion (10 mg in 250 mL of saline).
4. Increases in pulmonary artery pressure, which may lead to right ventricular failure, can be prevented by avoiding hypoxia, acidosis, and hypercarbia.

RECOMMENDED ANESTHETIC TECHNIQUE

I. Vaginal delivery: gradual-onset lumbar epidural anesthesia:
   A. Prevents marked increases in CO and heart rate (HR) secondary to pain.
   B. Requires careful attention to gradual prehydration (to avoid volume overload) and avoidance of epinephrine (to minimize the risk of tachycardia).
   C. Provides peripheral vasodilation, which helps to unload pulmonary circulation.
   D. Requires judicious use in patients with associated pulmonary hypertension.
   E. Prompts consideration of pulmonary artery catheterization to guide hemodynamic manipulation.
II. Cesarean section
   A. Establish lumbar epidural blockade slowly, following careful fluid preload; treat significant hypotension with fluids and metaraminol.

   B. In cases where general anesthesia is required:
     1. Avoid anticholinergics and pancuronium because of resultant increased heart rate.
     2. Induce with sodium thiopental, 3–4 mg/kg.
     3. Maintain with 0.5% halothane and 50% nitrous oxide and oxygen.
     4. Use fentanyl or alfentanil to deepen anesthesia pre-delivery despite possible fetal depression.
     5. Consider pulmonary artery catheterization to guide hemodynamic manipulation.

MITRAL OR AORTIC INSUFFICIENCY

Recommended anesthetic technique: regional anesthesia may reduce afterload for the left ventricle and therefore is the preferred technique for cesarean section and vaginal deliveries.

AORTIC STENOSIS

  I. Anesthetic considerations
    A. Avoid decreases in SVR.
    B. Avoid decreases in heart rate because CO depends on the heart rate secondary to the fixed stroke volume.
    C. Maintain venous return and left ventricular filling.
 II. Recommended anesthetic technique
    A. Regional techniques with local anesthetics may result in decreased SVR and decreased venous return. Epidural and subarachnoid narcotics are tolerated.
    B. Vaginal delivery may be accomplished by local infiltration or pudendal block, supplemented by small doses of narcotics.
    C. Balanced general anesthesia is preferred for cesarean section.

CONGENITAL HEART DISEASE

  I. Ventricular septal defect (similar considerations apply to other lesions with a left-to-right shunt):

A. Anesthetic considerations
   1. Avoid increases in SVR.
   2. Avoid increases in heart rate.
   3. With preexisting pulmonary hypertension, avoid increases in pulmonary vascular resistance and decreases in SVR or hypotension.

The recommended anesthetic technique is to use regional anesthesia, with a primary left-to-right shunt, for vaginal delivery and cesarean section. Epidural anesthesia effectively reduces SVR and eliminates the SVR increases associated with general anesthesia. However, if pulmonary vascular resistance is equal to or greater than systemic pressure, a systemic resistance decrease secondary to regional anesthesia could cause shunt reversal and a deterioration in oxygenation. Epidural fentanyl (alone or in combination with low concentrations of local anesthetics) or intrathecal morphine may be quite useful in these circumstances. Pudendal blocks may be required for vaginal delivery.

SUGGESTED READING

Clark SL, Phelan JP, Greenspoon J, et al. Labor and delivery in the presence of mitral stenosis: central hemodynamic observations. Am J Obstet Gynecol 1985;152:984.

Hankins GD, Wendell GD. Myocardial infarction during pregnancy: a review. Obstet Gynecol 1985;65:139.

APPENDIX 1
Useful Tables and Formulas

PART C: INFECTIOUS DISEASE

PART D: FETAL MEDICINE

PART A

Physiologic Tables and Formulas

Hemo-dynamics Abbreviation	Definition	Normal Value/Units
BSA	Body surface area	m^2
$\overline{\text{MAP}}$	Mean systemic arterial pressure	84–96 mm Hg
CVP	Central venous pressure	4–10 mm Hg
$\overline{\text{PA}}$	Mean pulmonary artery pressure	10–17 mm Hg
$\overline{\text{PCWP}}$	Mean pulmonary capillary wedge pressure	6–12 mm Hg
CO	Cardiac output	5.5–7.5 L/min
SVR	Systemic vascular resistance	1000–1400 dynes/sec/cm^{-5}
PVR	Pulmonary vascular resistance	55–100 dynes/sec/cm^{-5}
HR	Heart rate	75–95 beats/min
SV	Stroke volume	60–100 mL/beat
LVSWI	Left ventricular stroke work index	40–55 gmM/m^2
EF	Ejection fraction	0.67
EDV	End-diastolic volume	70–75 mL/m^2
COP	Colloid oncotic pressure	16–19 mm Hg
COP-PCWP	Colloid oncotic pressure-wedge pressure gradient	8–14 mm Hg
PAo_2	Mean partial pressure of oxygen in the alveolus	104 mm Hg
Pao_2	Partial pressure of oxygen in arterial blood	106–108 mm Hg (first trimester); 101–104 mm Hg (third trimester)
$P(A-a)o_2$	Alveolar-arterial, gradient	25–65 mm Hg with $Fio_2 = 1.0$
$PAco_2$	Partial pressure of carbon dioxide in the alveolus	40 mm Hg

(continued)

* Modified from Berk JL, Sampliner JE, eds. Handbook of Critical Care, Second Edition. Boston: Little, Brown and Co., 1982.

Normal third-trimester physiologic values *(continued)*

Hemo-dynamics Abbreviation	Definition	Normal Value/ Units
Pa_{CO_2}	Partial pressure of carbon dioxide in arterial blood	35 mm Hg
$P\bar{v}_{O_2}$	Partial pressure of oxygen in mixed venous blood	Varies, dependent upon cardiac output, FI_{O_2} and oxygen consumption from approximately 35–40 mm Hg
$P\bar{v}_{CO_2}$	Partial pressure of carbon dioxide in mixed venous blood	40–50 mm Hg
Sa_{O_2}	Oxyhemoglobin saturation of arterial blood	98% (room air)
$S\bar{v}_{O_2}$	Oxyhemoglobin saturation of mixed venous blood	75% (room air)
Ca_{O_2}	Arterial oxygen content	18–22 mL/dL
$C\bar{v}_{O_2}$	Mixed venous oxygen content	14–17 mL/dL
$C(a-v)_{O_2}$	Arteriovenous oxygen content difference	4–6 mL/100 mL
O_2 extraction ratio		0.25
V_{O_2}	Oxygen consumption	270–320 mL/min
V_{CO_2}	Carbon dioxide production	240–280 mL/min
R	Respiratory quotient	0.8
FRC	Functional residual capacity	2000 mL
VC	Vital capacity	65–75 mL/kg
Ventilation		11–13 L/min
IF	Inspiratory force	75–100 cm H_2O
EDC	Effective compliance	35–45 mL/cm H_2O

(continued)

Normal third-trimester physiologic values *(continued)*

Hemo-dynamics Abbreviation	Definition	Normal Value/ Units
V_D	Dead space	150 mL
V_T	Tidal volume	500 mL
V_D/V_T	Dead space to tidal volume ratio	0.30–0.35
$\dot{Q}_s/Q_t$	Right-to-left shunt (percent of cardiac output flowing past nonventilated alveoli or the equivalent)	3.3%
Flow volume loops (mean)		
$\dot{V}_{50}$	Instantaneous flow at 50% VC	3.5 L/sec
$\dot{V}_{25}$	Instantaneous flow at 25% VC	1.5 L/sec
$\dot{V}_{50R}$	Expiratory/inspiratory flow at 50% VC	1.0
$\dot{V}_{25R}$	Expiratory/inspiratory flow at 25% VC	0.5
$V_{50/25}$	Ratio of exp. flow at 50% VC to exp. flow at 25% VC	2.3

Useful formulas

$MAP = 2 \cdot$ (diastolic pressure) $+$ (systolic pressure)$/3$

$$CI \ (L/min/m^2) = \frac{Cardiac \ output \ (L/min)}{Body \ surface \ area \ (m^2)}$$

$$SVR \ (dynes \cdot sec \cdot cm^{-5}) = \frac{MAP \ [mm \ Hg] - CVP \ [mm \ Hg] \times 79.9}{(Cardiac \ output \ [L/min])}$$

$$PVR \ (dynes \cdot sec \cdot cm^{-5}) = \frac{MPAP \ [mm \ Hg] - PCWP \ [mm \ Hg] \times 79.9}{Cardiac \ output \ (L/min)}$$

$$SV \ (mL/beat) = \frac{Cardiac \ output}{Heart \ rate}$$

$$SVI \ (mL/min/m^2) = \frac{Stroke \ volume}{Body \ surface \ area}$$

$RVSWI \ (gmM/m^2) = SVI \times MPAP \ (mm \ Hg) \times 0.0136$

$LVSWI \ (gmM/m^2) = SI \times MAP \ (mm \ Hg) \times 0.0136$

$C(a-v)o_2 \ (mL/100 \ mL \ or \ vol\%) = Cao_2 - Cvo_2$

$\dot{V}o_2 \ (mL/min/m^2) = CI \times C(a-v)o^2 \times 10$

$$RQ = \frac{Vco_2}{\dot{V}o_2}$$

$O_2 \ avail \ (mL/min/m^2) = CI \times Cao_2 \times 10$

$$\dot{Q}s/\dot{Q}t \ (\%) = \frac{Cco_2 - Cao_2}{Cco_2 - Cvo_2} \times 100$$

$$\dot{Q}s/\dot{Q}t \ (\%) = \frac{0.0031 \times P(A-a)o_2}{[C(a-v)o_2 + (0.0031 \times P(A-a)o_2)]} \times 100$$

$$EDC \ (mL/cm \ H_2O) = \frac{Tidal \ volume \ (mL)}{Peak \ airway \ pressure \ (cm \ H_2O)}$$

$$VD/VT = \frac{Paco_2 - P\bar{E}co_2}{Paco_2}$$

$P(A-a)o_2$ (mm Hg) $= PAo_2 - Pao_2$

$Cao_2 = (Hgb)\ (1.34)\ Sao_2 + (Pao_2 \times 0.0031)$

$(Sao_2 =$ Arterial saturation)

$C\bar{v}o_2 = (Hgb)\ (1.34)\ S\bar{v}o_2 + (P\bar{v}o_2 \times 0.0031)$

$S\bar{v}o_2 =$ Percent saturation of mixed venous blood

$$\frac{\dot{Q}s}{Qt} = \frac{Cc'o_2 - Cao_2}{Cc'o_2 - C\bar{v}o_2}$$

$C\dot{c}o_2 = (1.34)\ (Hgb)\ 100\%$ saturation $+ 0.0031\ Pao_2$

$PAo_2 = (P_B - P_{H_2O})\ Fio_2 - P_{co_2}/0.8$

   $(P_{H_2O} =$ Water vapor pressure)

   $(P_B =$ Barometric pressure)

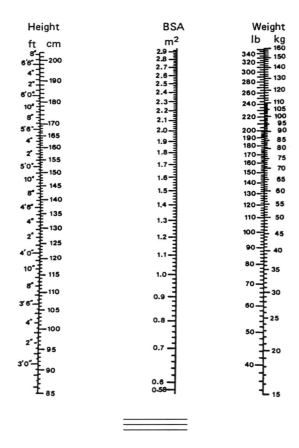

Body surface area calculation: DuBois nomogram for calculating the body surface area of adults. To find body surface of a patient, locate height in inches (or centimeters) on scale 1 and weight in pounds (or kilograms) on scale 3 and place straight edge (ruler) between these two points.

Serum osmolality calculation

$$\text{Osmolality (mosm/kg)} = 2\ [\text{Na(mEq/L)}$$

$$+ \text{K (mEq/L)}] + \frac{\text{Urea (mg/dL)}}{2.8} + \frac{\text{Glucose (mg/dL)}}{18}$$

EKG changes in pregnancy

	1TM	2TM	3TM	D	PP
Heart rate (bpm)	77	79	87	80	66
QT interval(s)	0.378	0.375	0.361	0.362	0.406
QT_c interval(s)	0.424	0.427	0.431	0.414	0.423
PR interval(s)	0.160	0.160	0.155	0.155	0.160
P wave					
Duration (s)	0.092	0.092	0.091	0.091	0.096
Amplitude (mm)	1.9	1.9	2.0	2.0	1.9
Axis (degrees)	40	38	38	41	35
QRS complex					
Duration (s)	0.074	0.074	0.074	0.076	0.077
Amplitude (mm)	11.5	11.5	12.4	12.2	11.2
Axis (degrees)	49	46	40	44	44
T wave					
Duration (s)	0.168	0.171	0.165	0.166	0.176
Amplitude (mm)	3.4	3.5	3.4	3.6	3.5
Axis (degrees)	27	25	22	33	34

1TM = first trimester; 2TM = second trimester; 3TM = third trimesters; D = 1–3 days after delivery; PP = 6–8 weeks postpartum.

Mean EKG measurements during normal pregnancy, delivery, and postpartum in 102 patients

(Reprinted with permission from Carruth JE, Mirvis SB, Brogan DR, et al. The electrocardiogram in normal pregnancy. Am Heart J 1981;6:1075.)

Thyroid function in pregnancy

	Total T$_4$	Free T$_4$	Total T$_3$	Free T$_3$	T$_3$ resin uptake	Free thyroxine index (T$_7$)
Normal nonpregnant	5–13 µg/100 ml	2.70 µg/100 ml	70–150 µg/100 ml	1.5 µg/100 ml	0.8–1.15	4.5–12
Normal pregnant	↑	↔	↑	↔	↓	4.5–12
Pregnant hyperthyroid	↑ to ↑↑↑	↑ to ↑↑	↑ to ↑↑↑	Not measured	Normal to ↑	↑↑↑
Pregnant hypothyroid	↔ to ↓	↓	↓	Not measured	↓ to ↓	Low

T$_4$ = thyroxine; T$_3$ = triiodothyronine; ↔ = stays the same.

(Reproduced with permission from Komins JI, et al. Hyperthyroidism in pregnancy. Obstet Gynecol Sur Baltimore: Williams & Wilkins, 1975;30:527.)

Modified Glasgow Coma Score (GCS)*

Sign	Evaluation	Score
Eye opening	Spontaneous	4
	To speech	3
	To pain	2
	None	1
Best verbal response	Oriented	5
	Confused	4
	Inappropriate	3
	Incomprehensible	2
	None	1
Best motor response	Obeys commands	6
	Localizes pain	5
	Withdrawal to pain	4
	Flexion to pain	3
	Extension to pain	2
	None	1

*GCS < 8 = severe brain injury; GCS < 7 = immediate intubation.

(Modified from Jennett B. Assessment of severity of head injury. J Neurol Neurolsurg Psychiatry 1976;39:647.)

Coagulation factor requirements for hemostasis

Coagulation factor	Requirement (% of normal)
Prothrombin	40
Factor V	10–15
Factor VII	5–10
Factor VIII	10–40
Factor IX	10–40
Factor X	10–15
Factor XI	20–30
Factor XII	0
Prekallikrein	0
High-molecular-weight kininogen	0
Factor XIII	1–5

(Reproduced with permission from Orland MJ, Saltmaur J, eds. Manual of medical therapeutics, 25th ed. Boston: Little, Brown, 1986: 277.)

Plasma coagulation factors in pregnancy

Factor	Name	Change in pregnancy
I	Fibrinogen	4.0–6.5 g/L
II	Prothrombin	100%–125%
IV	Ca^H	
V	Proaccelerin	100%–150%
VII	Proconvertin	150%–250%
VIII	Antihemophilic factor A (AHF)	200%–500%
IX	Antihemophilic B (Christmas factor)	100%–150%
X	Stuart Prower factor	150%–250%
XI	Antihemophilic factor C	50%–100%
XII	Hageman factor	100%–200%
XIII	Fibrin-stabilizing factor	35%–75%
	Antithrombin III	75%–100%
	Antifactor Xa	75%–100%

(Modified from Romero R. The management of acquired hemolytic failure in pregnancy. In: Berkowtiz RL, ed. Critical care of the obstetric patient. New York: Churchill Livingstone, 1983.)

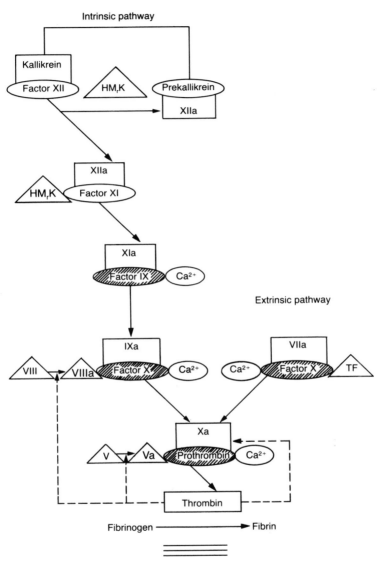

The coagulation cascade. Ovals represent inactive protease precursors. Rectangles represent active proteases. Nonenzymatic protein cofactors are represented by triangles. Hatched ovals represent factors which are felt to be activated on a tissue phospholipid surface. The feedback reactions accelerate the coagulation process. (Reproduced with permission from Orland MJ, Saltmaur J, eds. Manual of medical therapeutics, 25th ed. Boston: Little, Brown, 1986: 272.)

Anemia: differential diagnosis

Anemia Type	Peripheral Smear
Iron deficiency	Hypochromic microcytic
Anemia of chronic disease	Microcytic/normocytic
Thalassemia	Target cells, anisocytosis, microcytic
B_{12}/folate deficient	Macrocytic, hypersegmented PMNs
Microangiopathic hemolysis anemia	Normocytic schistocytes, helmet cells
Sickling disorders	Normocytic sickled cells

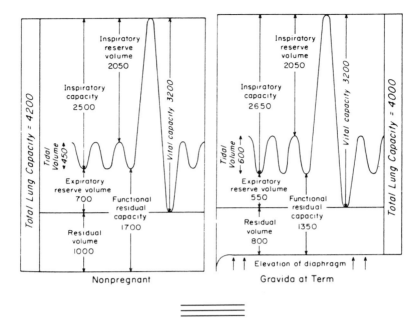

FIGURE A-3

Pulmonary function in pregnancy: Pulmonary volumes and capacities in the nonpregnant state and in the gravida at term. (Courtesy of Bonica J J. Principles and practice of obstetric analgesia and anesthesia. Philadelphia: F.A. Davis Company, 1967.)

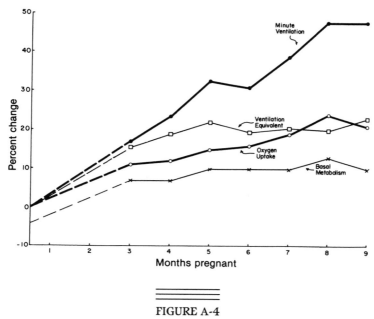

FIGURE A-4

Oxygenation throughout pregnancy: Percentage changes of minute
volume, oxygen uptake, basal metabolism, and the ventilation
equivalent for oxygen at monthly intervals throughout pregnancy.
(Reproduced by permission from Prowse CM, Gaensler EA. Respiratory and acid-base changes during pregnancy. Anesthesiology
1965;26:381.)

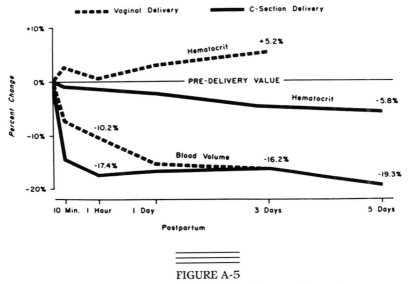

FIGURE A-5

Postpartum hematocrit and blood volume changes: Percentage changes in blood volume and venous hematocrit following vaginal delivery or cesarean section. (Reproduced by permission from Metcalfe J, Ueland K. Heart disease and pregnancy. In: Fowler NO, ed. Cardiac diagnosis and treatment, 3rd ed. Hagerstown, MD: Harper & Row, 1980:1153–1170.)

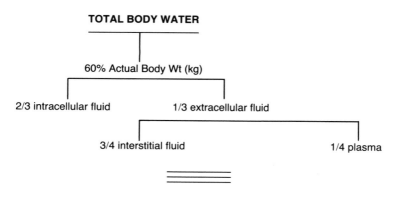

Body water distribution.

Electrolyte content of body fluids

Sweat or gastrointestinal secretion	Electrolyte concentration (mEq/L)				Replacement amount for each liter lost			
	Na^+	K^+	H^+	Cl^-	HCO_3^-	Isotonic saline (mL)	5% D/W (mL)	KCl* (mEq)	$NaHCO_3$[†] (mEq)
Sweat	30–50	5		45–55		300	700	5	
Gastric secretions	40–65	10	90[‡]	100–140		300	700	20[§]	
Pancreatic fistula	135–155	5		55–75	70–90	250	750	5	90
Biliary fistula	135–155	5		80–110	35–50	750	250	5	45
Ileostomy fluid	120–130	10		50–60	50–70	300	700	10	67.6
Diarrhea fluid	25–50	35–60		20–40	30–45		1000	35	45

*Caution should be used in administering potassium faster than 10 mEq/hour.

[†]One ampule of 7.5% $NaHCO_3$ contains 45 mEq HCO_3^- .

[‡]Variable (e.g., achlorhydria).

[§]Administration of more than the observed gastric loss of potassium is often required because of enhanced urinary potassium excretion in alkalosis.

(Reproduced with permission from Orland MJ, Saltmaur J, eds. Manual of medical therapeutics, 25th ed. Boston: Little, Brown, 1986: 43.)

PART B

Drugs, Devices, and Fluid Therapy

Guidelines for the institution and discontinuation of mechanical ventilation

Parameter	Normal range	Indication for ventilatory assistance	Indication for weaning
Mechanics			
Respiratory rate	12–20	>35	<30
Vital capacity (mL/kg of body weight)	65–75	<15	12–15
FEV_1 (mL/kg of body weight)	50–60	<10	>10
Inspiratory force	75–100	<25	>25
Oxygenation			
Pao_2 (mm Hg)	100–75 (room air)	<70 (on mask O_2)	—
$P(A-a)o_2$ (Fio_2 = 1.0)	25–65	450	<400
Ventilation			
$Paco_2$ (mm Hg)	35–45	>55	—
V_D/V_T	0.25–0.40	>0.60	<0.58

Oxygen delivery systems

Delivery	Common flow (L/min)	Inspired O_2 concentration (%)	Comments
Nasal cannula	1–6	24–44	Inspired O_2 concentration increases by approximately 4% for each 1 L/min flow; exact FIo_2 is uncertain.
Face mask	8–10	40–60	Oxygen flow should be higher than 5 L/min to avoid accumulation of exhaled air.
Face mask with oxygen reservoir	6–10	60–100	Inspired O_2 concentration increases by 10% for each 1 L/min flow.
Venturi mask	—	24,28,31 35,40,50	Provides constant controlled FIo_2.
Mouth-to-mouth	—	17	—
Mouth-to-mask	10–15	50–80	—

Vitamin requirements in pregnancy (compared with standard
intravenous vitamin preparation)

Vitamin	RDA	MVI-12
A	800 μg RE	3300 USP (retinol)*
D	400 IU (10 μg cholecalciferol)	200 USP units[†]
E (de-alpha-tocopheryl acetate)	10 mg a-TE	10 USP units*
Ascorbic acid	70 mg	100 mg
Thiamine (B_1)	1.5 mg	3.0 mg
Riboflavin (B_2)	1.6 mg	3.6 mg
Pyridoxine (B_6)	2.2 mg	4.0 mg
Niacin	17 mg	40.0 mg
Pantothenic acid	4–7 mg[‡]	15.0 mg
Biotin	30–100 μg[‡]	60 μg
Folic Acid	400 μg	400 μg
B_{12}	2.2 μg	5 μg
K	0.03–1.5 μg/kg (RDA)	—[§]

*Equivalent to RDA.

[†]May require additional supplementation for women with a history of poor intake.

[‡]Estimated safe and adequate daily dietary intakes in nonpregnant adults (RDA).

[§]Must be added to vitamin regimens.

(Reproduced with permission from Nutrition Support Dietetics, 2nd ed. American Society for Parenteral and Enteral Care, Silver Springs, MD, 1993.)

Mineral and trace element requirements in pregnancy

Mineral	Enteral Nutrition	Parenteral Nutrition
Calcium	1200 mg	200–250 mg (9.6–12.5 mEq)
Phosphorus	1200 mg (38 mm)	30–45 mm
Magnesium	450 mg (37.5 mEq)	10–15 mEq
Zinc	15 mg	2.55–3.0 mg
Copper	1.5–3.0 mg*	0.5–1.5 mg
Manganese	2.0–5.0 mg*	0.15–0.8 mg
Iodine	175 μg	50 μg†
Selenium	65 μg	20–40 μg‡
Iron	10 + 30–60 mg supplemental iron	3–6 mg
Chromium	0.05–0.2 mg*	10–15 μg

*Estimated safe and adequate daily intakes in nonpregnant adults.

†Assuming 80% absorption.

‡Recommended intravenous dose for stable adults.

(Reproduced with permission from Nutrition Support Dietetics, 2nd ed. American Society for Parenteral and Enteral Nutrition, Silver Springs, MD, 1993.)

Insulin preparations and properties

Type	Action (Hours)*		
	Onset	**Peak**	**Duration**
Rapid			
Regular (crystalline)	0.3–1	2–4	6–8
Semilente	0.5–1.0	2–6	10–12
Intermediate			
NPH	1–2	6–12	18–24
Lente	1–2	6–12	18–24
Slow			
Ultralente	3–8	18–24	36
Protamine zinc	3–8	14–24	36

*These are approximate figures. There is significant variation from patient to patient and from dose to dose in the same patient.

Topical corticosteroid preparations

Low potency
Hydrocortisone 0.5%
Hydrocortisone 1%
Desonide 0.05%

Medium potency
Triamcinolone acetonide 0.1%
Betamethasone dipropionate 0.05%
Betamethasone valerate 0.1%
Fluocinolone acetonide 0.025%
Flurandrenolide 0.05%

High potency
Fluocinonide 0.05%
Halcinonide 0.1%
Desoximetasone 0.25%

Glucocorticoids

Steroid action	Available tablet size (mg)	Relative anti-inflammatory effect	Relative mineralo-corticoid effect	Duration
Hydrocortisone	5, 10, 20	1.0	1.0	S
Prednisone	1, 2.5, 5, 10, 20, 50	4.0	0.8	I
Prednisolone	5	4.0	0.8	I
Methyl-prednisolone	2, 4, 8, 16, 24, 32	5.0	0.5	I
Dexamethasone	0.25, 0.5, 0.75, 1.5, 4, 6	25.0	0.0	L
Betamethasone	0.6	25.0	0.0	L

S = short; I = intermediate; L = long.

Narcotics: relative potency

Drug	Potency Relative to Morphine	Oral–Parenteral Potency
Hydromorphone	6.0	1:5
Morphine	1.0	1:6
Oxycodone	1.0	1:2
Pentazocine (Talwin)	0.25	1:3
Meperidine (Demerol)	0.15	1:3
Codeine	0.1	2:3

Commonly used antihypertensive agents

Drug	Indication	Oral Dose	Parenteral Dose
Alphamethyldopa	Chronic hypertension	250–500 mg b.i.d.–q.i.d.	
Hydralazine hydrochloride	Acute control of hypertensive crisis (IV) chronic hypertension (p.o.)	25–50 mg b.i.d.–q.i.d.	5–10 mg IV q 20 minutes
Atenolol	Chronic hypertension	50–100 mg p.o. q.i.d.	
Propranolol	Chronic hypertension	40–160 mg b.i.d.–q.i.d.	
Labetolol		200–400 mg b.i.d.	20–80 mg IV q 10 minutes
Nifedipine		10–20 mg q 6–8 h	

Commonly used agents for hemodynamic manipulation

Drug	Method of Preparation	Microdrop Concentration[†] μg/μgtt	Begin at Low Dosage[†] μg/kg/min	Progress to High Dosage[†] μg/kg/min	Comments
Dopamine (Inotropin) (Single Strength)	1 amp (200 mg) in 250 mL	13.3	5 (26)[‡]	20 (105)[‡]	Renal 0–3 Mixed renal/beta 3–7 Renal/beta/alpha > 7 μg/kg/min
Dopamine (Inotropin) (Double Strength)	2 amps (400 mg) in 250 mL	26.6	5 (13)[‡]	20 (52)[‡]	
Dobutamine (Dobutrex)	1 amp (250 mg) in 250 mL	16.6	5 (21)[‡]	—	NEJM 1979; 300:17.
Epinephrine	2 amps (2 mg) in 250 mL	0.13	0.01 (5)[‡]	0.20 (100)[‡]	Beta 0.01–0.03; mixed 0.03; alpha >0.15; μg/kg/ min
Isoproterenol (Isuprel)	1 large amp (1 mg) in 250 mL (or 5 small amps in 250 mL)	0.066	0.01 (10)[‡]	0.30 (300)[‡]	

(continued)

Commonly used agents for hemodynamic manipulation *(continued)*

Drug	Method of Preparation	Microdrop Concentration[†] $\mu g/\mu gtt$	Begin at Low Dosage[†] $\mu g/kg/min$	Progress to High Dosage[†] $\mu g/kg/min$	Comments
Phenylophrine (Neosynephrine)	1 amp (10 mg) in 250 mL	0.66	0.1 (11)[‡]	0.7 (74)[‡]	Practically, pure alpha
Norepinephrine (Levophed)	2 amps (8 mg) in 250 mL	0.53	0.05 (7)[‡]	1 (132)[‡]	
Phentolamine (Regitine)	1.5 amps (7.5 mg) in 250 mL	0.5	0.5 (70)[‡]	20 (2800)[‡]	
Nitroprusside (Nipride)	1 bottle (50 mg) in 250 mL	3.3	0.4 (8)[‡]	5 (106)[‡]	Toxic 8 $\mu g/kg/$ min; or acute toxicity 1.5 mg/ kg over 3 h period
Nitroglycerin	50 mg in 250 mL via millipore filter	3.3	0.4 (8)[‡]	1.5; may up to 5 in awake patients (106)[‡]	No known metabolic toxicity as yet

[†]Microdrop (μgtt) is provided by an infusion apparatus giving 60 drops per mL

[‡]Microdrops per minute for a 70 kg patient

Some guidelines are approximate and modulated by clinical response and indications

Blood component therapy

Product	Volume (mL)	Content	Life
Whole blood	450	All blood components	35 d No granulocytes or platelets after 24 hours. Decreased but functionally adequate levels of factors V and VIII for 1–2 weeks
Packed red blood cells	250	Red cells only	35 d
Fresh-frozen plasma	200–250	All stable and labile clotting factors	1 y
Cryoprecipitate	50	Factors V, VIII:c, VIII: Von Willibrand, XIII, fibronectin fibrinogen	1 y
Platelets	50 (per pack)	Platelets	5 d

Electrolyte equivalencies

	mg/mEq
NaCl	58
$NaHCO_3$	84
KCl	75
$KHCO_3$	100
$MgSO_4 \cdot 7H_2O$	123
$CaCO_3$	50
$CaCl_2 \cdot 2H_2O$	73
Ca gluconate$_2 \cdot 1H_2O$	224

Intravenous fluids

	Osmolality (mosm/kg)	Glucose concentration (g/L)	Na (mEq/L)	Cl (mEq/L)
5% dextrose/ water	252	50	—	—
10% dextrose/ water	505	100	—	—
50% dextrose/ water	2520	500	—	—
0.45% NaCl	154	—	77	77
0.9% NaCl	308	—	154	154
Lactated Ringer's solution	272	—	130	109

*Also contains K (4 mEq/L), Ca (3 mEq/L), and lactate (28 mEq/L)

======

Solution for total parenteral nutrition in pregnancy

PHARMACY ORDERS

Aminosyn 2, 8.5%	454.0 mL
Dextrose, 50%	516.0 mL
Lypholyte II	20.0 mL
Sodium phosphate (4.0 mEq/mL)	4.0 mL
MVI	5.5 mL
Trace elements*	0.7 mL

Make 2 bottles, send 500 mL of lipid emulsion 10%.

NURSING ORDERS

---

1. Run TPN bottles at 80 mL per hour.
2. Run lipid 10% emulsion at 125 mL per hour until 500 mL of lipid have been infused.
3. Routine monitoring (Weight, I&O, and Urinary Glucose q 6 h).

Each bottle of TPN (total volume 1000 mL) supplies the following:

Aminosyn 2, 8.5%	454 cc (38.6 gm protein)
Dextrose, 50%	516 cc (end concentration 25.8%) 1.03 cal/mL TPN
Sodium	51.0 mEq
Potassium	20.0 mEq
Calcium	4.5 mEq
Magnesium	5.0 mEq
Zinc	3.5 mg
Copper	0.7 mg
Manganese	0.4 mg
Chromium	7.0 mcg
Chloride	35.0 mEq
Acetate	29.5 mEq
Phosphate	24.0 mEq

*Add 800 μg folic acid and 6 mg iron to one bottle daily.

Sample TPN Solution in Pregnancy for 63-kg woman, height 168 cm, age 23.

(continued)

======

Solution for total parenteral nutrition in pregnancy *(continued)*

MVI-12	5.5 cc
Folic acid	800 mg
Iron	6 mg

Calories

Using the Harris–Benedict equation, these factors calculate a basal energy expenditure (BEE) of 1461 kcal/d. Since calorie and protein requirements parenterally are the same as for a pregnant woman being fed orally or enterally, we used the factor of 1.5 × BEE to calculate caloric need.

Pt's BEE (1461) × 1.5 − 2192 + additional kcals for 2nd + 3rd trimester (300 kcals/d) − 2500 kcals/d.

Protein

The current recommended dietary allowance (RDA) for protein has been reduced to an additional 10 g/d.

Feeding 1 g/kg/d would provide 63 g of protein for this patient on her ideal weight. An additional 10 g were added to her TPN for a total of 73 g or 1.2 g/kg/d.

Fats

The requirement for essential fatty acids (EFA) is slightly increased in pregnancy to 4.5% of total calories. It is important to use a fat emulsion that contains both linoleic and linolenic acids. Liposyn is the brand of fat emulsion used in this TPN order and it is composed of 60% essential fatty acids.

Electrolytes, trace elements

Most standard packs provide adequate amounts except for folate and iron. The iron can be safely infused intravenously, dependent upon rate and dosage.

PART C

Infectious Disease

Postexposure hepatitis prophylaxis

Hepatitis A:

0.02 mL/kg immune/globulin IM pre- or postexposure*

Hepatitis B:

Postexposure: 1. 0.06 mL/kg HBIG*†
2. Recombivax HB 1 mL (10 mg) or Engevix-B 1 mL (20 mg) at 0, 1 and 6 mos.

*Within 2 weeks of exposure, for postexposure prophylaxis.

†For percutaneous or mucous membrane exposure, dose is repeated in one mo.

Immunization during pregnancy

Agent	Type of Vaccine	Okay in Pregnancy
Measles	Live attenuated virus	No
Mumps	Live attenuated virus	No
Rubella	Live attenuated virus	No
Influenza	Inactivated virus	Yes
Hepatitis A	Inactivated virus	Yes
Hepatitis B	Recombinant virus	Yes
Polio	Live attenuated (OPV) or enhanced potency inactivated virus (e-IPV)	Yes, high-risk situation or travel to endemic areas
Pneumoccoccus	Polyvalent polysaccharide	Yes
Typhoid	Killed or live attenuated bacterial	Yes
Tetanus–Diptheria	Toxoid	Yes
Rabies	Killed virus	Yes

Antibiotic dosage for the treatment of serious infections in pregnancy*

Antibiotic	Total Daily Dose*	Usual Interval Between Doses (hours)*	Average Concentration (μg/mL) Needed to Inhibit Organism	
			Gram-Positive	Gram-Negative
Amikacin	15 mg/kg	8		1–16
Ampicillin	12 g	4	0.05–0.5	1–10
Carbenicillin	24–40 g	4	0.1–1.0	1–150
Cefamandole	6–12	4	0.05–1.0	1–16
Cefazolin	4–8 g	8	0.05–1.0	1–12
Cefoperazone	6–12 g	8–12	1–2	2
Cefotaxime	12–18 g	4	1	0.5–1
Cefoxitin	6–12 g	4	1–3	1–16
Cefuroxime	8–12 g	6–8	1–2	1–16
Cephalothin	8–12 g	4	0.05–1.0	1–16
Cephapirin	6–12 g	4	0.05–1.0	1–16
Chloramphenicol	50 mg/kg	6	0.5–2.0	1–10
Clindamycin	2–5 gm	6	0.02–1.5	anaerobes only
Colistimethate	5 mg/kg	6–8		0.5–2.0

(continued)

Antibiotic dosage for the treatment of serious infections in pregnancy* *(continued)*

Antibiotic	Total Daily Dose*	Usual Interval Between Doses (hours)*	Average Concentration Needed to Inhibit Organism (μg/mL)	
			Gram–Positive	Gram–Negative
Erythromycin	2–4 gm	6	0.05–1.0	
Gentamicin	3–6 mg/kg	8		1–5
Kanamycin	15 mg/kg	8–12		1–10
Lincomycin	4–8 g	6	0.5–1.0	
Metronidazole	3–4 g	8	0.8–4 (only anaerobes)	0.8–4
Mezlocillin	18 g	4–6	1†	5–10
Moxalactam	8–12 g	6–8	1–4	0.5–1
Nafcillin or Oxacillin	8–12 g	4–6	0.1–0.3	
Penicillin G	10–24 × 10⁶ MU	4	0.05–0.5	
Piperacillin	18 g	4–6	1†	5–10; 2–4 for Pseudomonas
Polymyxin B	2.5 mg/kg	6–8		0.5–2.0
Ticarcillin	12–18 g	4	0.1–1.0	1–100
Tobramycin	3–6 mg/kg	8		1–6
Vancomycin	2–4 g	6	0.5–6.0	

*Dosage intervals based on normal renal function.
†Nonpenicillinase–producing *S. aureus.*

Treatment of sexually transmitted diseases in pregnancy

Type or Stage	Drug of Choice	Dosage	Alternatives
Gonorrhea*			
Urethral, cervical, or rectal	Ceftriaxone	125–250 mg I.M. once	Spectinomycin 2 g I.M. once
Pharyngeal	Ceftriaxone	125–250 mg I.M. once	Spentinomycin 2 g I.M. once
Ophthalmia	Ceftriaxone	1 g I.M. once plus saline irrigation	Ceftriaxone 1 g IV or I.M. daily × 5 days, plus saline irrigation
Bacteremia and arthritis	Ceftriaxone	1 g IV daily × 7–10 days	Ceftizoxime or cefotaxime, 1 g IV q8h for 2–3 d or until improved, followed by cefuroxime axetil 500 mg orally bid to complete 7–10 d total therapy[†]
Meningitis	Ceftriaxone	2 g IV daily for at least 10 days	Penicillin G at least 10 million U IV daily for at least 10 days[‡]
			Chloramphenicol 4–6 g/d IV for at least 10 days[‡]

*Since a high percentage of pregnant women with gonorrhea have coexisting *Chlamydia trachomatis* infection, these patients should also receive a seven-day course of erythromycin as recommended for treatment of *Chlamydia*.

[†]If the infecting strain of *N. gonorrhoeae* is known to be susceptible to penicillin, treatment may be changed to penicillin G 10 million U IV daily, or amoxicillin 500 mg orally q.i.d.

[‡]If infecting strain of *N. gonorrhoeae* is known to be susceptible.

(continued)

Treatment of sexually transmitted diseases in pregnancy *(continued)*

Type or Stage	Drug of Choice	Dosage	Alternatives
Endocarditis	Ceftriaxone	2 g IV daily for at least 3 to 4 weeks	Penicillin G at least 10 million U IV daily for at least 3 to 4 weeks‡
Chlamydia trachomatis§			
Urethritis or cervicitis	Erythromycin 500 mg oral q.i.d. × 7 d		
Oculogenital syndrome	Erythromycin 500 mg oral q.i.d. × 7 d		
Proctitis	Erythromycin 500 mg oral q.i.d. × 7 d		
Lymphogranuloma venereum	Erythromycin 500 mg oral q.i.d. × 21 d		
Pelvic inflammatory disease			
—hospitalized patients	Cefoxitin or	2 g IV q6h	Clindamycin 600 mg IV q6h plus gentamicin 2 mg/kg IV once followed by gentamicin 1.5 mg/kg IV q8h until improved followed by doxycycline‖ 100 mg oral b.i.d. to complete 10–14 d#
(non-pregnant)	Cefotetan either one plus Doxycycline followed by Doxycycline‖	2 g IV q12h 100 mg IV q12h until improved 100 mg oral b.i.d. to complete 10–14 days	

§Includes clinical syndromes that mimic chlamydial infection, such as nongonococcal urethritis.

‖Or tetracycline 500 mg oral q.i.d.

#Or clindamycin 450 mg oral q.i.d. to complete 10–14 days.

—outpatients	Cefoxitin plus probenecid	2 g I.M. once	
	or	1 g oral once	
	Ceftriaxone either one followed by	250 mg I.M. once	
	Doxycycline	100 mg oral b.i.d. × 10–14 days	
(non-pregnant)			
Vaginal infection			
Trichomoniasis	Metronidazole	2 g oral once or 500 mg oral b.i.d. × 7 d**	
Bacterial vaginosis	Metronidazole	500 mg oral b.i.d. × 7 d	Clindamycin 300 mg oral b.i.d. × 7 d
Vulvovaginal candidiasis	Miconazole nitrate	200 mg suppository intravaginally hs × 3 d	Miconazole nitrate (100 mg suppository or 5 g 2% cream) intravaginally hs × 7 d
	or		
	Clotrimazole	200 mg vaginal tablet intravaginally hs × 3 d	Clotrimazole (100 mg vaginal tablet or 5 grams 1% cream) intravaginally hs × 7 d
	or		
	Butoconazole	5 g of 2% cream intravaginally hs × 3 d	Butoconazole (5 g of 2% cream) intravaginally hs × 6 d
	or		
	Terconazole	80 mg suppository intravaginally hs × 3 d	Terconazole (0.4% cream) 5 g intravaginally hs × 7 d
Syphilis			
Early (Primary, secondary, or latent less than one year)	Penicillin G benzathine	2.4 million U I.M. once	Ceftriaxone 250 mg I.M. once daily × 10 days††

**Metronidazole should be avoided during pregnancy but, for pregnant women with severe symptoms, 2 g oral (single dose) may be given after the first trimester.

††Limited experiences; use only if compliance and follow-up are assured.

(continued)

Treatment of sexually transmitted diseases in pregnancy *(continued)*

Type or Stage	Drug of Choice	Dosage	Alternatives
Late (more than one year's duration, cardiovascular, gumma, late-latent)	Penicillin G benzathine	2.4 million U I.M. weekly × 3 weeks	No proven effective alternative; allergic patients should be desensitized
Neurosyphilis	Penicillin G or Penicillin G procaine plus probenecid	2 to 4 million U IV q4h × 10–14 d 2.4 million U I.M. daily 500 mg q.i.d. orally both × 10–14 d	No proven effective alternative; allergic patients should be desensitized
Chancroid	Erythromycin or Ceftriaxone	500 mg oral q.i.d. × 7 d 250 mg I.M. once	Trimethoprim–sulfamethoxazole 160/800 mg oral b.i.d. × 7 d#
Herpes simplex			
First Episode Genital (non-pregnant)	Acyclovir	400 mg oral t.i.d. × 7–10 d	Acyclovir 200 mg oral 5 times/day × 7–10 d
First Episode Proctitis (non-pregnant)	Acyclovir	800 mg oral t.i.d. × 7–10 d	Acyclovir 400 mg oral 5 times/day × 7–10 d
Severe	Acyclovir	5 mg/kg IV q8h × 5–7 d	
Prevention of Recurrences (non-pregnant)	Acyclovir	200 mg oral 2–5 times d	Acyclovir 400 mg b.i.d.

#Resistance has been reported, especially outside the USA.

Aminoglycoside dosing: normal and renal failure

Aminoglycoside	Usual Loading Doses	Expected Peak Serum Levels
Tobramycin	1.5 to 2.0 mg/kg	4 to 10 μg/mL
Gentamicin		
Amikacin	5.0 to 7.5 mg/kg	15 to 30 μg/mL
Kanamycin		

1. Select loading dose in mg/kg (ideal weight) to provide peak serum levels in range listed in the table for desired aminoglycoside.

2. Select maintenance dose (as percentage of chosen loading dose) to continue peak serum levels indicated in the table, according to desired dosing interval and the patient's corrected creatinine clearance.*

*Calculate corrected Creatinine Clearance $Cl_{(C)_{CR}}$ as:
$Cl_{(C)_{CR}}$ male = 140 − age/serum creatinine
$Cl_{(C)_{CR}}$ female = $0.85 \times Cl_{(C)_{CR}}$ male

(Reproduced by permission from Hull, JH, Sarubbi, FA. Amikacin serum concentrations: prediction of levels and dosage guidelines. Ann Intern Med 1978;89:612.)

Percentage of loading dose required for dosage interval selected

$CL_{(C)_{CR}}$ (mL/min)	Half-life* (hours)	8 hours (%)	12 hours (%)	24 hours (%)
90	3.1	84	—	—
80	3.4	80	91	—
70	3.9	76	88	—
60	4.5	71	84	—
50	5.3	65	79	—
40	6.5	57	72	92
30	8.4	48	63	86
25	9.9	43	57	81
20	11.9	37	50	75
17	13.6	33	46	70

(continued)

Percentage of loading dose required for dosage interval selected
(continued)

$CL_{(C)_{CR}}$ (mL/min)	Half-life* (hours)	8 hours (%)	12 hours (%)	24 hours (%)
15	15.1	31	42	67
12	17.9	27	37	61
10	20.4	24	34	56
7	25.9	19	28	47
5	31.5	16	23	41
2	46.8	11	16	30
0	69.3	8	11	21

*Alternatively, half the chosen loading dose may be given at an interval approximately equal to the estimated half-life.

(Reproduced by permission from Hull, JH, Sarubbi, FA. Amikacin serum concentrations: prediction of levels and dosage guidelines. Ann Intern Med 1978; 89:612.)

Dialysis and antibiotic blood levels

	Effect on Blood Levels		Added Dose Given After Dialysis	
	Peritoneal Dialysis	**Hemodialysis**	**Peritoneal Dialysis**	**Hemodialysis**
Penicillins:				
Penicillin G	Slight	Yes	Variable	Yes
Ampicillin–Amoxicillin	Slight	Yes	Variable	Yes
Carbenicillin–Ticarcillin	Slight	Yes	Variable	Yes
Methicillin	No	Yes	Variable	Yes
Oxacillin				
Nafcillin				
Cloxacillin	No	No	Variable	Yes
Dicloxacillin				
Piperacillin	Slight	Yes	Variable	Yes
Cephalosporins:				
Cephalothin	Variable	Yes	Variable	Variable
Cephapirin	Variable	Yes	Variable	Yes, usually
Cefazolin	Variable	Yes	Variable	0.5–1.0 g
Cephalexin	Variable	Yes	Variable	
Cephradine	Variable	Yes	Variable	

(continued)

Dialysis and antibiotic blood levels *(continued)*

| | Effect on Blood Levels | | Added Dose Given After Dialysis | |
	Peritoneal Dialysis	Hemodialysis	Peritoneal Dialysis	Hemodialysis
Cefoxitin	Variable	Yes	Variable	
Cefamandole	Variable	Yes	Variable	
Moxalactam	Variable	Yes	Variable	1.0 g after dialysis
Cefotaxime	Variable	Yes	Variable	15 mg/kg after dialysis
Cefoperazone	Unknown	Yes	Unknown	Yes
Aminoglycosides:				
Gentamicin	Yes	Yes	Additional	$\frac{1}{2} - \frac{3}{4}$ loading dose for these three amino-glycosides
Tobramycin	Yes	Yes	parenteral dose given with caution if antibiotic added to dialysate.	
Amikacin	Yes	Yes	Blood level must be checked.	

Operative wound classification—infection risk

Class 1—Clean

Nontraumatic
No inflammation encountered
No break in technique
Respiratory, alimentary,
    genitourinary tracts not
    entered

Reported infection rates are usually 1 to 4%. In general, no antibiotics are needed unless the host's defenses are suppressed or unless the consequences of infection are catastrophic: heart value replacement, etc. Drains are not used unless blood or fluid must be evacuated.

Class 2—Clean–Contaminated

Gastrointestinal or respiratory
    tracts entered without
    significant spillage
Appendectomy—not
    perforated—no cloudy peri-
    toneal exudate
Prepared oropharynx or va-
    gina entered
Genitourinary or biliary tracts
    entered in absence of in-
    fected urine or bile
Minor break in technique

Reported infection rates are 5 to 15%. Here the surgeon must use judgment about using preoperative antibiotic. One hopes that it will not be necessary to use antibiotics in most cases of biliary or small intestinal surgery unless the host's defenses are suppressed. Cases in which consequences of infection are trivial (anal and minor mouth procedures) do not require antibiotics. Delayed primary closure may be considered.

Class 3—Contaminated

Major break in technique
Gross spillage from gastrointes-
    tinal tract
Traumatic wound, fresh
Entrance of genitourinary or
    biliary tracts in presence of
    infected urine or bile
Colon entered, with any spill
    of content

Reported infection rates are about 16 to 25%, although many centers are reporting less with preventive antibiotics. In this category, most patients need antibiotic supplementation unless the operation is trivial, as in anal surgery. Delay of primary or secondary closure techniques should be used frequently.

(continued)

Operative wound classification—infection risk *(continued)*

Class 4—Dirty and Infected

Acute bacterial inflammation or pus encountered

Transection of "clean" tissue for the purpose of surgical access to a collection of pus

Perforated viscus entered

Traumatic wound with retained devitalized tissue, foreign bodies, fecal contamination and/or delayed treatment, or from dirty source

Infection rates mean little here, but are often over 25%. Here, either secondary closure of skin and subcutaneous tissues or antibiotics or both should be used. Antibiotics are not usually necessary for drainage of a small abscess.

Reproduced by permission from Altemeier, WA ed. Manual on control of infection in surgical patients. Philadelphia: Lippincott, 1976.

Common antimicrobial drug interactions

Antibiotic Antimicrobial*	Interacting Drug	Unwanted Effect	Probable Mode of Action
Aminoglycosides	Cephalosporin: Only reported with Cephalothin	Nephrotoxic	Unknown
	Curariform neuromuscular blockers	Neuromuscular paralysis	Both exert additive effect
	Ethacrynic acid, Furosemide	Eighth–nerve toxicity	Additive effect
	Methoxyflurane	Kidney damage	Unknown
	Digoxin	Decreased absorption	Malabsorption
	Beta lactam antibiotics: Penicillins Cephalosporins	Inactivate each other. Decreased aminoglycoside activity important when drugs mixed together	Binding to charged groups
Isoniazid (INH)	Alcohol	Greater tendency to hepatitis; decreased INH action	Unknown, enhanced INH metabolism by chronic alcohol intake
	Antacids	Decreased INH effects	Interference with INH absorption in gut

(continued)

Common antimicrobial drug interactions *(continued)*

Antibiotic Antimicrobial*	Interacting Drug	Unwanted Effect	Probable Mode of Action
	Disulfiram	Psychosis; neurological disorders	Disturbance in metabolism of catecholamines
	Phenylhydantoin	Enhanced potential for phenylhydantoin toxicity	Isoniazid inhibits detoxification by microsomes
Sulfonamides	Oral anticoagulants	Enhanced action of anticoagulant	Displacement of anticoagulant from protein binding site
	Oral hypoglycemics	Increased hypoglycemia	Unknown: sulfonamides and sulfonylureas have structural similarities
	Methotrexate	Neutropenia	Not known
Tetracyclines	Oral antacids; calcium rich foods	Decreased anti–microbial effect	Tetracycline chelate divalent ions. Leads to decreased absorption of both
	Barbiturates	Doxycycline loses effect	Barbiturate-induced hepatic breakdown of doxycycline
	Carbamazepine	Doxycycline loses effect	Carbamazepine induces hepatic breakdown of doxycycline

Drug	Interacting agent	Effect	Mechanism
Lincomycin or Clindamycin	Methoxyflurane	Kidney damage	Unknown
	Kaolin–pectin	Decreased antibiotic effect	Interference with gastrointestinal absorption of lincomycin
	Curariform agents	Neuromuscular paralysis	Both drugs are neuromuscular blockers, giving additive effects
Rifampin	Oral anticoagulants	Less anticoagulant action	Detoxification enzymes induced by rifampin
	Oral contraceptives	Greater pregnancy risk	Estrogen breakdown induced by rifampin
	Probenecid	Rifampin toxicity increased	Disturbance of hepatic metabolism of rifampin
	Corticosteroids	Decreased steroid effect	

Toxicity of antimicrobial agents

Agent	Mechanism	Signs
Hematologic:		
Chloramphenicol	Inhibit protein synthesis	Reversible anemia; leukopenia
	Damage stem cell	Aplastic anemia
Sulfonamide	G6PD deficiency	Hemolytic anemia
Carbenicillin*	Platelet aggregation decreased	Bleeding
Ticarcillin		
Piperacillin		
Mezlocillin		
Moxalactam	Vitamin K absorption, or metabolism	Bleeding responsive to vitamin K
Cefamandole		
Cefoperazone		
Nervous System:		
Aminoglycosides	Binding hair cells of organ of corti	Deafness
		Vertigo
	Binding vestibular cells	Respiratory paralysis
	Competitive neuromuscular blockade	
Erythromycin	Effect on auditory portion of 8th cranial nerve	After I.V. use, deafness may be reversible
Polymyxin	Non-competitive neuromuscular blockade	Respiratory paralysis
Penicillin	Cortical stimulation	Myoclonic seizures
Cephalosporin*		
Nalidixic Acid	Unknown	Peripheral neuritis
Metronidazole		
Gastrointestinal:		
Rifampin	Liver cell damage	Hepatitis
Isoniazid		
Neomycin	Villous damage	Malabsorption
Clindamycin	Stool overgrowth with *Clostridium difficile*	Diarrhea
Lincomycin		Pseudomembranous colitis
Ampicillin and Cephalosporin		
Most antibiotics		

(continued)

Toxicity of antimicrobial agents *(continued)*

Agent	Mechanism	Signs
Renal:		
Amphotericin B	Tubular damage Bone marrow depression	Azotemia Alkaline urine; pancytopenia
Penicillins (Methicillin most common)	Interstitial nephritis	Fever, eosinophilia, azotemia, eosinophiluria
Cephaloridine	Tubular damage	Azotemia
Aminoglycoside	Tubular damage	Cylindruria, azotemia
Polymyxin	Tubular damage	Azotemia
Fetal:		
Ciprofloxacin	Possible cartilage erosion in weight-bearing joints	
Tetracycline	Adverse effects on teeth and bones	

*With high serum levels associated with renal insufficiency.

Common antifungal agents

Drug	Organisms Inhibited	Route	Dose
Amphotericin B	Aspergillus, candida, blastomyces, coccidioides, cryptococci, histoplasma, phycomyces, paracoccidioides, sporotrichum, leishmania	I.V. p.o. irrigation	Test 1 mg; 0.6–1 mg/kg/d, or q.o.d. 5 mg, variable
Nystatin	As above	p.o. topical vaginal inserts	10,000 U-10^6U q6h apply b.i.d.
5-Fluorocytosine	Cryptococci, candida, torulopsis, chromo-blastomyces	p.o.	150 mg/kg/d in 3–4 doses
Clotrimazole	Dermatophytes, molds, cryptococci, candida	topical vaginal	b.i.d.
Ketoconazole	Dermatophytes, candida, histoplasma, blastomyces, coccidioides immitis, cryptococci	p.o.	200 mg/d Serious infections 400 mg/d
Miconazole	Dermatophytes, cryptococci, candida, coccidioides	I.V. topical	200–400 mg t.i.d. b.i.d.
Griseofulvin	Dermatophytes	p.o.	Adults: 0.5–1.0 g/d

| Serum T½ | | Duration | Some Common Side Effects/ |
Normal h	Oliguria h		Comments
24	24	Unknown 1.0–2.0 g empiric	Low renal excretion. Rapid infusion produces hypotension. Fever, arrhythmias, hypokalemia, increased SGOT, anemia, azotemia common. Reversible blood dyscrasias. Soluble only in water—comes out of solution in saline. Avoid reactions by pretreating with salicylates, antihistamines, or hydrocortisone. Has been used at lower dosages—0.4 mg/kg/24 h with 5–FC to treat cryptococcal infection.
—	—	While on antibiotics 7–10 d	Use in immunosuppressed patients, patients on long–term broad spectrum antibiotics.
5	60	Unknown	Coadminister with amphotericin-B; leukopenia, diarrhea. Adjust dose in renal failure. Lower dose for renal candidiasis, 50 mg/kg/day.
—	—	7–10 d	Very effective in mixed candidas— dermatophyte infections.
Biphasic: 2 for 1st 10 h, then 8	27	variable	Hepatotoxicity may be fatal; must monitor hepatic function. Poor diffusion into CSF.
—	—	While infection persists 7–10 d	Liver, lipoprotein, CNS effects. Failures of cryptococcosis and coccidioidomycosis.
12	12	Variable, 2–8 w	Follow liver enzymes; alters anticoagulation, rashes.

Common parasitic infections*

Parasite	Drug	Dose
Amoeba	Metronidazole	750 mg t.i.d. × 10 d
Ascaris	Pyrantel pamoate	11 mg/kg, single dose
Babesia microti	Clindamycin and	1.2 g b.i.d. parenteral
	Quinine	650 mg t.i.d. oral × 7 d
Cryptosporidium	TMP/SMX	TMP: 20 mg/kg/d SMX: 100 mg/kg/d
Enterobius	Pyrantel pamoate	11 mg/kg, repeat in 2 wks
Giardia lamblia	Metronidazole	250 mg. t.i.d. for 5 d
Hookworm	Mebendazole	100 mg. b.i.d. × 3 d
Iaspora belli	TMP/SMX	160 mg TMP, 800 mg q.i.d. × 10 d, then b.i.d. × 3 wks
Lice	1% Permethrin	Topically
Malaria	Chloroquine	1 g, then 500 mg 6 h later, then 500 mg/d × 2 d
Pneumocystis carinii	TMP/SMX	TMP: 20 mg/kg/d × 14–21 d SMX: 100 mg/kg/d × 14–21 d
Scabies	5% permethrin	Apply topically
Schistosoma mansoni	Oxamniquine Praziquantel	15 mg/kg/d, 1 dose 40 mg/kg/d, 1 dose
Strongyloides	Thiabendazole	25 mg/kg/b.i.d. × 2 d
Taenia	Niclosamide	Adult—2 g single dose Child—11–34 mg/kg single dose

(continued)

Common parasitic infections *(continued)*

Parasite	Drug	Dose
Toxoplasma gondii	Spiramycin	3–4 g/d, until delivery
Trichuris trichiura	Mebendazole	100 mg b.i.d. × 3 d

*Caution: None of these agents has been studied extensively during pregnancy, although available evidence does not suggest significant teratogenic potential. A careful assessment of risks vs. benefits is mandatory prior to use in pregnancy.

Common antituberculosis drugs

Drug	Adult Dosage (daily)	Pediatric Dosage (daily)	Main Adverse Effects
Isoniazid*/† (I.N.H., and others)	300 mg	10–20 mg/kg (max. 300 mg)	Hepatic toxicity
Rifampin*/‡	600 mg	10–20 mg/kg (max. 600 mg)	Hepatic toxicity, flu-like syndrome
Pyrazinamide§	1.5 to 2.5 g p.o.	same as adult	Hepatic toxicity, hyperuricemia
Ethambutol‖ (Myambutol)	15–25 mg/kg p.o.	same as adult	Optic neuritis
OTHER DRUGS			
Capreomycin (Capastat)	15 mg/kg (about 1 g)	15–30 mg/kg	Auditory and vestibular toxicity, renal damage
Kanamycin (Kantrex, and others)	15 mg/kg I.M. or I.V.	15–30 mg/kg	Auditory toxicity, renal damage
Streptomycin#	15 mg/kg I.M.**	20–40 mg/kg IM	Vestibular toxicity, renal damage

| Cycloserine (Seromycin, and others) | 250–500 mg b.i.d.†† | 15–20 mg/kg | Psychiatric symptoms, seizures |
| Ethionamide (Trecator-SC) | 250–500 mg b.i.d. | 15–20 mg/kg | Gastrointestinal and hepatic toxicity |

*Rifamate (containing rifampin 300 mg plus isoniazid 150 mg) is also available.

†Can be given orally or parenterally. Pyridoxine should be given to prevent neuropathy in malnourished or pregnant patients and those with alcoholism or diabetes. For intermittent use after a few weeks to months of daily dosage, the dosage is 15 mg/kg twice per wk (max. 900 mg).

‡Available orally or intravenously. For intermittent use after a few weeks to months of daily dosage, the dosage is 600 mg twice per wk.

§For intermittent use after a few weeks to months of daily dosage, the dosage is 40–50 mg/kg twice per wk (max. 3 g).

‖Daily dosage should be 25 mg/kg/d if organism isoniazid-resistant or during first 1 to 2 mos; decrease dosage if renal function diminished. For intermittent use after a few wks to mos of daily dosage, the dosage is 50 mg/kg twice per wk.

#Temporarily not available in the USA.

**For patients > 40 years old, 500 to 750 mg/day or 20 mg/kg twice/week; decrease dosage if renal function is diminished. Some clinicians change to lower dosage at 60 rather than 40 years old.

††Some authorities recommend pyridoxine 50 mg for every 250 mg of cycloserine to decrease the incidence of adverse psychiatric effects.

PART D

Fetal Medicine

Fetal transfusion formulas

Intraperitoneal: Use fresh O negative, washed, tightly packed red blood cells.

Volume = [Gestational age (weeks) − 20] × 10 mL

Intravascular: Use fresh O negative, washed, tightly packed, red blood cells.

$$V_T = V_F \frac{(40 - Hct_F)}{(Hct_D - 40)}$$

V_T = volume to be transfused
V_F = fetal blood volume, based upon estimated weight and assuming 80 cc/kg
Hct_F = initial fetal hematocrit
Hct_D = donor cells hematocrit

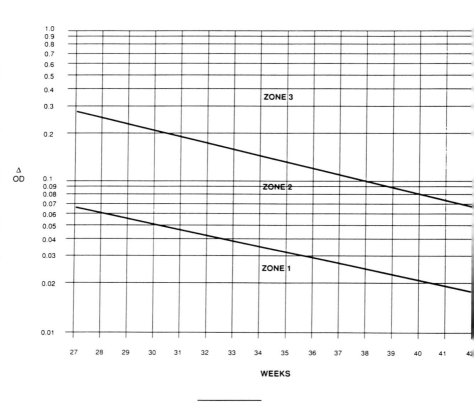

The Liley Curve: Liley graph used to depict degrees of sensitization. (Reproduced by permission from Liley AW. Liquor amnii analysis in management of pregnancy complicated by rhesus sensitization. Am J Obstet Gynecol 1961;82(6):1359–1370.)

A.

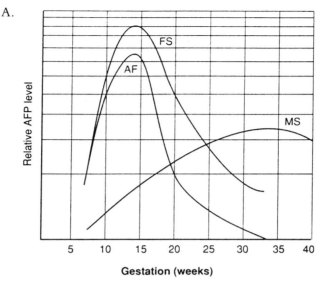

Gestation (weeks)

B.

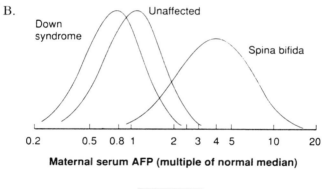

Maternal serum AFP (multiple of normal median)

Alphafetoprotein Curves

A. Relative levels of AFP in fetal serum (FS), amniotic fluid (AF), and maternal serum (MS) throughout a normal singleton pregnancy. (Modified from Milunsky A, ed. Genetic disorders and the fetus: diagnosis, prevention, and treatment. 2nd ed. New York: Plenum Press, 1986:459.)

B. AFP levels in maternal serum at 16-18 weeks of gestation in singleton pregnancies. (Modified from Wald N, Cuckle H. AFP and age screening for Down syndrome. Am J Med Genet 1988;31:197–209.)

APPENDIX 2
Management Protocols and ACLS Protocols

PART A: MANAGEMENT PROTOCOLS

PART B: ACLS PROTOCOLS

PART A

Management Protocols

Severe valvular cardiac disease*

Goals of Therapy

Avoid hypotension, hypoxia, fluid overload.

Management Protocol

1. Admit patient at term with favorable cervix.
2. Place pulmonary artery catheter and optimize hemodynamics × 24 hours.
3. Oxytocin induction of labor.
4. Labor on left or right side.
5. Administer O_2 at 4–6 L/min.
6. I.V. 5% dextrose solution.
7. Use epidural anesthesia.
8. Intrapartum hemodynamic manipulation.
   A. Mitral stenosis: no pulmonary hypertension.
      1. Keep heart rate below 100 bpm with oral/I.V. beta blocker.
      2. Diuresis to wedge pressure 12 to 14 mm Hg.[†]
   B. Aortic stenosis or pulmonary hypertension: Adjust wedge pressure to approximately 16 mm Hg.[‡]
9. Bacterial endocarditis prophylaxis.

Critical Laboratory Tests

Arterial blood gas, complete blood count, electrolytes, electrocardiogram, chest x-ray.

Consultation

Cardiology.

---

*For patients who are NYHA Class I or II throughout pregnancy, without prior myocardial infarction or pulmonary hypertension, steps 1–3 and 8 may be omitted.

†This must be done with careful attention to maintenance of blood pressure and cardiac output. In some patients, this optimal level cannot be achieved.

‡To maintain a margin of safety against unexpected hypotension or blood loss.

Anticoagulation during pregnancy of patients with prosthetic heart valves

Goals of Therapy

To prevent valvular thrombosis or arterial thromboembolism.

Management Protocol

1. Sodium heparin, 2500–5000 units intravenously, followed by 1000 units/hour via infusion pump *or* sodium heparin, 8000–14,000 units every 12 hours, subcutaneously. (Use heparin with a concentration of at least 20,000 units/mL. Use insulin U—100 syringes.)
2. Adjust dose to achieve aPTT 1.5–2.0 times control at midinterval (6 hours after the heparin is injected). This corresponds to a heparin plasma concentration of 0.2–0.4 IU/mL plasma.
3. Withhold heparin when labor begins or prior to cesarean delivery. Check aPTT.
4. If the aPTT is prolonged prior to delivery, delay if possible. If delay not possible, administer protamine sulfate. Immediately following I.V. heparin injection, 1.0 mg protamine sulfate will neutralize 100 units of heparin. After 30 minutes, only one-half the aforementioned protamine dose is used. Several hours after subcutaneous injection, begin with small doses (5–10 mg) and titrate according to aPTT response. (In some laboratories, a protamine titration test may be available.)
5. Resume heparin 6–12 hours following vaginal delivery or 12–24 hours following cesarean delivery. Use an intravenous continuous infusion of heparin, and titrate the dose so that the patient is fully anticoagulated (the aPTT is 1.5–2 times the control).
6. Begin oral anticoagulant, and adjust the dose so that the prothrombin time INR is 3.0–4.5. This corresponds to a prothrombin time ratio of 1.6–1.8 when rabbit brain thromboplastin is used. Discontinue heparin infusion when the prothrombin time is therapeutic for at least 4 days after beginning oral anticoagulants.
7. When switching from intravenous to subcutaneous doses, given one-half of the total 24-hour intravenous dose subcutaneously, every 12 hours.

(continued)

Anticoagulation during pregnancy of patients with prosthetic heart valves *(continued)*

Critical Laboratory Tests

aPTT (or heparin assay).

Consultation

Hematology, cardiology.

Deep venous thrombosis in pregnancy

Goals of Therapy

1. Promotion of thrombus resolution.
2. Prevention of thrombus extension and recurrence.

Management Protocol

1. Immediately begin therapy, based on strong clinical suspicion, pending complete diagnostic work-up.
2. Administer heparin (5,000 U I.V.) followed by 1,000–2,000 U/h via infusion pump.
3. Adjust heparin infusion to achieve aPTT 1.5–2 times that of control.
4. Maintain full anticoagulation for 7 days.
5. Continue anticoagulation with adjusted-dose subcutaneous heparin, initially 8,000–12,000 U twice or three times daily (antepartum or postpartum) or oral anticoagulation (only if postpartum) until 6 weeks postpartum.
6. Implement bed rest, elastic hose, and extremity elevation if source of embolus is the leg.

Critical Laboratory Tests

aPTT, complete blood count (CBC), with platelet count.

Consultation

Hematology.

Pulmonary embolism in pregnancy

Goals of Therapy

1. Maintenance of oxygenation and cardiac output.
2. Promotion of thrombus resolution.
3. Prevention of thrombus extension and recurrence.

Management Protocol

1. Immediately begin therapy, based on strong clinical suspicion, pending complete diagnostic work-up.
2. Administer O_2 via mask, 6 L/min.
3. Administer heparin (5,000–10,000 U I.V.) followed by 1,000–2,000 U/h via infusion pump.
4. Adjust heparin infusion to achieve aPTT 1.5–2 times that of control.
5. Maintain full anticoagulation for 7–10 days.
6. Continue anticoagulation with adjusted-dose subcutaneous heparin, initially 8,000–12,000 U twice or three times daily (antepartum or postpartum) or oral anticoagulation (only if postpartum) until 6 weeks postpartum.
7. Implement bed rest, elastic hose, and extremity elevation if source of embolus is the leg.

Critical Laboratory Tests

ABG, aPTT, complete blood count (CBC) with platelet count, chest x-ray, electrocardiogram (EKG), invasive or noninvasive diagnostic tests, as indicated.

Consultation

Pulmonary medicine, hematology.

Hypovolemic shock

Goals of Therapy

1. Maintain the following:
   A. Systolic pressure ≥ 90 mm Hg,
   B. Urine output ≥ 25 mL/h,
   C. Normal mental status.
2. Eliminate source of hemorrhage.
3. Avoid overzealous volume replacement that may contribute to pulmonary edema.

Management Protocol

1. Establish two large-bore intravenous lines.
2. Place patients in Trendelenburg position.
3. Rapidly infuse 5% dextrose in lactated Ringer's solution while blood products are obtained.
4. Infuse fresh whole blood or packed red blood cells, as available.
5. Infuse platelets and FFP only as indicated by documented deficiencies in platelets (<50,000/mL) or clotting parameters (fibrinogen, PT, PTT).
6. Search for and eliminate source of hemorrhage.
7. Use invasive hemodynamic monitoring if patient fails to respond to clinically adequate volume replacement.

Critical Laboratory Tests

Complete blood count (CBC), platelet count, fibrinogen, PT, PTT, arterial blood gases.

Postpartum hemorrhage

Management Protocol

(To be undertaken simultaneously with management of hypovolemic shock.)

1. Examine uterus to rule out atony.
2. Examine vagina and cervix to rule out lacerations—repair if present.
3. Explore uterus and perform curettage to rule out retained placenta.
4. For uterine atony:
   A. Firm bimanual compression.
   B. Oxytocin infusion, 40 units in 1 L of D_5RL.
   C. 15-methyl prostaglandin $F_{2\alpha}$, 0.25–0.50 mg I.M.; may be repeated.
   D. Bilateral uterine artery ligation.
   E. Bilateral hypogastric artery ligation (if patient clinically stable and future childbearing of great importance).
   F. Hysterectomy.

Sickle-cell crisis

Goals of Therapy

1. Relief of symptoms.
2. Minimize maternal and fetal morbidity/mortality.

Management Protocol

1. Hospitalize. Administer mild sedation and analgesia.
2. Monitor the fetal heart rate carefully if gestational age is sufficient to consider intervention for fetal well-being.
3. Vigorously hydrate with warm fluids if there are no signs of congestive heart failure, infusing 1 L of Ringer's lactate solution or normal saline over a 2-h period and continuing fluid replacement at 125–175 mL/h based on maternal size and such clinical conditions.
4. Record fluid intake and output.
5. Administer acetaminophen if mild analgesia is needed, acetaminophen with codeine for moderate pain, or intravenous morphine or butorphanol for severe pain. In severe crisis pain situation, continuous morphine administration by standard intravenous infusion or by patient-controlled administration pump should be considered.
6. If physical findings and laboratory test results suggest a crisis-associated infection, obtain appropriate cultures and begin antibiotics immediately. Otherwise, prophylactic antibiotic use is discouraged.
7. If the pregnant gravida in crisis is in labor, has evidence of a respiratory infection or a partial pressure of oxygen less than 70 mm Hg, or a hemoglobin saturation <94%, begin oxygen at 6–8 L/min by mask. Hyperoxia should be avoided in order to avert acute suppression of erythropoiesis.
8. Institute partial exchange transfusion. Several considerations apply:
   A. Continuous automated erythrocytophoresis utilizing an IBM 2997 Cell Separator is optimal. Closely monitor withdrawal and return rates to protect the patient and her fetus from volume overload or hypovolemia. This is particularly important for the patient in crisis who also has congestive heart failure or acute renal failure. Six units of packed red cells are exchanged by this process, generally with rapid alleviation of crisis pain, as well as a decrease in Hgb S concentration, blood viscosity, and sickling.
   B. A partial exchange transfusion using a manual protocol may also be performed.

(continued)

Sickle-cell crisis *(continued)*

    C. A simple manual transfusion is helpful when the patient's initial packed red cell volume is dangerously low (hematocrit <15% or hemoglobin <6 g/dL).

9. At the conclusion of blood transfusion therapy, measure the complete blood count as well as the Hgb A concentration (which should be greater than 50%).

Critical Laboratory Tests

1. Arterial blood gas or Sao_2 by pulse oximetry, complete blood count with differential count, chemistry panel, lactic dehydrogenase isoenzymes 1 and 2, hemoglobin electrophoresis, type and cross-hatch of 6 units of packed red blood cells, HIV/hepatitis screen.
2. Consider chest x-ray, electrocardiogram or pulmonary function tests if clinically indicated.

Consultation

Hematology, anesthesiology.

Sympathomimetic-associated pulmonary edema

Goals of Therapy

1. Relief of symptoms.
2. Maintenance of adequate oxygenation ($Pao_2 > 60$ mm Hg or $Sao_2 > 90\%$).
3. Diuresis of excess fluid.
4. Avoid problem by avoiding fluid overload and infusing D_5W, as opposed to isotonic crystalloid solutions.

Management Protocol

1. Discontinue sympathomimetic agent.
2. O_2 by mask.
3. Furosemide 20–40 mg I.V.
4. Morphine sulfate 10 mg I.V.
5. Foley catheter for hourly output determinations.
6. Insert pulmonary artery catheter if clinical response to steps 1–4 is not prompt. Additional hemodynamic manipulations (preload optimization [5–14 mm Hg] or inotropic support) as indicated by hemodynamic indices.

Laboratory Tests

Arterial blood gas, chest x-ray, serum electrolytes, electrocardiogram.

Monitoring Techniques

1. Pulse oximetry.
2. Foley catheter.
3. Pulmonary artery (PA) catheter.

Possible Consultation

Pulmonary medicine, cardiology, respiratory therapy.

PIH: Hypertensive crisis

Goals of Therapy

1. Diastolic BP < 110 mm Hg.
2. Systolic BP < 180–200 mm Hg.

Management Protocol

1. Assure adequate intravascular volume. Consider 500–1000 cc NS fluid load.
2. Hydralazine hydrochloride 5 mg I.V., followed by 10 mg I.V. as often as every 20 minutes to achieve blood pressure goals.
   or
   Labetolol 10 mg I.V. followed by progressively increasing doses (20, 40, 80 mg) every 10 minutes to achieve blood pressure goals or to total dose of 300 mg.
3. If hydralazine or labetolol is ineffective, place arterial line and possibly pulmonary artery catheter, and consider nitroglycerine or nitroprusside. Nitroglycerine: 10 mg/min, doubling dose every 5 minutes to achieve blood pressure goals. Nitroprusside: 0.25 mg/kg/min, increasing by same dose every 5 minutes to achieve blood pressure goals.
4. Fetal monitoring.
5. Initiate delivery.

Critical Laboratory Tests

Hematocrit and red blood cell morphology, platelet count, aspartate aminotransferase (AST), alanine aminotransferase (ALT).

Septic shock

Goals of Therapy

1. Systolic BP > 90 mm Hg.
2. Urine output > 25 mL/h.
3. Cardiac output > 4 L/min.
4. Arterial Po_2 > 60 mm Hg.
5. Normal mental status.
6. Eradication of source of infection.

Management Protocol

1. Rapid volume expansion with D_5RL (1000–2000 mL, followed by 150–200 mL/h).
2. Administer O_2 to maintain Po_2 > 60 mm Hg.
3. Initiate empiric antibiotic therapy: Gentamicin 1.5 mg/kg, then 1 mg/kg I.V. every 8 hours. Clindamycin 900 mg I.V. every 9 hours. Penicillin 3,000,000 units I.V. every 4 hours.
4. Search for surgically correctable origin of infection (abscess, appendicitis, etc.).
5. Use pulmonary artery catheterization if no clinical response to initial volume loading. Optimize preload, with PCWP of 14–15 mm Hg.
6. After optimal preload achieved, begin dopamine if necessary (starting dose 2–5 μg/kg/min), titrated to hemodynamic and clinical response.
7. Consider digitalization or other inotropic support if invasive monitoring parameters—left ventricular stroke work index (LVSWI)—indicated myocardial failure.
8. Control overt hyperthermia with acetaminophen or cooling blanket.

Critical Laboratory Tests

Complete blood count (CBC), platelet count, urinalysis, fibrinogen, prothrombin time, partial thromboplastin time, fibrin split products, electrolytes, blood urea nitrogen (BUN), creatinine, serum glutamic-pyruvic transaminase (SGPT), serum glutamic-oxalocetic transaminase (SGOT), arterial blood gas, urine and blood cultures, other cultures as clinically indicated, serum lactate, chest x-ray, pelvic/abdominal computed tomography scan or MRI if abscess suspected. Monitor mixed venous oxygen saturation or arterial-venous O_2 content difference.

Consultation

Infectious disease.

Anaphylactic shock in pregnancy

Goals of Therapy

1. Maintain airway and oxygenation.
2. Support blood pressure.
3. Eliminate exposure to inciting agent.
4. Decrease release of vasoactive substances.
5. Monitor fetus, if viable ex utero.

Management Protocol

1. Maintain airway-intubation or tracheostomy if necessary.
2. Administer oxygen.
3. Epinephrine, 0.5 mg (5 mL of 1:10,000 solution) I.V. or endotracheal q 5–10 minutes (severe reactions). Epinephrine 0.5 mg (0.5 mL of 1:1000 solution) subcutaneous, q 20–30 minutes (mild reactions).
4. Volume expand with normal saline.
5. Hydrocortisone sodium succinate 500 mg I.V. q 6 hours.
6. Diphenhydramine hydrochloride 50 mg I.V. or p.o.
7. Delay absorbtion (if possible):
   A. For oral antigen, Ipecac 30 cc p.o., then activated charcoal.
   B. For parenteral antigen, venous torniquet proximal to injection site.
8. Support blood pressure as necessary with volume and dopamine.
9. Careful fetal heart rate monitoring if viability has been achieved.

Thyroid storm in pregnancy

Goals of Therapy

1. Control of synthesis and release of thyroid hormone.
2. Reversal of peripheral effects of hyperthyroidism.
3. Prevention or treatment of hypotension, extreme hyperthermia, severe tachycardia, cardiac dysrhythmias, or congestive heart failure.
4. Identification and treatment of precipitating factors.

Management Protocol

1. Tranfer to intensive care unit.
2. Judicious hydration with crystalloid solution.
3. Cooling blanket.
4. Acetaminophen 325 mg rectally every 3 hours.
5. Electrocardiographic monitoring.
6. Sodium iodine 0.5–1 g I.V. every 8 hours.
7. Propylthiouracil 1000 mg orally, then 300 mg every 6 hours.
8. Propranolol 1 mg/min I.V. titrated to achieve maternal heart rate of 100–120
   or
   Propranolol 40–80 mg orally every 4 hours.
9. Hydrocortisone 100 mg I.V. every 8 hours.
10. Search for precipitating cause, especially infection. Treat with broad spectrum antibiotics (pending culture).

Critical Laboratory Tests

CBC, electrolytes, blood and urine cultures, thyroid function tests.

Consultation

Medical endocrinology, intensivist, cardiologist.

Diabetic ketoacidosis in pregnancy

Goals of Therapy

1. Rehydration.
2. Restoration of electrolyte homeostasis.
3. Correction of acidemia.
4. Normalization of serum glucose.
5. Elimination of underlying cause.
6. Return of maternal-fetal homeostasis.

Management Protocol

1. Infuse 0.9 saline, 1000 mL over first hour, 1000 mL over subsequent 2 hours, 250 mL/h thereafter.
2. Change I.V. solution to D_5NS as serum glucose falls below 250 mg/dL.
3. Add KCl 20–40 mEq/L to I.V. fluids after adequate urine output is established.
4. A. Administer regular insulin 0.1 U/kg I.V. push.
   B. Begin an infusion of 5–10 U/h.
   C. Double infusion rate if serum glucose has not decreased by 25% in 2 hours.
   D. Reduce infusion to 1–2 U/h as serum glucose falls below 150 mg/dL.
5. Administer sodium bicarbonate 44 mEq I.V. in 1000 mL 0.45 NS for arterial pH <7.10.
6. Search for underlying cause, such as infection.

Critical Laboratory Tests

Serum electrolytes, glucose, arterial blood gas, complete blood count (CBC), bicarbonate, blood urea nitrogen (BUN), ketones.

Consultation

Internal medicine.

Adult respiratory distress syndrome (ARDS)

Goals of Therapy

1. To identify and eliminate the causal agent.
2. To achieve:
   Pao_2 >60 mm Hg or 90% hemoglobin saturation,
   Pvo_2 >30 mm Hg,
   $Paco_2$ 35–40 mm Hg.

Management Protocol

1. Identify that a lung injury has been sustained and eliminate the causal agent.
2. Assess pulmonary function:
   A. $Pao_2 \div Fio_2$:
      >3 = good function,
      <3 = suspect injury.
   B. 100% oxygen × 2 minutes.
      Pao_2 400 mm Hg: probably hypoventilation. Aggressive pulmonary toilet and/or incentive spirometry.
      Pao_2 300–400 mm Hg: possible early ARDS. Aggressive pulmonary toilet; supplemental mask oxygen; monitor with pulse oximetry. Reevaluate immediately if there is any clinical, laboratory deterioration.
      Pao_2 300 mm Hg: probable ARDS. Intubate, ventilate.
3. Maximize oxygen delivery to tissue. Correct anemia, hypothermia, and alkalosis. Optimize cardiac output via pulmonary artery catheter guided hemodynamic manipulation.
4. Avoid therapeutic pitfalls:
   A. Fluid overload: daily weights, intake and output balance, invasive hemodynamic monitoring.
   B. Oxygen toxicity: use minimum Fio_2 required to achieve a Pao_2 of 60 mm Hg or a 90% hemoglobin saturation.
   C. Barotrauma: limit by use of "best" PEEP.
   D. Iatrogenic lung injury: administration of colloid, mannitol, and hetastarch in the setting of a permeability lung injury should be avoided.
   E. Nosocomial infections: sinus infections in intubated patients, urinary tract infections resulting from indwelling catheter, and phlebitis from peripheral and central lines should be identified. Central and peripheral intravenous lines should be changed every 72 hours.

(continued)

Adult respiratory distress syndrome (ARDS) *(continued)*

Goals of Therapy

Critical Laboratory Tests

Arterial blood gases, mixed venous blood gases, complete blood count (CBC), electrolytes, chest x-ray.

Consultation

Respiratory therapy, pulmonary medicine, intensivists.

Amniotic fluid embolism

Goals of Therapy

1. To maintain systolic blood pressure >90 mm Hg, urine output >25 mL/h and arterial Po_2 >60 mm Hg or SaO_2 >90.
2. To correct coagulation abnormalities.

Management Protocol

1. Initiate cardiopulmonary resuscitation if indicated.
2. Administer oxygen at high concentrations. If the patient is unconscious, she should be intubated and ventilated with 100% Fio_2.
3. AFE is often associated with and, in fact, may be heralded by fetal distress. Therefore, the fetal heart rate should be monitored carefully if gestational age is sufficient to warrant intervention for fetal distress.
4. Hypotension is usually secondary to cardiogenic shock. Treatment involved optimization of cardiac preload by rapid volume infusion. Subsequent dopamine infusion would be appropriate if the patient remains hypotensive.
5. Pulmonary artery catheterization may be helpful in guiding hemodynamic management.
6. After correction of hypotension, fluid therapy should be restricted to maintenance levels to minimize pulmonary edema due to developing ARDS.
7. Administer fresh whole blood or packed red blood cells and fresh-frozen plasma to treat bleeding secondary to disseminated intravascular coagulation.

Critical Laboratory Tests

Arterial blood gas, complete blood count (CBC), platelet count, fibrinogen, fibrin split products, prothrombin time (PT), partial thromboplastin time (PTT).

Consultation

Pulmonary medicine, hematology.

Acute renal failure (ARF) in pregnancy

Goals of Therapy

1. Maintain euvolemia.
2. Avoid hyperkalemia, acidosis, hyponatremia, hypocalcemia.
3. Maintain adequate nutrition.
4. Avoid severe hypertension.
5. Institute dialysis early, if necessary.
6. Assess fetal well-being.
7. Identify and eliminate or treat cause of ARF.

Management Protocol

1. Volume status.
   A. Consider pulmonary artery catheterization for closer assessment of volume status.
   B. Fluid intake: 6–8 mL/kg + urine output.
   C. Lasix 40–500 mg I.V., to assist in fluid balance.
   D. Dialysis if volume overload occurs.
2. Hyperkalemia:
   A. K+ >8.0 mEq/L or EKG changes (other than peaked T waves).
      1. Calcium gluconate 10–20 mL of 10% solution.
      2. 10 units of regular insulin and 50 mL of 50% glucose.
      3. Sodium bicarbonate 50–150 mEq (if the patient is not volume overloaded).
      4. Dialysis.
      5. Cardiac monitor.
   B. K+ 6.8–7.0 mEq/L.
      1. 10 units of regular insulin and 50 mL of 50% glucose.
      2. Sodium bicarbonate 50–150 mEq/L (if the patient if not volume overloaded).
      3. Kayexalate 20–30 g every 2–4 hours orally, 50–100 g rectally.
      4. Dialysis.
      5. Cardiac monitor.
   C. K+ 5.6–6.8 mEq/L.
      1. Kayexalate as in step B, *and/or*
      2. Dialysis.
3. Acidosis: Maintain bicarbonate above 15 mEq/L and pH above 7.2.
   A. Euvolemic patient: sodium bicarbonate dose to achieve desired increase in bicarbonate × 0.6 body weight.
   B. Volume overloaded, hypernatremic, or severely catabolic patient: dialysis with high bicarbonate dialysate.

(continued)

Acute renal failure (ARF) in pregnancy *(continued)*

4. Hyponatremia.
    A. Serum sodium >125 mEq/L: restrict free water.
    B. Serum sodium 120–125 mEq/L: dialysis.
    C. Serum sodium <120: dialysis with high-sodium dialysate; administration of hypertonic saline during dialysis.
5. Hypocalcemia: administer calcium intravenously only if positive Chvostek sign or carpal pedal spasm is present. Oral supplements to maintain serum calcium above 7.5 mg% and to keep phosphorus below 5.5 mg%.
6. Nutrition.
    A. Management without dialysis: at least 100 g of glucose, 25–50 kcal/day, 0.6 g of protein/kg ideal body weight, up to 1.5 g/kg if BUN can be kept less than 100 mg% or if the patient is still pregnant.
    B. Management with dialysis.
        1. Oral intake: 1–5 g of protein/kg; 25–50 kcal to prevent catabolism, potassium 50 mEq, sodium 2 g in the form of food or enteral-elemental diet preparation; supplemental multivitamins.
        2. TPN: total parenteral nutrition, 25–50 kcal day, 70% as glucose with 1–1.5 g protein as essential amino acids; maximum lipid is 500 mL of a 10% intralipid solution, supplemental multivitamins; electrolytes added indicated by lab values.
7. Adjust drug doses for renal failure.
8. Indications for dialysis:
    A. Uremia: BUN >100 mg% or uremic symptoms.
    B. Volume overload.
    C. Hyperkalemia.
    D. Acidosis with volume overload or hypernatremia.
    E. Pericarditis.
    F. Need for TPN, blood products, or other fluid in excess of what can be tolerated with conservative therapy.

Critical Laboratory Tests

Serum electrolytes (including HCO_3; bicarbonate), BUN, creatinine, total serum protein and albumin, calcium, phosphorus, creatinine clearance, arterial blood gases, serum osmolality, urine sodium–osmolality, chest x-ray.

Consultation

Nephrology.

Adult TTP/HUS syndrome

Goals of Therapy

1. To improve neurologic and renal status (serum creatinine, creatinine clearance).
2. To control hypertension.
3. To reverse thrombotic microanigopathy (stable hematocrit, platelet count >100,000/mL, LDH <500 IU/mL).

Management Protocol

1. Transfer to tertiary care facility.
2. Mild aTTP-aHUS: infuse 30 mL/kg fresh-frozen plasma over 24 hours (6–8 units in divided administrations) and follow with 15 mL/kg daily.
3. Moderate to severe aTTP-aHUS: initiate plasma exchange therapy, 40 mL/kg in exchange daily, days 1–5, and follow with 30 mL/kg in exchange, days 7 and 9. Use a continuous automated erythro-cytapheresis procedure if equipment is available.
4. Perform concurrent dialysis if necessary to control renal failure.
5. Initiate antihypertensive therapy for diastolic BP >110 mm Hg.
6. Transfuse as necessary to maintain the hemoglobin above 10 g%.
7. Following clinical response, administer dipyridamole 50 mg p.o. t.i.d., aspirin 325 mg P.O. b.i.d., prednisone 100 mg p.o. q.d., multivitamin, and folate.
8. If above modalities fail, consider splenectomy, prostacyclin infusions, and vincristine sulfate.
9. Careful fetal monitoring is crucial, with intervention for standard obstetric criteria only.

Critical Laboratory Tests

CBC with platelet count and red cell morphology, LDH, bilirubin, BUN, creatinine, electrolytes, PT and PTT, thrombin clotting time, fibrinogen, fibrin split products, direct and indirect Coomb's test, uric acid, urinalysis, antiplatelet antibody testing. LE prep/antinuclear antibody and serum complement levels. Bone marrow, gingival, or petechial skin biopsy in suspected aTTP.

Consultation

Nephrology, hematology, neurology.

Acute fatty liver of pregnancy

Goals of Therapy

1. To normalize liver function tests, electrolytes, clotting profile, and serum ammonia.
2. To prevent renal failure.
3. To maintain serum glucose >60 mg%.
4. To return patient to normal mental status.
5. To deliver the fetus.

Management Protocol

1. Hospitalize in intensive care unit.
2. If the patient is comatose, provide a secure airway and maintain effective ventilation and oxygenation.
3. Provide optimal nutrition. Administer 2000–2500 calories per 24 hours. Administer most of the calories in the form of concentrated glucose solutions.
4. Decrease endogenous ammonia production. Restrict protein intake during acute phase of illness. Evacuate colonic contents by administering magnesium citrate orally or by instilling Fleet enema solutions via rectum. Administer oral neomycin, 6–12 g/24 h, to decrease production of ammonia by intestinal bacteria.
5. Avoid use of medications that require hepatic metabolism.
6. Correct electrolyte and metabolic derangements.
7. Identify and correct coagulation abnormalities. Administer vitamin K, fresh-frozen plasma, or platelets as indicated.
8. Maintain surveillance for nosocomial infection, especially pneumonia, urosepsis, bacteremia.
9. Prevent gastrointestinal hemorrhage.
10. Deliver the patient promptly after the diagnosis is established.

Critical Laboratory Tests

Complete blood count (CBC), platelet count, partial thromboplastin time (PTT), prothrombin time (PT), fibrinogen, fibrin split products, serum glutamic pyruvic transaminase (SGPT), serum glutamic oxaloacetic transaminase (SGOT), alkaline phosphatase, total and direct bilirubin, blood urea nitrogen (BUN), creatinine, serum electrolytes, serum ammonia, liver biopsy (if coagulopathy is not present).

(continued)

Acute fatty liver of pregnancy *(continued)*

Consultation

Internal medicine, gastroenterology.

Multiple trauma in pregnancy

Goals of Therapy

1. To stabilize maternal condition.
2. To undertake thorough diagnostic evaluation.
3. To evaluate fetal condition.
4. To administer definitive therapy.

Management Protocol

1. Determine cardiopulmonary status.
2. Initiate resuscitation if necessary.
3. Control hemorrhage.
4. Place the patient in a lateral decubitus position.
5. Maintain maternal Po_2 >60 mm Hg to achieve adequate fetal oxygenation.
6. Start one or two large-bore intravenous lines.
7. Implement volume replacement; stabilize vital signs.
8. Initiate fetal monitoring.
9. Insert Foley catheter.
10. Use nasogastric or orogastric tube if warranted.
11. Administer tetanus prophylaxis with or without tetanus-immune globulin.
12. Apply antibiotic coverage as appropriate.
13. Use definitive therapy.

Critical Laboratory Tests

CBC, type and cross-match, arterial blood gas, serum electrolytes, serum amylase, urinalysis; peritoneal lavage and radiographic studies, as appropriate.

Consultation

General surgery, urology, neurosurgery.

Intracranial hemorrhage in pregnancy

Goals of Therapy

1. To prevent cerebral ischemia.
2. To reduce intracranial pressure (ICP).
3. To minimize cerebral edema.
4. To correct lesions surgically when and where appropriate.

Management Protocol

1. Ruptured aneurysm: Grades I, II, and III—Early surgical intervention Grades IV and V; stabilization and conservative management.
   A. Bed rest, quiet environment.
   B. Sedative, analgesic support, supplemented by a stool softener.
   C. Surgery after stabilization.
2. Arteriovenous malformation (AVM): Early surgical intervention versus embolization labor and delivery after repair.
   A. Cesarean for obstetric indications only.
   B. Labor with epidural anesthesia.
   C. Outlet forceps to shorten second stage of labor.
3. Cerebral edema: Mannitol 12.5–50 g I.V. (serum osmolality not to exceed 315 mosm/L).

Critical Laboratory Tests

MRI or CT scan of head, lumbar puncture, cerebral angiography, prothrombin time, partial thromboplastin time, fibrinogen, platelets.

Consultation

Neurosurgery, neurology, intensivist.

Molar gestation

Goals of Therapy

1. To completely evacuate the uterus.
2. To avoid volume overload and cardiorespiratory compromise.
3. To avoid or be prepared to treat massive hemorrhage.

Management Protocol

1. Administer I.V. D_5RL (5% dextrose in lactated Ringer's solution), at 125 mL/h (16- to 18-gauge angiocath).
2. Consider pulmonary artery catheter if clinically unstable.
3. Carefully use suction/curettage.
4. Match intake and output.
5. Observe carefully for evidence of respiratory distress.

Critical Laboratory Tests

CBC, quantitative beta-HCG, type and cross-match 2–4 units PRBC, platelet count, fibrinogen, PT, PTT, chest x-ray, arterial blood gas.

Hemolytic transfusion reactions

Goals of Therapy

1. To maintain blood pressure.
2. To avoid respiratory failure.
3. To prevent renal shutdown and maintain urine output >100 mL/ hour.

Management Protocol

1. Stop the transfusion.
2. Maintain an open line with normal saline.
3. Support blood pressure (with dopamine starting dose 2–5 mg/kg/ min, titrated to hemodynamic response) and respiration.
4. Maintain urine output with mannitol, 20–25 mg I.V. over 5 minutes. May be repeated up to 4 times within 24 hours.
5. Check container and patient labels to detect misidentification of patient or blood.
6. Send blood container, transfusion set, and I.V. solutions used with new sample of patient blood to blood bank.
7. Inspect recipient's postreaction plasma for hemolysis; compare with prereaction plasma when available. Pink plasma indicates at least 20 mg/dL of free hemoglobin.

Critical Laboratory Tests

Review labels and records; centrifuge plasma and urine for hemoglobin; direct antiglobulin test on postreaction sample, and compare with prereaction sample.

Consultation

Blood bank, hematology, pulmonary medicine.

.

PART B

ACLS Protocols

Asystole (cardiac standstill)

If rhythm is unclear and possibly ventricular
fibrillation, defibrillate as for VF. If asystole is present:*
↓
Continue CPR.
↓
Establish IV access.
↓
Epinephrine, 1:10,000, 0.5–1.0 mg IV push.†
↓
Intubate when possible.‡
↓
Atropine, 1.0 mg IV push (repeated in 5 min).
↓
(Consider bicarbonate).‡
↓
Consider pacing.

Flow of algorithm presumes asystole is continuing. VF =
ventricular fibrillation; IV = intravenous.

*Asystole should be confirmed in two leads.

†Epinephrine should be repeated every 5 minutes.

‡Value of sodium bicarbonate is questionable during cardiac
arrest, and it is not recommended for the routine cardiac arrest sequence. Consideration of its use in a dose of 1 mEq/kg
is appropriate at this point. Half of original dose may be repeated every 10 minutes if it is used.

(Reprinted with permission. Textbook of advanced cardiac
life support. American Heart Association, 1987.)

Ventricular fibrillation (and pulseless ventricular tachycardia)*

Witnessed arrest   Unwitnessed arrest
↓   ↓
Check pulse. If no pulse: Check pulse. If no pulse:
↓
Precordial thump
↓
Check pulse. If no pulse:

↓
CPR until a defibrillator is available.
↓
Check monitor for rhythm. If VF or VT:
↓
Defibrillate, 200 joules.†
↓
Defibrillate, 200–300 joules.†
↓
Defibrillate with up to 360 joules.†
↓
CPR if no pulse.
↓
Establish IV access
↓
Epinephrine, 1:10,000, 0.5–1.0 mg IV push.‡
↓
Intubate if possible.
↓
Defibrillate with up to 360 joules.†
↓
Lidocaine, 1 mg/kg IV push.
↓
Defibrillate with up to 360 joules.†
↓
Bretylium, 5 mg/kg IV push.‡
↓
(Consider bicarbonate).§
↓
Defibrillate with up to 360 joules.†
↓
Bretylium, 10 mg/kg IV push.‡
↓
Defibrillate with up to 360 joules.†
↓

(continued)

Repeat lidocaine or bretylium.
↓
Defibrillate with up to 360 joules.†

Flow of algorithm presumes that VF is continuing. CPR = cardiopulmonary resuscitation.

*Pulseless VT should be treated identically to VF.

†Check pulse and rhythm after each shock. If VF recurs after transiently converting (rather than persists without ever converting), use whatever energy level has previously been successful for defibrillation.

‡Epinephrine should be repeated every 5 minutes.

§Value of sodium bicarbonate is questionable during cardiac arrest sequence. Consideration of its use in a dose of 1 mEq/kg is appropriate at this point. Half of original dose may be repeated every 10 minutes if it is used. (Reprinted with permission. Textbook of advanced cardiac life support, copyright American Heart Association, 1987.)

Electromechanical dissociation

Continue CPR.
↓
Establish I.V. access.
↓
Epinephrine, 1:10,000, 0.5–1.0 mg I.V. push.
↓
Intubate when possible.
↓
(Consider bicarbonate).[†]
↓
Consider hypovolemia,
cardiac tamponade,
tension pneumothorax,
hypoxemia,
acidosis,
pulmonary embolism.

Flow of algorithm presumes that electromechanical dissociation is continuing. CPR = cardiopulmonary resuscitation; IV = intravenous.

[*]Epinephrine should be repeated every 5 minutes.

[†]Value of sodium bicarbonate is questionable during cardiac arrest, and it is not recommended for the routine cardiac arrest sequence. Consideration of its use in a dose of 1 mEq/kg is appropriate at this point. Half of original dose may be repeated every 10 minutes if it is used.

(Reprinted with permission. Textbook of advanced cardiac life support. American Heart Association, 1987.)

Sustained ventricular tachycardia (VT)

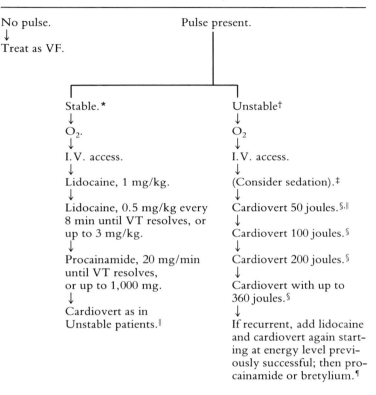

No pulse.
↓
Treat as VF.

Pulse present.

Stable.*
↓
O₂.
↓
I.V. access.
↓
Lidocaine, 1 mg/kg.
↓
Lidocaine, 0.5 mg/kg every
8 min until VT resolves, or
up to 3 mg/kg.
↓
Procainamide, 20 mg/min
until VT resolves,
or up to 1,000 mg.
↓
Cardiovert as in
Unstable patients.‖

Unstable†
↓
O₂
↓
I.V. access.
↓
(Consider sedation).‡
↓
Cardiovert 50 joules.§,‖
↓
Cardiovert 100 joules.§
↓
Cardiovert 200 joules.§
↓
Cardiovert with up to
360 joules.§
↓
If recurrent, add lidocaine
and cardiovert again start-
ing at energy level previ-
ously successful; then pro-
cainamide or bretylium.¶

Flow of algorithm presumes that VT is continuing. VF indicates ventricular fibrillation.

*If patient becomes unstable (see footnote † for definition) at any time, move to "Unstable" arms of algorithm.

†"Unstable" indicates symptoms (e.g., chest pain or dyspnea), hypotension (systolic blood pressures < 90 mm Hg), congestive heart failure, ischemia, or infarction.

‡Sedation should be considered for all patients, including those defined in foot-note † as "unstable," except those who are hemodynamically unstable (e.g., hypotensive, in pulmonary edema, or unconscious).

§If hypotension, pulmonary edema, or unconsciousness is present, unsynchronized cardioversion should be done to avoid delay associated with synchronization.

(continued)

‖In the absence of hypotension, pulmonary edema, or unconsciousness, a precordial thump may be employed prior to cardioversion.

¶Once VT has resolved, begin intravenous (I.V.) infusion of antiarrhythmic agent that has aided resolution of VT. If hypotension, pulmonary edema, or unconsciousness is present, use lidocaine if cardioversion alone is unsuccessful, followed by bretylium. In all other patients, recommended order of therapy is lidocaine, procainamide, and then bretylium.

(Reproduced with permission. Textbook of advanced cardiac life support. American Heart Association, 1987.)

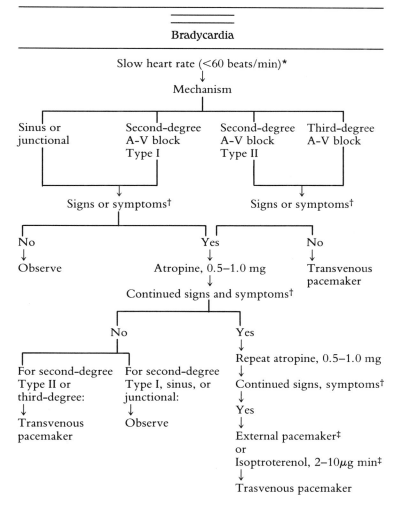

A-V = atrioventricular.

*A solitary chest thump or cough may stimulate cardiac electrical activity and result in improved cardiac output and may be used at this point.

†Hypotension (blood pressure <90 mm Hg), premature ventricular contractions, altered mental status or symptoms (e.g., chest pain or dyspnea), ischemia, or infarction.

‡Temporizing therapy.

(Reproduced with permission. Textbook of advanced cardiac life support. American Heart Association, 1987.)

Ventricular ectopy: acute suppressive therapy

Assess for need for
acute suppressive therapy
↓

→Rule out treatable cause.
→Consider serum
  potassium.
→Consider digitalis level.
→Consider bradycardia.
→Consider drugs.

Lidocaine, 1 mg/kg.
↓
If not suppressed,
repeat lidocains, 0.5 mg/kg every 2–5 min,
until no ectopy, or up to 3 mg/kg given.
↓
If not suppressed,
procainamide 20 mg/min
until no ectopy, or up to 1000 mg given.
↓
If not suppressed,
and not contraindicated,
bretylium, 5–10 mg/kg over 8–10 min.
↓
If not suppressed,
consider overdrive pacing.

Once ectopy resolved, maintain as follows:
   After lidocaine, 1 mg/kg: lidocaine drip, 2 mg/min.
   After lidocaine, 1–2 mg/kg: lidocaine drip, 3 mg/min.
   After lidocaine, 2–3 mg/kg: lidocaine drip, 4 mg/min.
   After procainamide: procainamide drip, 1–4 mg/min (check blood level).
   After bretylium: brethylium drip, 2 mg/min.

(Reproduced with permission. Textbook of advanced cardiac life support. American Heart Association, 1987.)

Paroxysmal supraventricular tachycardia (PSVT)

Unstable	Stable
↓	↓
Synchronous cardioversion 75–100 joules	Vagal maneuvers
↓	↓
Synchronous cardioversion 200 joules	Verapamil, 5 mg I. V.
↓	↓
Synchronous cardioversion 360 joules	Verapamile, 10 mg I. V.
↓	(in 15–20 min)
Correct underlying abnormalities	↓
↓	Cardioversion, digoxin,
Pharmacological therapy + cardioversion	β-blockers

Flow of algorithm presumes that PSVT is continuing. If conversion occurs but PSVT recurs, repeated electrical cardioversion is not indicated. Sedation should be used as time permits.

(Reproduced with permission. Textbook of advanced cardiac life support. American Heart Association, 1987.)

Neonatal resuscitation

Ventilation rate:	40–60 minute
Compression rate:	120/minute
Medications:	Heart rate <80/minute despite adequate ventilations with 100% O_2 and chest compressions

Medication	Concentration	Dose
Epinephrine	1:10,000 (0.1 mg/mL)	0.01–0.03 mg/kg
Sodium Bicarbonate	0.5 mEq/mL	2 mEq/kg

Weight	Epinephrine (total mL)	Bicarbonate (total mL)	ET/Suction Catheter	Larying Blade
1 kg	0.1–0.3 mL	4 mL	2.5/5 Fr	0
2 kg	0.2–0.6 mL	8 mL	3.0/8 Fr	0
3 kg	0.3–0.9 mL	12 mL	3.5/8 Fr	0–1

INDEX